# Digital Forensics in Next-Generation Internet of Medical Things

This book provides a comprehensive exploration of the security challenges and solutions with digital sustainability in the rapidly evolving digital landscape of digital forensics. It explores the details of protecting Internet of Medical Things (IoMT) environments, where the medical data, patient data, and machine data are at high risk with the digital experiences. The book seeks to provide researchers, medical practitioners, and IT specialists with important information. It aims to set the stage for a future in which security and efficiency in IoMT smoothly blend through real-world case studies. Key themes cover IoMT-specific forensic techniques, the difficulties of striking a balance between environmental responsibility and security, and creative solutions that combine the two viewpoints.

# Digital Forensics in Next-Generation Internet of Medical Things

## Balancing Security and Sustainability

Edited by
Hemant Kumar Saini, Sita Rani,
Mariya Ouaissa, Mariyam Ouaissa,
Zakaria Abou El Houda,
and Hajar Moudoud

CRC Press
Taylor & Francis Group
Boca Raton London New York

CRC Press is an imprint of the
Taylor & Francis Group, an **informa** business

Designed cover image: Shutterstock

First edition published 2026
by CRC Press
2385 NW Executive Center Drive, Suite 320, Boca Raton FL 33431

and by CRC Press
4 Park Square, Milton Park, Abingdon, Oxon, OX14 4RN

*CRC Press is an imprint of Taylor & Francis Group, LLC*



ISBN: 978-1-041-07046-7 (hbk)
ISBN: 978-1-041-07400-7 (pbk)
ISBN: 978-1-003-64032-5 (ebk)

DOI: 10.1201/9781003640325

Typeset in Sabon
by Newgen Publishing UK

# Contents

*Preface* vii
*Editor biographies* xi
*List of contributors* xv

**1 The role of artificial intelligence and machine learning in safeguarding IoMT security and privacy** 1
ABDELGHANI EL CHEDDADI, HAJAR MOUDOUD, AND STÉPHANE GAGNON

**2 Federated learning in healthcare: privacy-preserving collaboration for medical advancements** 18
MAROUA CHERIFI AND ZAKARIA ABOU EL HOUDA

**3 Secure authentication and authorization in the internet of medical things** 35
ARYENDRA DALAL

**4 Threat-aware circular security in smart healthcare** 55
I. SAKTHIDEVI AND G. FATHIMA

**5 Unveiling IoMT architecture: a deep dive into the technology stack for next-gen healthcare** 86
AKASHBHAI ASHOKBHAI DAVE

**6 SecureHealth: a blockchain-based framework for privacy-preserving healthcare data management in health centers** 102
RACHID ED-DAOUDI

7 Digital forensics in next-generation internet of medical things for sustainable telehealthcare 121

MARIAPPAN RAMASAMY

8 AI-driven forensics in IoMT: strengthening security, legal compliance, and ethical governance 149

VIJAISHREE DUBEY PANDEY, VIJETA VERMA, RITURAJ SINHA, AND SHASHANK SOLANKI

9 AI-driven cyber forensics for critical healthcare infrastructure security 170

SAINAG NETHALA

10 Sustainable forensics: energy efficiency and resource management for the future 192

P. SUDHEER, M. SARAVANAN, IMMANUEL ANUPALLI, AND S. ASHMAD

11 Awareness and training for attaining sustainable forensics in secure IoMT 208

PELLATE ANOUSHKA, C. KISHOR KUMAR REDDY, PRANAV SRINIVASAN, AND SRINATH DOSS

12 Educational transformations for IoMT forensics: challenges and opportunities 239

SOUFIANE OUARIACH, FATIMA ZAHRA OUARIACH, INAM ULLAH KHAN, MARIYA OUAISSA, AND MARIYAM OUAISSA

*Index* 263

# Preface

The Internet of Medical Things, or IoMT, is a leading healthcare technology that is transforming patient care through sophisticated monitoring and treatment techniques. However, this digital revolution also presents a new problem: sensitive medical data is now easily vulnerable to profitable cyberattacks. The majority of attacks occur on individual patient EHRs, which means that data owners must also be assured of privacy when diagnosing patients. Running a tight ship in the IoMT ecosystem is dependent on digital forensic analysis, which looks into ways to defend IoMT devices against potential breaches by investigating dubious threats like ransomware, botnets, data exfiltration, and data tampering. To guarantee a trustworthy reaction to any misconduct, forensic policies need to be revised to cooperate with broader policies and procedures. The interconnected structure of IoMT creates a huge attack surface when delving deeply into privacy issues related to medical devices and suspicious activity. An entire network of medical devices may be compromised by a breach in one device, increasing the damage and endangering the entire healthcare system. A further illustration of cybercriminals may be able to take advantage of the inherent vulnerabilities in many IoMT equipments, including infusion pumps and pacemakers. This directly jeopardizes patient safety because hacked devices could result in inaccurate diagnoses or inappropriate treatment administration.

IoMT digital forensics sheds light on the ecosystem's future. Its goals are many, ranging from using cryptography techniques to protect medical data and diagnoses to figuring out the complexities of the health chain. The advantages and difficulties of using forensic analysis in healthcare are discussed in the book, with a focus on the network of IoMT devices. Through an examination of the possibilities of federated learning (FL) and digital forensics techniques in enhancing privacy and protecting better healthcare, the book seeks to provide researchers, medical practitioners, and IT specialists with important information. It aims to set the stage for a future in which security and efficiency in IoMT smoothly blend through real-world case studies. Key themes will cover IoMT-specific forensic techniques, the difficulties of striking a balance between environmental responsibility and security, and creative solutions that combine the two viewpoints.

This book provides a comprehensive exploration of the security challenges and solutions with the digital sustainability in the rapidly evolving digital landscape of digital forensics. It explores the details of protecting IoMT environments, where the medical data, patient data, and machine data are at high risk with the digital experiences.

Let's take a closer look at the specific themes and contributions of each chapter:

**Chapter 1** explores how AI and ML enhance security and privacy in IoMT environments. It covers real-time threat detection, automated anomaly identification, and privacy-preserving AI techniques, ensuring compliance with regulations like HIPAA and GDPR.

**Chapter 2** discusses its applications in IoMT, benefits for privacy, challenges in implementation, and its role in secure medical research collaborations.

**Chapter 3** addresses authentication and authorization challenges in IoMT. It covers biometric authentication, multifactor authentication (MFA), blockchain-based identity management, and access control models to prevent unauthorized access to medical devices and data.

**Chapter 4** introduces the concept of circular security, where continuous monitoring, threat intelligence, and adaptive security mechanisms work together to protect IoMT environments. It discusses proactive threat detection, risk assessment, and mitigation strategies.

**Chapter 5** describes a comprehensive look at IoMT architecture, covering hardware components, communication protocols, cloud and edge computing, and interoperability. It highlights vulnerabilities at each layer and their forensic implications.

**Chapter 6** presents blockchain as a solution for secure medical data exchange. It explains smart contracts, decentralized storage, and cryptographic techniques to ensure data integrity, access control, and tamper-proof medical records.

**Chapter 7** focuses on forensic investigation techniques for remote healthcare services. It covers data collection, analysis of cyber incidents, forensic readiness, and compliance with healthcare regulations.

**Chapter 8** demonstrates how AI enhances digital forensic investigations in IoMT. Topics include AI-powered evidence analysis, legal and regulatory compliance (HIPAA, GDPR), and ethical concerns related to automated forensic tools.

**Chapter 9.** provides a deep dive into AI's role in cyber forensic investigations within critical healthcare infrastructure. It covers intrusion detection, malware analysis, digital evidence preservation, and case studies on AI-driven forensic investigations in hospital networks.

**Chapter 10** examines energy-efficient forensic methodologies and sustainable computing practices. It discusses green forensics, carbon footprint reduction in IoMT security operations, and balancing security with resource constraints.

**Chapter 11** investigates the educational programs, cybersecurity training for medical staff, and best practices for sustainable forensic investigations.

**Chapter 12** analyzes how integrating IoMT forensics into academic curricula and professional training programs. It discusses the skills gap, challenges in forensic education, and opportunities for interdisciplinary research and development.

# Editor biographies

**Hemant Kumar Saini** works as an academic in Lincoln University, Malaysia and the School of Computer Science Engineering at Bennett University (The Times Group), India. He earned his Ph.D. in Computer Science and Engineering from Manipal University in 2023. He had been honored for his research work in Master's degree from Governor of Rajasthan in 2015. He has more than 14 years of teaching experience. He is an active member of ISTE, IEEE, and IAENG, CSI. He has demonstrated his research prowess by publishing articles in the renowned SCI and Scopus journals and conference proceedings. He has published several national and international articles and authored, edited, and coedited 18 books. Dr Saini has delivered many expert talks in ATAL-sponsored Faculty Development Programs and keynote talks in many national and international conferences. He is a member of editorial board and reviewer of many international journals of repute. His research interest includes wireless networks, soft computing, deep and machine learning, Internet of Things (IoT), Industry 4.0, and smart contract. His contributions to these fields have been well-recognized, and he continues to push the boundaries of scientific knowledge.

**Sita Rani** works in the Department of Computer Science and Engineering at Guru Nanak Dev Engineering College, Ludhiana. She earned her Ph.D. in Computer Science and Engineering from I.K. Gujral Punjab Technical University, Kapurthala, Punjab, in 2018. She has also completed Post Graduate Certificate Program in Data Science and Machine Learning from Indian Institute of Technology, Roorkee, in 2023. She has completed her Postdoc from Big Data Mining and Machine Learning Lab, South Ural State University, Russia in August, 2023. She has more than 21 years of teaching experience. She is an active member of ISTE, IEEE, and IAENG. She is the receiver of ISTE Section Best Teacher Award-2020 and International Young Scientist Award-2021. She has contributed to the various research activities while publishing articles in the renowned SCI and Scopus journals and conference proceedings. She has published several national and international patents and authored, edited, and coedited nine books. Dr Rani has delivered many expert talks in A.I.C.T.E.-sponsored Faculty Development Programs and keynote talks in many national and international conferences. She has also organized many international conferences during her 20 years of teaching experience. She is a member of editorial board and reviewer of many international journals of repute. She is also the vice president of SME and MSME (UT Council), Women Indian Chamber of Commerce and Industry (WICCI) from last 3 years. Her research interest includes parallel and distributed computing, data science, machine learning, Internet of Things (IoT), Industry 4.0, and Smart Healthcare.

**Mariya Ouaissa** is currently a professor in cybersecurity and networks at Faculty of Sciences Semlalia, Cadi Ayyad University, Marrakech, Morocco. She is a Ph.D. graduated in 2019 in Computer Science and Networks from ENSAM-Moulay Ismail University, Meknes, Morocco. She is a networks and telecoms engineer, graduated in 2013 from National School of Applied Sciences Khouribga, Morocco. She is a cofounder and IT consultant at IT support and consulting center. She was working for School of Technology of Meknes Morocco as a visiting professor from 2013 to 2021. She is a member of the International Association of Engineers and International Association of Online Engineering, and since 2021, she is an "ACM Professional Member". She is an expert reviewer with Academic Exchange Information Centre (AEIC) and Brand Ambassador with Bentham Science. She has served and continues to serve on technical program and organizer committees of several conferences and events and has organized many symposiums/workshops/conferences as a general chair, also as a reviewer of numerous international journals. Dr Ouaissa has made contributions in the fields of information security and privacy, Internet of Things security, and wireless and constrained networks security. Her main research topics are IoT, M2M, D2D, WSN, cellular networks, and vehicular networks. She has published over 80 papers (book chapters, international journals, and conferences/workshops), 30 edited books, and 10 special issues as guest editor.

**Mariyam Ouaissa** is currently an assistant professor in networks and systems at ENSA, Chouaib Doukkali University, El Jadida, Morocco. She received her Ph.D. degree in 2019 from National Graduate School of Arts and Crafts, Meknes, Morocco, and her Engineering Degree in 2013 from the National School of Applied Sciences, Khouribga, Morocco. She is a communication and networking researcher and practitioner with industry and academic experience. Dr Ouaissa's research is multidisciplinary that focuses on Internet of Things, M2M, WSN, vehicular communications and cellular networks, security networks, congestion overload problem, and the resource allocation management and access control. She is serving as a reviewer for international journals and conferences including *IEEE Access, Wireless Communications and Mobile Computing*. Since 2020, she is a member of "International Association of Engineers IAENG" and "International Association of Online Engineering", and since 2021, she is an "ACM Professional Member". She has published more than 60 research papers (this includes book chapters, peer-reviewed journal articles, and peer-reviewed conference manuscripts), 20 edited books, and 6 special issue as guest editor. She has served on program committees and organizing committees of several conferences and events and has organized many symposiums/workshops/conferences.

**Zakaria Abou El Houda** is currently Professor at INRS, University of Quebec, Canada. He was a researcher at the Department of Computer Science and Operations Research, Université de Montréal, Montréal, Canada. He received the M.Sc. degree in Computer Networks from Paul Sabatier University, Toulouse, France, the Ph.D. degree in Computer Science from the University of Montréal, Canada, and the Ph.D. degree in Computer Engineering from the University of Technology of Troyes, Troyes, France. He has made contributions in the fields of information security, intrusion detection/prevention system, and security in software-defined network. His current research interests include ML/DL-based intrusion detection, federated learning, and blockchain. He has also served and continues to serve on technical program committees and as a reviewer of several international conferences and journals, including IEEE ICC, IEEE Globecom, and IEEE transactions.

**Hajar Moudoud** is currently Professor with the Department of Computer Science and Engineering of the Université du Québec en Outaouais (UQO), Canada. She received the B.Eng. degree in software engineering from the Mohammadia School of Engineers, Rabat, Morocco, in 2018, the Ph.D. degree in Computer Engineering from the University of Sherbrooke, Canada, and the Ph.D. degree in Computer Engineering from the University of Technology of Troyes, France, both in 2022. She is currently a professor with the Department of Computer Science and Engineering of the Université du Québec en Outaouais (UQO), Canada. Prior to joining UQO, she served as a research scientist in various institutions, contributing to significant research projects on the security of the networks based on machine learning models. Her research interests include the security of the Internet of Things, applied machine/deep learning for intrusion detection systems, and leveraging blockchain to enhance the security of next-generation networks.

# Contributors

**Pellate Anoushka**
Stanley College of Engineering & Technology for Women, Hyderabad, India

**Immanuel Anupalli**
Audisankara College of Engineering, Gudur, Nellore, Andhra Pradesh, India

**S. Ashmad**
Sreenivasa Institute of Technology and Management Studies, Chittoor, Andhra Pradesh, India

**Abdelghani El Cheddadi**
Université du Québec en Outaouais, Canada – Global Affairs Canada

**Maroua Cherifi**
Institut National de la Recherche Scientifique Centre Énergie, Matériaux, et Télécommunications (INRS-EMT), Gatineau, Canada

**Aryendra Dalal**
Middle Georgia State University, Macon, GA, USA

**Akashbhai Ashokbhai Dave**
The CVM University, Anand, India

**Srinath Doss**
The Independent Institute of Education, IIEMSA, South Africa – Faculty of Engineering and Technology, Botho University, Botswana,

**Rachid Ed-daoudi**
Ibn Tofail University, Kenitra Morocco

**Zakaria Abou El Houda**
Institut National de la Recherche Scientifique Centre Énergie, Matériaux, et Télécommunications (INRS-EMT), Gatineau, Canada

**G. Fathima**
Adhiyamaan College of Engineering (Autonomous), Hosur, TN, India

**Stéphane Gagnon**
Université du Québec en Outaouais, Canada

**Inam Ullah Khan**
Multimedia University, Cyberjaya, Malaysia

**Hajar Moudoud**
Université du Québec en Outaouais, Canada

**Sainag Nethala**
Cisco Systems, USA

**Mariya Ouaissa**
Cadi Ayyad University, Marrakech, Morocco

**Mariyam Ouaissa**
Chouaib Doukkali University, El Jadida, Morocco

**Fatima Zahra Ouariach**
Abdelmalek Essaadi University, Tanger, Morocco

**Soufiane Ouariach**
Abdelmalek Essaadi University, Tanger, Morocco

**Vijaishree Dubey Pandey**
Christ University, India, Bengaluru, Karnataka, India

**Mariappan Ramasamy**
School of Computer Science and Engineering, Vellore Institute of Technology, India

**C. Kishor Kumar Reddy**
Stanley College of Engineering & Technology for Women, Hyderabad, India

**I. Sakthidevi**
Adhiyamaan College of Engineering (Autonomous), Hosur, TN, India

**M. Saravanan**
Sreenivasa Institute of Technology and Management Studies, Chittoor, Andhra Pradesh, India

**Rituraj Sinha**
Christ University, India, Bengaluru, Karnataka, India

**Shashank Solanki**
Christ University, India, Bengaluru, Karnataka, India

**Pranav Srinivasan**
Mahatma Gandhi Medical College and Research Institute, Pondicherry, India

**P. Sudheer**
Sreenivasa Institute of Technology and Management Studies, Chittoor, Andhra Pradesh, India

**Vijeta Verma**
Christ University, India, Bengaluru, Karnataka, India

Chapter 1

# The role of artificial intelligence and machine learning in safeguarding IoMT security and privacy

*Abdelghani El Cheddadi, Hajar Moudoud, and Stéphane Gagnon*

## 1.1 INTRODUCTION

The healthcare sector is experiencing significant evolution, fueled by breakthroughs in artificial intelligence (AI), the Internet of Medical Things (IoMT), and cutting-edge communication technologies [1]. These advancements are revolutionizing conventional approaches, facilitating more accurate diagnostics, tailored treatments, and integrated patient care, all while striving to enhance resource efficiency and lower operational expenses. Yet, realizing these transformative objectives is hindered by pressing issues such as data security, scalability, and interoperability. A key factor propelling this shift is the growing incidence of chronic illnesses and the aging population worldwide. Chronic ailments like diabetes, heart disease, and respiratory disorders are responsible for 60% of global deaths, according to the World Health Organization (WHO) [2]. These conditions impose a substantial strain on healthcare systems, leading to escalated costs, extended hospitalizations, and a heightened need for specialized services. The aging demographic further intensifies these challenges, with the United Nations forecasting that by 2050, one in six individuals globally will be 65 or older, up from 1 in 11 in 2019 [3]. This trend significantly amplifies the pressure on healthcare infrastructure and personnel. Additionally, the shortage of healthcare workers presents a critical obstacle to addressing these escalating demands. The WHO predicts a global deficit of over 18 million healthcare professionals by 2030, with low- and middle-income nations likely to be the most affected. This gap highlights the pressing necessity for technological solutions that can improve efficiency and reduce the workload on healthcare staff. For example, AI-driven tools that automate administrative duties and IoMT systems that enable continuous patient monitoring can help mitigate workforce shortages while ensuring quality care.

AI has emerged as a groundbreaking force in the healthcare sector, revolutionizing areas such as diagnostics, treatment planning, patient monitoring, and operational efficiency [4]. By harnessing advanced machine learning (ML) techniques, natural language processing, and computer vision,

DOI: 10.1201/9781003640325-1

AI-powered systems are addressing some of the most critical challenges in healthcare. In diagnostics, AI has demonstrated exceptional precision, particularly in identifying conditions like diabetic retinopathy, breast cancer, and lung diseases. Trained on vast datasets, ML models have achieved diagnostic accuracy rates of up to 90%, often outperforming human clinicians in specific, well-defined tasks [5]. For instance, AI tools analyzing mammograms or retinal scans can detect early disease indicators that might elude even seasoned specialists. This not only enhances patient outcomes through early detection but also helps meet the rising demand for diagnostic services in resource-limited areas.

Beyond diagnostics, AI is driving advancements in personalized medicine and treatment optimization [6]. By evaluating patient-specific data, including genetic information, medical histories, and lifestyle factors, AI platforms can recommend customized treatment plans that improve effectiveness while reducing side effects. In fields like oncology, AI is being utilized to determine the best drug combinations and dosages for individual patients, enabling more targeted and efficient therapies. AI is also transforming patient monitoring and predictive analytics. With the ability to process real-time data from wearable devices and IoT-enabled sensors, AI algorithms can identify irregularities or predict health risks before they escalate. For example, AI-based systems can notify healthcare providers of early warning signs of conditions like heart failure or sepsis, allowing for prompt intervention and minimizing complications.

In addition to optimizing treatment, AI is used to optimize healthcare pathways, especially for patients with comorbidity and chronic conditions [7]. Complex care requires numerous health service encounters, whether with the treating physician or specialists, and with various services such as testing centers, rehabilitation services, etc. Scheduling each service requires careful monitoring of ongoing chronic conditions and rapid response to reschedule services as needed. In addition, coordination among multiple providers requires seamless information exchange while preserving patient privacy and assuring care quality. Hence, AI can be used to extract service rules from patient records, which are then fed back into a hybrid rule-based and inference-based knowledge graph (KG) to enable reasoning by agents for rescheduling [8].

Compliance management plays a crucial role in ensuring the security and privacy of the IoMT, particularly as regulatory frameworks evolve to address emerging cyber threats. ML and AI enhance compliance by automating security monitoring, threat detection, and risk assessment processes [9]. These technologies enable organizations to proactively identify vulnerabilities, enforce security policies, and ensure adherence to regulations such as HIPAA, GDPR, and FDA guidelines. By leveraging AI-driven anomaly detection and predictive analytics, healthcare institutions can maintain real-time compliance with security standards while minimizing the risk of data breaches and unauthorized access to sensitive medical information.

Moreover, AI and ML streamline compliance documentation and auditing by automating the classification of medical data and verifying adherence to established security protocols [10–12]. These technologies assist in generating detailed audit logs, conducting continuous compliance checks, and responding to regulatory changes dynamically. AI-driven compliance solutions can also enhance patient data privacy by implementing advanced encryption techniques, access controls, and identity verification mechanisms. By integrating AI-powered compliance management into IoMT security frameworks, healthcare providers can ensure both regulatory adherence and robust protection of patient information, ultimately fostering trust and reliability in connected medical devices.

The main contributions of this paper can be summarized as follows:

- We present a systematic overview of AI/ML models for threat detection, anomaly identification, and adaptive security in IoMT ecosystems.
- We synthesize and compare global data protection regulations (GDPR, HIPAA, PIPEDA). First, we provide actionable implementation guidelines for IoMT stakeholders. We then identify regulatory gaps in current healthcare IoT frameworks.
- We present a use case study evaluating federated learning (FL) as a privacy-preserving solution for IoMT. Using a breast cancer dataset, we assess FL's performance in decentralized medical data analysis, achieving high accuracy (98%) while maintaining patient privacy.

## 1.2 ROLE OF ARTIFICIAL INTELLIGENCE TO SECURE THE IOMT

### 1.2.1 Overview of the IoMT

The IoMT is a specialized subset of the Internet of Things (IoT) designed for healthcare applications [13]. It consists of interconnected medical devices, sensors, and systems that collect, transmit, and analyze health-related data. To understand its architecture, the IoMT is often divided into layers, each serving a specific function in the data lifecycle. The perception layer captures health metrics through wearables, implants, and medical sensors, while the network layer ensures secure data transmission using protocols like Bluetooth, 5G, or LPWAN. The edge layer processes data locally to reduce latency, enabling real-time responses in critical scenarios. In the cloud layer, data are stored and analyzed at scale, integrating with electronic health records and AI-driven diagnostic tools. The application layer delivers actionable insights to healthcare providers and patients through telemedicine platforms or remote monitoring systems. Across all layers, the security and compliance layer safeguards sensitive data, adhering to regulations like HIPAA and GDPR.

### 1.2.2 AI-powered threat detection and anomaly identification

AI enhances IoMT security by identifying cyber threats in real time through advanced anomaly detection techniques. Traditional security measures often struggle to keep up with the dynamic nature of cyber threats targeting medical devices [14]. AI-driven threat detection systems analyze massive streams of data from connected IoMT devices, identifying unusual patterns that may indicate potential cyberattacks. These systems use ML models to detect deviations from normal device behavior, such as unauthorized access attempts, irregular data transmission, or unexpected software modifications. By continuously monitoring device activity, AI ensures that threats are identified and addressed before they can compromise patient safety or healthcare operations.

In addition to detecting known threats, AI-powered security solutions can identify previously unseen or zero-day attacks. Since AI models learn from historical attack patterns, they can recognize subtle indicators of compromise and flag suspicious activities that might otherwise go undetected. This proactive approach minimizes false positives while ensuring that genuine threats receive immediate attention. By integrating AI-driven anomaly detection into IoMT security frameworks, healthcare organizations can significantly reduce the risk of cyberattacks and ensure the integrity of patient data and medical devices.

### 1.2.3 Automated risk assessment and predictive analytics

Risk assessment is a critical component of IoMT security, as medical devices are increasingly targeted by cybercriminals [15]. AI enables automated risk evaluation by analyzing real-time and historical data to assess vulnerabilities and predict potential threats. ML algorithms examine network traffic, device logs, and system configurations to identify weak points that could be exploited. This allows security teams to take preventive measures, such as patching software vulnerabilities or reinforcing authentication mechanisms, before an attack occurs. AI-driven risk assessment tools provide continuous monitoring and real-time risk scoring, enabling healthcare providers to prioritize their security efforts based on the severity of potential threats.

Predictive analytics further enhances IoMT security by forecasting emerging cyber threats and attack trends. By analyzing threat intelligence feeds and past security incidents, AI can anticipate future attack methods and recommend strategies to mitigate risks. For instance, AI can predict when a ransomware campaign might target healthcare institutions and advise organizations on strengthening their defenses accordingly. By leveraging AI-powered risk assessment and predictive analytics, IoMT environments can transition from a reactive security posture to a proactive one, significantly reducing the chances of successful cyberattacks.

### 1.2.4 Adaptive security and self-learning defense mechanisms

IoMT security must continuously evolve to combat sophisticated cyber threats, and AI-driven adaptive security systems provide a dynamic approach to protection. Unlike traditional security measures that rely on static rules, AI-based security frameworks adjust and refine their defense strategies based on real-time threat intelligence. Self-learning AI models analyze new attack patterns, update security protocols, and autonomously strengthen defenses without human intervention. This ensures that IoMT networks remain resilient against emerging threats, including advanced persistent threats and zero-day exploits [16].

Self-learning AI mechanisms also play a crucial role in reducing false positives and improving response accuracy. By analyzing past security incidents and refining its detection models, AI minimizes alert fatigue and ensures that security teams focus on genuine threats. Additionally, AI-powered defense systems can deploy automated countermeasures, such as isolating compromised devices or enforcing stricter access controls in response to detected anomalies. This ability to adapt in real time enhances the overall security posture of IoMT environments, making them more resilient to cyber threats.

### 1.2.5 AI-driven compliance monitoring and regulatory enforcement

Ensuring compliance with healthcare security regulations is essential for protecting patient data and maintaining trust in IoMT systems. AI simplifies compliance management by automating security monitoring and regulatory enforcement. AI-powered compliance tools continuously scan IoMT networks for noncompliant behaviors, such as unsecured data transmissions, unauthorized device access, or outdated security configurations. These tools generate real-time reports and alerts, enabling healthcare organizations to promptly address compliance gaps and avoid regulatory penalties. By automating routine compliance checks, AI reduces the burden on IT and security teams while ensuring continuous adherence to industry standards such as HIPAA, GDPR, and FDA cybersecurity guidelines.

## 1.3 PRIVACY IN THE IOMT: OVERVIEW OF COMPLIANCE MONITORING

Developed nations have established data privacy and protection laws to ensure the secure handling of citizens' personal information. This section briefly examines some of these regulations, highlighting their objectives and characteristics. By comparing these laws, we can understand how they offer security at various levels within the proposed healthcare framework.

Law enforcement bodies in America, Europe, and other leading countries are striving to find common solutions to healthcare data privacy challenges while enhancing existing legal frameworks. An effective legal framework should empower users by raising awareness and giving them control over IoT healthcare products and services. Aligning with international data privacy standards further strengthens this framework. Implementing IoT data privacy regulations is crucial for legal compliance, upholding human rights, and maintaining social norms. Typically, these regulations aim to support core privacy principles such as fairness, purpose fulfillment, proportionality, and accountability. Collaboration between government agencies and private organizations can help achieve these goals [17, 18].

### 1.3.1 Personal information protection and electronic documents act

Introduced by the Canadian federal government in 2001, the Personal Information Protection and Electronic Documents Act (PIPEDA) aims to give individuals some control over their personal information. It mandates that organizations handling and disclosing the personal information of Canadian citizens adhere to specific policies. These policies require informing citizens about the personal information being processed or disclosed and ensuring that this information is protected with adequate security measures.

PIPEDA applies to all personal data, including healthcare data and other private information. Organizations that collect data are responsible for protecting it. However, PIPEDA is not universally applicable across Canada; each province can enforce its own rules and policies, provided they align with PIPEDA.

PIPEDA offers basic guidelines for organizations collecting and processing personal information for business purposes. Interconnected devices should adhere to the data privacy principles and security standards outlined in PIPEDA.

Although Canada currently lacks IoT-specific legislation, the Office of the Privacy Commissioner (OPC) issued privacy guidelines for IoT device manufacturers on August 20, 2020 [19]. These guidelines, informed by federal investigations, outline essential and recommended practices for device makers. While aimed at manufacturers, other IoT stakeholders involved in deploying IoT solutions should also review these guidelines. We summarize the key points of PIPEDA as follows:

- Regulatory Compliance: IoT device data collection must be carefully examined. The regulator notes that metadata may be considered personal information, subjecting it to federal privacy legislation like PIPEDA or relevant provincial laws. Additionally, manufacturers must adhere to the Canada Consumer Product Safety Act (CCPSA), which prohibits the manufacture, import, advertising, or sale of products posing health or safety risks.
- Privacy Accountability: Establishing a privacy management program is crucial for monitoring personal information and ensuring legal compliance, including mandatory breach reporting. Manufacturers remain responsible for data even after device sales, and conducting privacy impact assessments during product development is recommended.
- Meaningful Information Handling: Data collection should have a clear purpose, with use, collection, and disclosure limited to that purpose. Consent must be meaningful and aligned with reasonable expectations, especially concerning children's personal information in smart toys and educational products.
- Access, Accuracy, and Safeguarding: Consumers have the right to access and correct their information. Manufacturers should provide user-friendly mechanisms for data deletion and ensure robust safeguards, including encryption and firmware updates, to protect personal information throughout the device's lifecycle.

The OPC Guidance 3: Privacy Guidance on the Internet of Things for Manufacturers and Canadians [19], published by the Office of the Privacy Commissioner of Canada in August 2020, emphasizes the importance of complying with existing privacy and product liability regulations for IoT solutions in Canada. Additionally, institutions procuring IoT solutions should prioritize the protection of personal information as a fundamental aspect of their digital transformation initiatives.

### 1.3.2 Office of privacy commissioner's guidance of internet of things devices

Organizations must implement robust privacy practices to protect personal information under their control. This begins with accountability, ensuring that policies and procedures are in place to manage personal data responsibly. Additionally, organizations must identify the purposes for collecting personal information before gathering any data, ensuring transparency and compliance.

Consent plays a critical role in privacy protection. Organizations must obtain informed and meaningful consent from individuals before collecting, using, or disclosing their personal information. They should also adopt a limiting collection approach, designing devices to gather only the data necessary for the stated purposes. Similarly, the use, disclosure, and retention of personal data should be restricted to the original purpose of collection.

To maintain data integrity, organizations must ensure accuracy, keeping personal information up-to-date and complete, particularly when making decisions about individuals or sharing their data. Implementing appropriate safeguards—such as encryption and password protection—is essential to protecting personal information from unauthorized access.

Transparency is another key principle. Organizations should practice openness by informing individuals about their information management policies and practices. They must also provide individual access, allowing people to review their information and request corrections if necessary. Furthermore, organizations should establish procedures for challenging compliance, enabling individuals to raise concerns about privacy practices.

Special attention must be given to children's information, ensuring limited collection, use, sharing, and retention of their data. Additionally, technological safeguards, including encryption and secure authentication methods, should be employed to enhance data security. To strengthen privacy protections, organizations should adopt transparent privacy policies tailored to specific devices. These policies should outline data collection practices, including a list of sensors used and the duration of security updates. User notifications should be implemented to inform individuals when data is being collected and provide options to limit this collection.

Risk assessments are vital for identifying and mitigating potential privacy and security risks associated with devices and information handling. Additionally, password management practices should encourage users to create strong, unique passwords to enhance security.

Consumers should be given data deletion options that allow them to permanently remove their personal information, with clear instructions on the process. Lastly, organizations must ensure that firmware updates are available and accessible, allowing users to update or patch their devices to maintain security over time.

### 1.3.3 General data protection regulation

In May 2018, the General Data Protection Regulation (GDPR) replaced Directive 95/46/EC, consolidating and enhancing data protection rules across the European Union. The GDPR is more comprehensive and introduces internal compliance mechanisms that were previously absent. It applies to all economic sectors, broadly defined personal data, and any sector that controls or processes data. The regulation ensures protective standards throughout the data lifecycle, empowering individuals to better control their personal information.

The GDPR addresses inconsistencies in the 1995 EU Data Protection Directive, ensuring uniform application across all EU member states. Its impact is particularly significant for healthcare organizations, hospitals, and other entities processing healthcare data. Under GDPR, these organizations must demonstrate accountability for how healthcare data is processed. Both data controllers and processors are responsible for compliance and any data breaches that occur.

Healthcare organizations must be transparent and vigilant in managing data processing activities and must ensure that staff maintain a secure data flow.

### 1.3.4 Health insurance portability and accountability act

In the United States, there is no universally recognized standard for privacy concerning big data sets used in precision medicine. The primary federal law governing health information is the Health Insurance Portability and Accountability Act (HIPAA) [19, 20]. This law applies to "covered entities," including healthcare providers, health plans, and health information clearinghouses, as well as their business associates.

HIPAA serves three main purposes related to medical information:

- Establishing frameworks for the disclosure of protected health information (PHI).
- Creating security standards for patient information, whether stored or in transit.
- Specifying a common format and data structure for the electronic exchange of health information.

PHI encompasses any individually identifiable health information created or collected by a covered entity or business associate.

The privacy rule within HIPAA governs how health information can be disclosed, both with and without patient consent. It allows the disclosure of PHI without consent for treatment, payment, and routine healthcare operations. Additionally, consent is not required for mandatory reporting to public health agencies, informing law enforcement or national security, and determining eligibility for public benefits. The privacy rule aims to minimize the potential harm that can result from disclosing sensitive health information, recognizing the particular sensitivity of such data for many patients.

### 1.3.5 Health information technology for economic and clinical health act

The HITECH Act, enacted as Title XIII of the American Recovery and Reinvestment Act of 2009, reinforced many HIPAA regulations.

It introduced stricter enforcement guidelines and increased civil and criminal penalties for violations of HIPAA's security and privacy rules. The law expanded HIPAA's reach to include business associates and contractors of covered entities, making them directly accountable for compliance. Key provisions of the HITECH Act include the following:

- Breach Notification: Mandated practices for covered entities, business associates, and contractors to notify and publicly disclose breaches of PHI.
- Federal Standards: Established federal health data breach standards that complement state laws and pre-empt contradictory state regulations.
- Audit Program: Initiated by the HHS Office for Civil Rights (OCR) in 2012, the HIPAA compliance audit program assesses organizations' adherence to HIPAA privacy, security, and breach notification regulations, including those added or amended by HITECH.

Prior to 2012, HIPAA compliance audits were conducted only in response to formal complaints or notifications alleging violations. The HITECH-mandated audit program aims to proactively ensure compliance. To assist covered entities and business associates in preparing for potential audits, OCR publishes a detailed audit protocol outlining each criterion, assessment methods, and specific procedures used by auditors.

Several aspects of the Internet of Healthcare Things (IoHT) are not addressed by existing legislative initiatives [21]. Next, we overview some major challenges that need to be addressed:

- Security and Privacy: Integrating healthcare data raises significant security and privacy concerns. Patient information is processed at varying security levels in data centers. While many American organizations have HIPAA certification, this does not ensure the safety of patient records, as HIPAA focuses more on security policies than implementation.
- Data Transmission: Transmitting large datasets from different locations adds complexity to processing and storage. Traditional security solutions are insufficient for handling large, dynamic datasets.
- Cloud Solutions: The rise of cloud healthcare solutions introduces additional security challenges, with no specific policies outlined in current healthcare data protection laws.
- Data Governance: Effective data governance is crucial for managing healthcare data, especially as the industry shifts toward a value-based business model. This requires a common data representation that encompasses various security standards (e.g., ICD, CPT, LOINC).

- Diverse Data: The healthcare industry generates diverse data, necessitating a robust governance model. However, there are currently no policies for standardizing and normalizing healthcare data to ensure proper governance.

## 1.3.6 Privacy-preserving analytics in healthcare

The healthcare industry is increasingly adopting IoT devices to monitor and transmit vital signs to healthcare clouds, necessitating ad hoc, decentralized data processing and analysis. However, executing resource-intensive operations while preserving privacy poses significant challenges. As healthcare data analytics gain traction, existing privacy laws need revision, and new legislation should be drafted to address the comprehensive use of patients' private data.

### *1.3.6.1 Privacy violations in IoT-based devices*

Privacy can be compromised when third parties collect data without user awareness or consent. Unauthorized data collection can lead to potential breaches and misuse of sensitive personal information, raising significant privacy concerns.

Unauthorized use and sharing of private data further exacerbate these risks. When personal information is distributed without proper safeguards, individuals lose control over their data, which can be exploited for commercial, insurance, or other unintended purposes.

In many cases, newly generated data is combined with existing patient information, often without the user's knowledge. This process, known as data aggregation, enhances the commercial value of data for organizations that rely on data-driven insights. However, it also increases privacy risks, as more comprehensive data profiles can be created without patient consent.

Automated medical devices generate the majority of healthcare data, necessitating a higher level of trust compared to manually entered information. Insurance companies increasingly use these devices to monitor health conditions and assess risks, highlighting the need for robust security measures. To protect patient privacy, legislative controls must be in place to regulate data usage, including restrictions on geolocation tracking and unauthorized data access.

### *1.3.6.2 Data and context quality*

Data quality is highly dependent on the environment in which it is collected. Variations in environmental conditions can impact the accuracy and reliability of data, potentially leading to inconsistencies or errors. Additionally, incomplete or contradictory context information can create ambiguity, increasing the risk of confidentiality breaches and misinterpretation of data.

The sensitivity of context quality, including changes in contextual information, further underscores the need for strict privacy protections. Unauthorized access to or misuse of this information can expose individuals to security risks and privacy violations.

IoT devices rely heavily on contextual data and often do not provide users with straightforward options to shut down or disconnect. This persistent connectivity raises significant privacy concerns, emphasizing the need for enhanced privacy measures to protect users from unauthorized data collection and potential misuse.

#### *1.3.6.3 Enhancing transparency in healthcare systems*

To improve transparency in healthcare systems, it is crucial to manage both the data propagated from various devices and the data automatically generated by healthcare devices. Despite the importance of this issue, there is currently no legislation addressing it. A combined approach, integrating technical standards and existing regulatory frameworks, is necessary to ensure data transparency.

#### *1.3.6.4 Privacy concerns in IoT-based healthcare applications*

Interactive devices such as heartbeat monitors, geo-tracking devices, and automated insulin pumps require continuous interaction with patients. These devices collect highly sensitive information through sensors and medical readings, which, when exchanged across different systems, can pose significant privacy threats. Unauthorized access to this data can lead to security breaches and misuse of personal health information. In smart cities, data transmission must be carefully managed to protect patient privacy. Queries for healthcare services should not inadvertently disclose personal information, for example, requesting directions to a health clinic should remain private and not be publicly visible. Additionally, medical devices must encrypt data during transmission to prevent unauthorized access and ensure the confidentiality of sensitive health data.

#### *1.3.6.5 Privacy risks during life cycle transitions*

Privacy is at risk when IoT devices disclose sensitive information during their life cycle transitions. Many healthcare devices store vital sign readings, drug dosages, and actuator functions, making the data they hold highly sensitive. Any unauthorized disclosure during updates, repairs, or disposal can lead to privacy breaches.

Even seemingly simple usage data, such as location, duration, and frequency of device use, can reveal critical details about individuals' lifestyles. This type of data, when aggregated, can expose behavioral patterns and personal health conditions, further highlighting the need for strict privacy controls.

A major challenge in healthcare IoT is the outdated "buy-once-own-forever" model, where privacy solutions are often limited to complete memory wipes or physical destruction of devices. This approach is neither flexible nor sustainable, emphasizing the urgent need for improved privacy management mechanisms throughout the entire life cycle of healthcare devices. Addressing these concerns requires the implementation of robust and adaptable privacy solutions that safeguard sensitive information at every stage of a device's use.

## 1.4 USE CASE STUDY: FEDERATED LEARNING TO ENABLE SECURITY AND PRIVACY IN THE IOMT

Numerous studies have explored the application of privacy-preserving techniques, such as FL, to improve data security and operational efficiency in healthcare systems. In this section, we propose evaluating the security and privacy of IoMT. We propose using a FL model and evaluate it on a medical dataset [7, 22–24]. First, we outline the experimental parameters and performance metrics. Subsequently, we analyze the results of our ranking-based resource providers approach and compare their performance with other existing methods.

### 1.4.1 Simulation parameters and metrics

To evaluate our proposal, we used a breast cancer dataset. Tables 1.1 and 1.2 present a description of the dataset.

### 1.4.2 Simulation results

In Figure 1.1, we evaluate the performance of a classification model using the receiver operating characteristic (ROC) curve. The plot illustrates

*Table 1.1* Breast cancer dataset description

| *Classes* | 2 |
|---|---|
| Samples per class | 212(M),357(B) |
| Samples total | 569 |
| Dimensionality | 30 |
| Features | Real, positive |

*Table 1.2* Quantitative evaluation of federated learning on breast cancer dataset

| *Classification* | *Precision* | *Recall* | *F1-Score* | *Support* |
|---|---|---|---|---|
| 0 | 0.91 | 1.00 | 0.95 | 39 |
| 1 | 1.00 | 0.97 | 0.98 | 132 |
| Accuracy | | | 0.98 | 171 |
| Macro avg | 0.95 | 0.98 | 0.97 | 171 |
| Weighted avg | 0.98 | 0.98 | 0.98 | 171 |

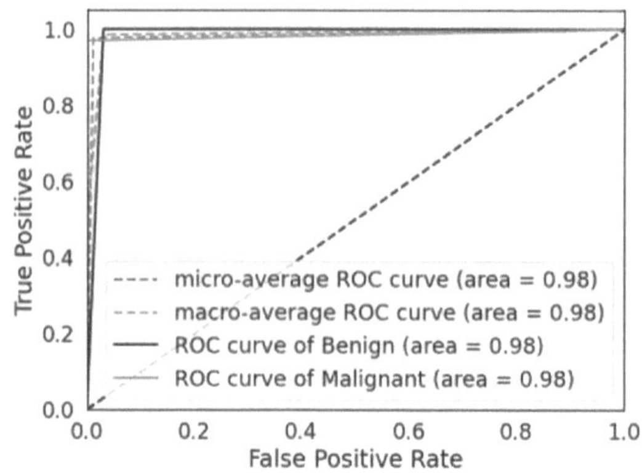


*Figure 1.1* ROC curve comparison.

the trade-off between the true positive rate and the false positive rate for different scenarios, including micro-average, macro-average, and individual class curves (benign and malignant). The high area under the curve value of 0.98 across all curves indicates excellent model performance, demonstrating strong discrimination between the two classes. The diagonal dashed line represents a random classifier, while the curves lying significantly above it confirm the model's effectiveness in distinguishing between benign and malignant cases.

In Figure 1.2, we evaluate the model's accuracy over multiple training rounds. The plot demonstrates a rapid increase in accuracy during the initial rounds, followed by a plateau as the model converges toward its optimal performance. The accuracy stabilizes at a high level, indicating that the model quickly learns from the training data and achieves consistent performance. The trend suggests that additional training rounds may provide minimal improvements, highlighting the model's efficiency in reaching high accuracy within a few iterations.

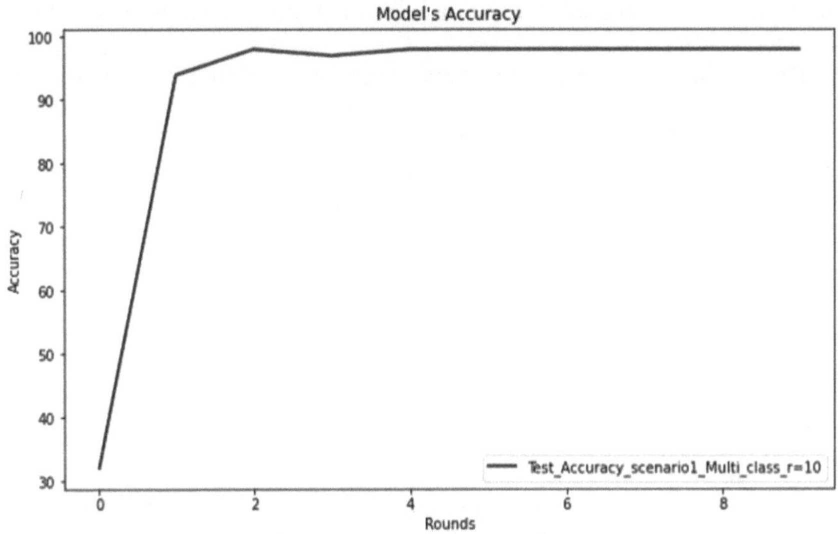


*Figure 1.2* Model accuracy per number of rounds.

## 1.5 CONCLUSION

The integration of AI and ML into the IoMT represents a transformative advancement in healthcare, offering unparalleled opportunities to enhance diagnostics, treatment personalization, and operational efficiency. However, this evolution also brings significant challenges, particularly in safeguarding data security and privacy. AI-driven solutions, such as real-time threat detection, adaptive security mechanisms, and automated compliance monitoring, provide robust defenses against cyber threats while ensuring adherence to stringent regulations like HIPAA, GDPR, and PIPEDA.

As healthcare services are increasingly more diverse and patients require more complex care, AI will become determinant in ensuring services remain efficient and effective. There will be a greater role of ML in rule discovery to optimize service delivery. KGs will also become standard in ensuring AI remains conforming to formal conditions to guide services. The impact of IoMT on healthcare outcomes will be greater as all information sources are adequately integrated within a more intelligent and autonomic digital health framework.

The chapter highlights the critical role of FL in preserving privacy by enabling decentralized data analysis without compromising sensitive patient information. Experimental results on a breast cancer dataset demonstrate the efficacy of FL, achieving high accuracy and strong performance metrics, as evidenced by the ROC curve and training accuracy trends. These findings underscore the potential of FL to balance data utility with privacy in IoMT environments.

Despite these advancements, gaps remain in legislative frameworks and data governance, particularly for emerging technologies like cloud-based healthcare solutions and IoT devices. Addressing these challenges requires a collaborative effort among policymakers, healthcare providers, and technology developers to establish standardized protocols and enhance transparency.

## REFERENCES


[1] Vishnu, S., S. R. Jino Ramson, and R. Jegan. "Internet of medical things (IoMT)-An overview." *2020 5th international conference on devices, circuits and systems (ICDCS)*. IEEE, 2020.

[2] Mathers, C. D., T. Boerma, and D. M. Fat. "Global and regional causes of death." *British Medical Bulletin*, 2009; 92(1): 7–32.

[3] Pilleron, S., et al. "Estimated global cancer incidence in the oldest adults in 2018 and projections to 2050." *International Journal of Cancer*, 2021; 148 (3): 601–608.

[4] Saraswat, D., et al. "Explainable AI for healthcare 5.0: opportunities and challenges." *IEEE Access*, 2022; 10: 84486–84517.

[5] Chugh, G., S. Kumar, and N. Singh. "Survey on machine learning and deep learning applications in breast cancer diagnosis." *Cognitive Computation*, 2021; 13 (6): 1451–1470.

[6] Asif, S., et al. "Advancements and prospects of machine learning in medical diagnostics: unveiling the future of diagnostic precision." *Archives of Computational Methods in Engineering* 2024; 32: 1–31.

[7] Scheplitz, T., M. Burwitz, and T. Weimann, "PathwAI systems in healthcare – a framework for coupling AI and pathway-based health information systems." *Hawaii International Conference on System Sciences 2022 (HICSS-55)*, Jan. 2022 [Online]. Available: https://aisel.aisnet.org/hicss-55/hc/process_mining/3

[8] Dwyer, O. P., T. Baldazzi, J. Davies, E. Sallinger, and A. Vlad, "Reasoning over health records with Vadalog: a rule-based approach to patient pathways." 2023. Accessed: Apr. 04, 2025. [Online]. Available: https://ora.ox.ac.uk/objects/uuid:e6aa3977-71b2-4f67-8ef0-9b608a0d7c59

[9] Rasool, R. Ur, et al. "Security and privacy of internet of medical things: A contemporary review in the age of surveillance, botnets, and adversarial ML." *Journal of Network and Computer Applications*, 2022; 201: 103332.

[10] Moudoud, H., S. Cherkaoui, and L. Khoukhi. "Towards a secure and reliable federated learning using blockchain." *2021 IEEE global communications conference (GLOBECOM)*. IEEE, 2021.

[11] Abou El Houda, Z., H. Moudoud, and B. Brik. "Federated deep reinforcement learning for efficient jamming attack mitigation in O-RAN." *IEEE Transactions on Vehicular Technology*, 2024; 73 (7): 9334–9343.

[12] Abou El Houda, Z., et al. "Securing federated learning through blockchain and explainable AI for robust intrusion detection in IoT networks." *IEEE INFOCOM 2023-IEEE Conference on Computer Communications Workshops (INFOCOM WKSHPS)*. IEEE, 2023.

[13] Si-Ahmed, A., M. A. Al-Garadi, and N. Boustia. "Survey of machine learning based intrusion detection methods for internet of medical things." *Applied Soft Computing* 2023; 140: 110227.

[14] Zachos, G., et al. "An anomaly-based intrusion detection system for internet of medical things networks." *Electronics*, 2021; 10 (21): 2562.

[15] Alsubaei, F., A. Abuhussein, and S. Shiva. "Security and privacy in the internet of medical things: taxonomy and risk assessment." *2017 IEEE 42nd conference on local computer networks workshops (LCN workshops)*. IEEE, 2017.

[16] Thomasian, N. M. and E. Y. Adashi. "Cybersecurity in the internet of medical things." *Health Policy and Technology*, 2021; 10 (3): 100549.

[17] Porambage, P., M. Ylianttila, C. Schmitt, P. Kumar, A. Gurtov, and A. V. Vasilakos. "The quest for privacy in the internet of things." *IEEE Cloud Computing*, 2016; 3, 36–45.

[18] Shahid, J., R. Ahmad, A. K. Kiani, T. Ahmad, S. Saeed, and A. M. Almuhaideb. "Data protection and privacy of the internet of healthcare things (IoHTs)." *Applied Sciences*, 2022; 12, 1927. https://doi.org/10.3390/app12041927)

[19] Office of the Privacy Commissioner of Canada. Privacy guidance on the Internet of Things for manufacturers and Canadians, August, 2020.

[20] Klonoff, D. C., and W. N. 2nd. Price. "The need for a privacy standard for medical devices that transmit protected health information used in the precision medicine initiative for diabetes and other diseases." *Journal of Diabetes Science and Technology*, 2017; 11(2), 220–223. doi:10.1177/1932296816680006

[21] Elbasi, E. "B-DCT based watermarking algorithm for patient data protection in IoMT." *2020 International Conference on Information Security and Cryptology (ISCTURKEY)*. IEEE, 2020.

[22] Moudoud, H., and S. Cherkaoui. "Federated learning meets blockchain to secure the metaverse." *2023 International Wireless Communications and Mobile Computing (IWCMC)*. IEEE, 2023.

[23] Abou El Houda, Z., H. Moudoud, and L. Khoukhi. "Secure and efficient federated learning for robust intrusion detection in IoT networks." *GLOBECOM 2023–2023 IEEE Global Communications Conference*. IEEE, 2023.

[24] Moudoud, H., Z. A. El Houda, and B. Brik. "Advancing security and trust in WSNs: A federated multi-agent deep reinforcement learning approach." *IEEE Transactions on Consumer Electronics* 2024; 70, 6909–6918.

Chapter 2

# Federated learning in healthcare

## Privacy-preserving collaboration for medical advancements

*Maroua Cherifi and Zakaria Abou El Houda*

## 2.1 INTRODUCTION

Artificial intelligence (AI) has significantly impacted various sectors, with healthcare being one of the most transformative. AI technologies have enhanced the ability of healthcare professionals to diagnose and treat diseases more accurately and efficiently. Despite these advances, the adoption of AI in healthcare faces challenges due to the difficulty in accessing large, diverse, and up-to-date medical datasets, which are essential for developing effective AI models [1–3]. This challenge is primarily due to the sensitive nature of medical data in terms of privacy, making it difficult for healthcare providers to share patient information. To address these challenges, this article presents an innovative federated learning (FL) architecture that ensures patient data confidentiality while promoting effective collaboration among different stakeholders in the medical field. FL is a decentralized method that allows the training of machine learning models on datasets distributed across multiple sites, eliminating the need to centralize the data. FL enables each healthcare provider to train a local model using their data and then share only the model updates with a central server. This approach ensures that sensitive patient data remains local, reducing the risk of data breaches and ensuring compliance with privacy regulations. In our paper, we leverage three medical datasets, namely: brain tumors, breast cancer, and dermatology data. The brain tumor data comes from MRI scans and includes images classified into two categories: the presence or absence of a tumor. These data are crucial for developing models capable of early detection of brain tumors and improving patient survival rates [4–6]. The breast cancer data includes mammograms labeled to indicate the presence of benign or malignant tumors. This type of data is essential for training breast cancer detection models, which can help diagnose the disease at a treatable stage [7, 8]. Regarding dermatology data, skin samples were taken for the evaluation of 22 histopathological characteristics, whose values are determined by analyzing the samples under a microscope. These dermatology data comprise six different classes, each representing a specific skin

 DOI: 10.1201/9781003640325-2

condition. For the brain tumor and breast cancer datasets, which are binary and consist of two classes, we distributed the data nonspecifically among different clients. This general approach allowed us to evaluate the performance of our models without focusing on the intricacies of data distribution. In contrast, we employed a more structured distribution strategy for the dermatology dataset. Each class within this dataset was assigned to a specific client during the training phase. This method aimed to simulate real-world scenarios where data might be separated by different institutions or departments, each specializing in certain types of cases. By assigning each class to a distinct client, we were able to examine the impact of this data partitioning on model performance [9]. We then applied various algorithms, including convolutional neural networks (CNN), VGG16, Decision Tree, and Random Forest, to these datasets. Our primary objective was to measure the differences in terms of accuracy and F1 score across these methods. This comprehensive evaluation helps identify the most effective techniques for improving diagnostic accuracy while maintaining data confidentiality in a FL environment [10–44].

## 2.2 SYSTEM ARCHITECTURE

The system architecture of the FL model used in this study is designed to ensure data privacy and security while enabling collaborative learning across multiple medical institutions. The architecture is built upon a decentralized learning model where the data remains at the local sites (medical institutions), and only model updates are shared with a central server. This ensures that sensitive patient data, such as medical images and diagnostic information, never leave their respective locations, thereby maintaining strict compliance with privacy regulations like HIPAA.

### 2.2.1 Overview of federated learning in healthcare

The architecture follows the general FL workflow, as shown in Figure 2.1. In this architecture, several clients (medical institutions) independently train their local machine learning models on local datasets and then send only the updated model parameters to a central server. The central server aggregates the model updates using algorithms such as federated averaging (FedAvg) to create a global model, which is then sent back to the clients for further training. This iterative process continues until the model achieves convergence.

### 2.2.2 Components of the system architecture

1. **Local clients (medical institutions):**
   - **Data locality:** The client institutions (hospitals, clinics) maintain their own datasets, including medical images (e.g., MRI

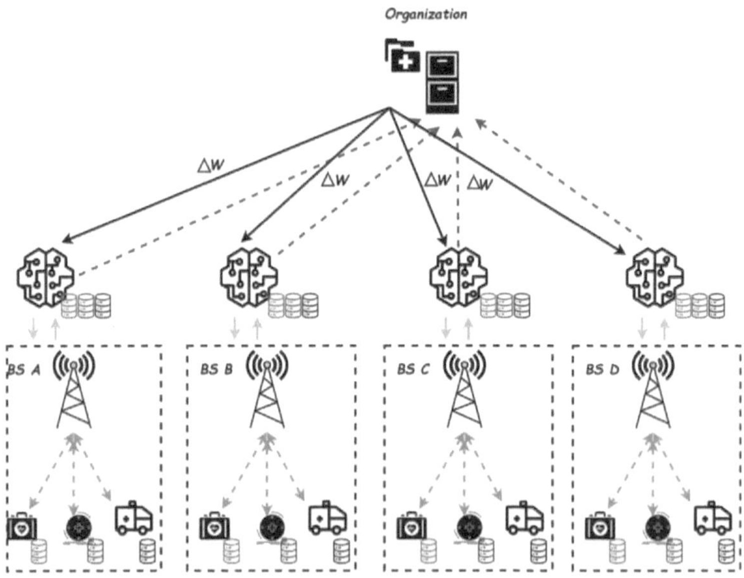


*Figure 2.1* System architecture.

scans, mammograms) and other patient information (e.g., dermatological histopathological data). These datasets are never centralized or transferred to the server, ensuring data privacy.

- **Local model training:** Each client trains a local machine learning model using the data it holds. In our case, various models, such as CNN, VGG16, Decision Trees, and Random Forest, are applied to local datasets (brain tumor, breast cancer, dermatology datasets).
- **Model update:** After training on the local data, each client sends only the updated model parameters (weights) and gradients to the central server. These data are minimal and do not expose sensitive patient information.

2. **Central server:**
   - **Model aggregation:** The central server receives model updates from the clients and performs aggregation, typically using the federated averaging (FedAvg) algorithm. This ensures that the server builds a global model without ever having access to the raw data.
   - **Global model distribution:** Once the aggregation process is complete, the server sends the updated global model back to the clients for further training. This ensures the learning process is

decentralized while benefiting from the knowledge gained from multiple sites.

- **Privacy preservation:** The central server only receives model weights and parameters, never raw data, thus maintaining the privacy and confidentiality of the sensitive medical information.

### 2.2.3 Flow of the federated learning process

The FL process unfolds as follows:

1. **Initialization:** The server initializes a global model with random weights and sends it to all participating clients.
2. **Local training:** Each client trains the model on its local dataset and calculates the local gradients.
3. **Model update:** Clients send the local model updates (gradients/weights) back to the central server.
4. **Aggregation:** The central server aggregates the local updates using the FedAvg algorithm to create a new global model.
5. **Iteration:** The global model is sent back to the clients for further training, and this cycle continues until the model reaches an acceptable level of performance.

This architecture not only enables AI-based medical diagnosis but also ensures that sensitive data remains secure throughout the process, fostering trust and compliance with privacy standards.

## 2.3 SYSTEM EVALUATION

In this section, we provide a comprehensive overview of the methodologies and frameworks employed to evaluate the performance of our system. Specifically, we discuss the datasets used, the experimental setup, and the algorithms that form the core of our evaluation process.

### 2.3.1 Datasets

We utilized three distinct and well-known medical datasets in our study, each representing a different domain of healthcare: brain tumor imaging, breast cancer detection, and dermatological disease classification. The brain tumor dataset contains MRI scans of patients with various types of brain tumors, providing a foundation for analyzing medical image processing and tumor detection methods. The breast cancer dataset includes patient data and diagnostic features related to breast cancer, offering a platform for evaluating classification models that distinguish between malignant and benign tumors. Lastly, the dermatology dataset consists of images and clinical information of various skin lesions, enabling the development and testing of algorithms for the automatic identification of dermatological conditions, such as melanoma and other skin cancers. Together, these diverse datasets provide a comprehensive evaluation framework, allowing us to test the generalizability and effectiveness of our proposed system across different medical conditions and data types.

Figure 2.2 presents a visual overview of the datasets used in this study. Figure 2.2a illustrates the distribution of brain tumor types, highlighting the class imbalance that may influence model performance. Figure 2.2b shows the feature distribution within the breast cancer dataset, emphasizing the distinction between malignant and benign tumors. Lastly, Figure 2.2c depicts the categories of skin diseases in the dermatology dataset, displaying the respective sample sizes for each class. This visualization highlights the variability within the dataset, which contains six distinct classes.

### 2.3.2 Experimental setup

The implementation was carried out using Flower and PyTorch. These powerful libraries provide a flexible and efficient platform for building and optimizing deep learning models. Data preprocessing and analysis were conducted using the Pandas and NumPy libraries, which facilitated smooth data manipulation and numerical operations. Pandas helped in organizing and cleaning the dataset, while NumPy enabled efficient handling of arrays and mathematical operations, ensuring the datasets were properly prepared for input into the machine learning models. The datasets were distributed among different clients in a FL environment. For the brain tumor and breast cancer datasets, the data were distributed in a nonspecific manner among the clients, ensuring varied data points across the network. In contrast, for the dermatology dataset, a more structured distribution approach was employed, assigning each class to a dedicated client. This structure was implemented to simulate real-world scenarios where data is often segregated by class or other factors in healthcare applications.

We evaluated the performance of each algorithm using the following metrics:

- Accuracy: This metric measures the ratio of correctly predicted instances to the total number of instances in the dataset. It provides an overall sense of the model's performance, though it may be influenced by class imbalance in the data.
- F1 Score: The harmonic mean of precision and recall, the F1 score provides a balanced metric, especially in situations where both false positives and false negatives are critical to consider. It is especially useful when dealing with imbalanced datasets, as it ensures that both precision and recall are adequately accounted for.

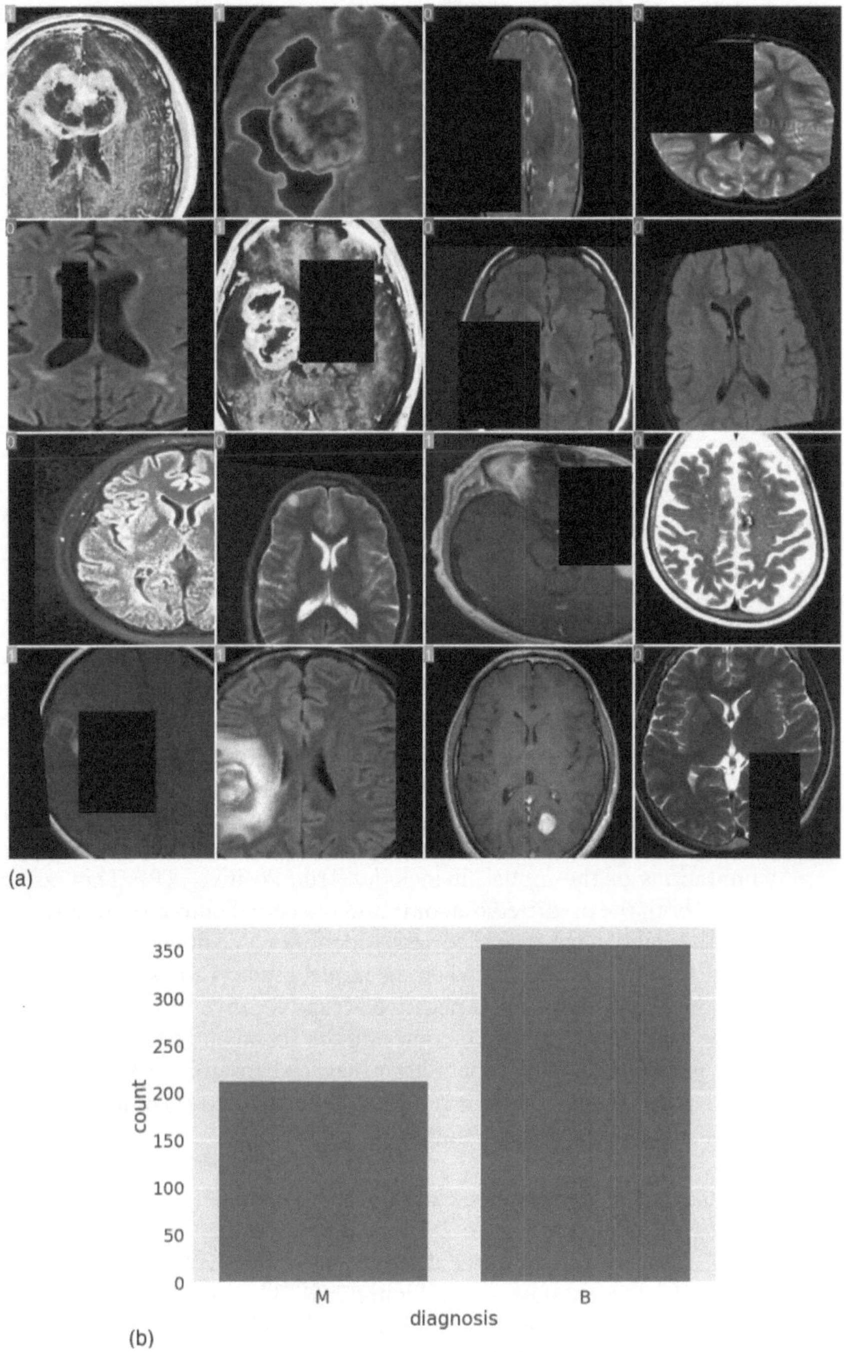


*Figure 2.2* Distribution and characteristics of the datasets used in this study.

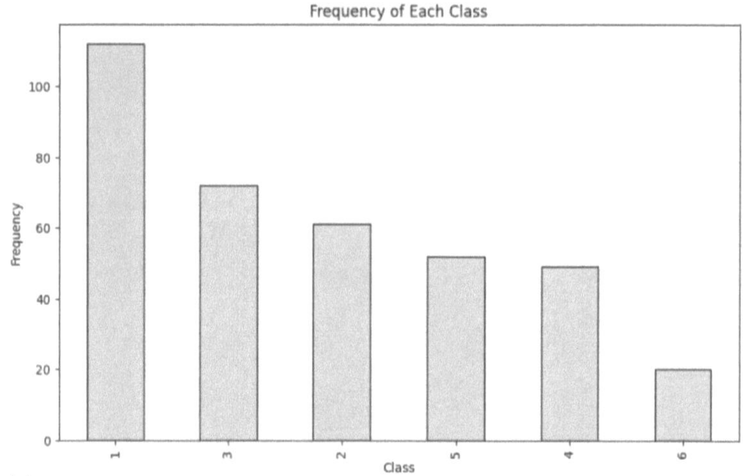


(c)

*Figure 2.2* (Continued)

- Loss: Loss refers to the difference between the predicted and actual values, providing a quantitative measure of the model's error. A lower loss value indicates that the model's predictions are closer to the actual outcomes. This metric is commonly used during model training to guide the optimization process.
- Confusion Matrix: To assess the effectiveness of the system's model, we used confusion matrix. These metrics categorize predictions into four distinct outcomes, which help us understand the accuracy and limitations of the model. It includes True Positive (TP): This occurs when both the predicted outcome and the actual outcome are positive. In other words, the model correctly identifies a positive instance. False Positive (FP): This occurs when the model predicts a positive outcome, but the actual outcome is negative. True Negative (TN): This occurs when both the predicted outcome and the actual outcome are negative. The model successfully identifies a negative instance. False Negative (FN): This occurs when the model incorrectly predicts a negative outcome, despite the actual result being positive.

We evaluated the performance of our system model in terms of loss for the three datasets (see Figure 2.3), accuracy for the three datasets (see Figure 2.4), F1-score for the three datasets (see Figure 2.5), and confusion matrices for the three datasets (see Figure 2.6). The loss values decreased consistently over the course of training, which indicates that our models were effectively learning and improving their predictions. Figure 2.3 depicts

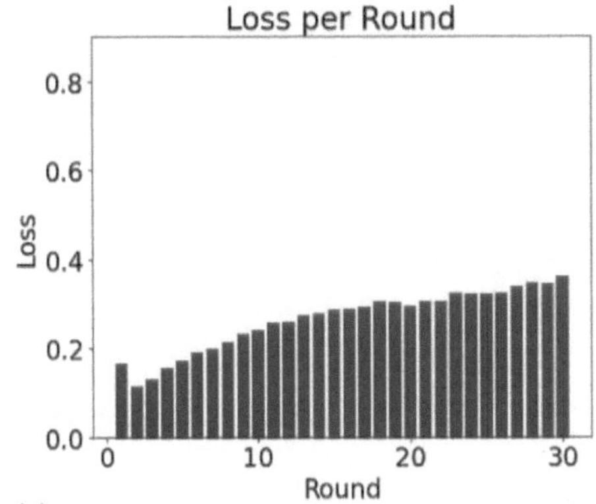


(a)

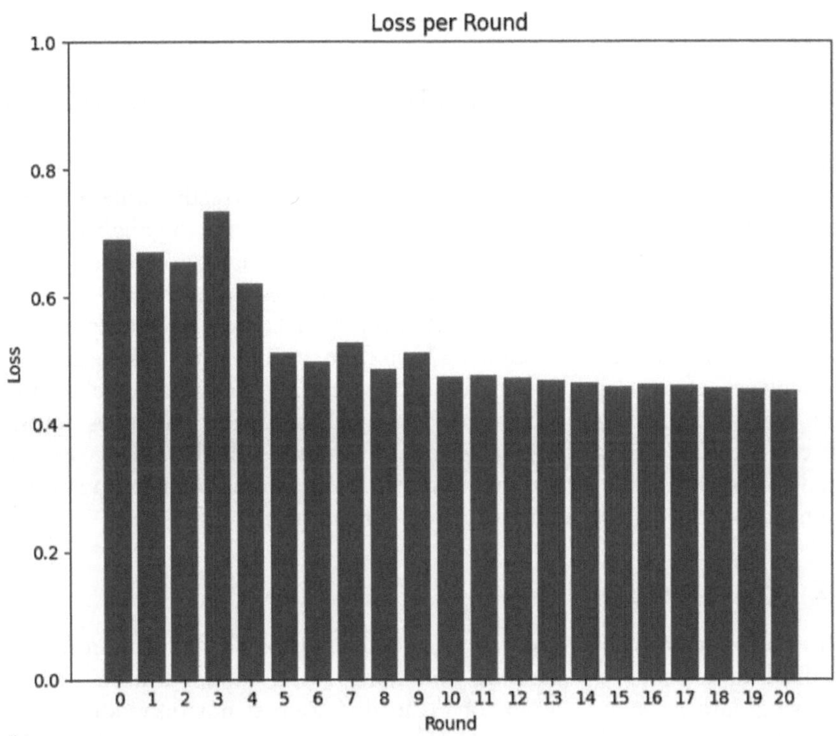


(b)

*Figure 2.3* Loss curves for the (a) dermatology, (b) brain tumor, and (c) breast cancer datasets.

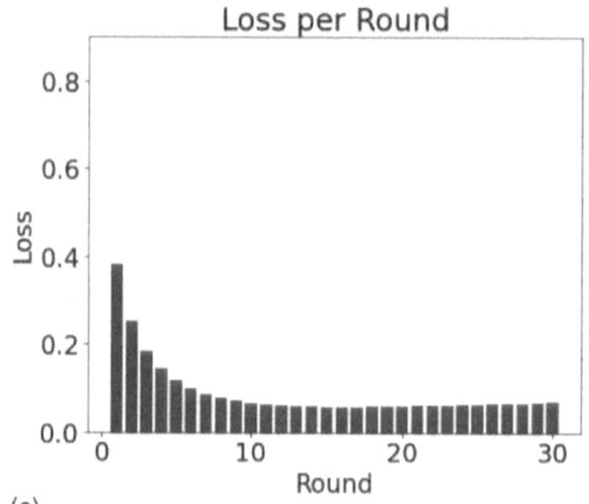


(c)

*Figure 2.3* (Continued)

the loss curves for the three datasets. The gradual and steady decline in loss demonstrates how our models refine their predictions with each training round, moving steadily toward more accurate classifications.

Figure 2.4 illustrates the progression of accuracy across the same training period. We observe a clear upward trend in this metric, highlighting the models' growing ability to enhance their decision-making capabilities as training continues. Figure 2.5 presents the F1-scores for each dataset. This consistent rise in F1-scores signifies that the models are successfully balancing precision and recall, minimizing both false positives and false negatives to achieve robust classification results. Figure 2.6 showcases the confusion matrices, providing a detailed view of classification outcomes across all classes. The strong diagonal elements confirm a high rate of correct predictions, while the few remaining misclassifications point to potential avenues for further fine-tuning or data augmentation.

## 2.4 CONCLUSION

This paper demonstrates the promising potential of FL in revolutionizing medical diagnostics by enabling collaborative AI model training while ensuring data privacy. The use of FL in this context not only adheres to stringent privacy regulations but also facilitates the development of robust, high-performing models across decentralized medical institutions. By leveraging data without compromising patient confidentiality, FL opens the door for more widespread adoption of AI-driven solutions in healthcare.

However, challenges such as the handling of non-IID data, communication efficiency, and model interpretability need to be addressed to fully unlock

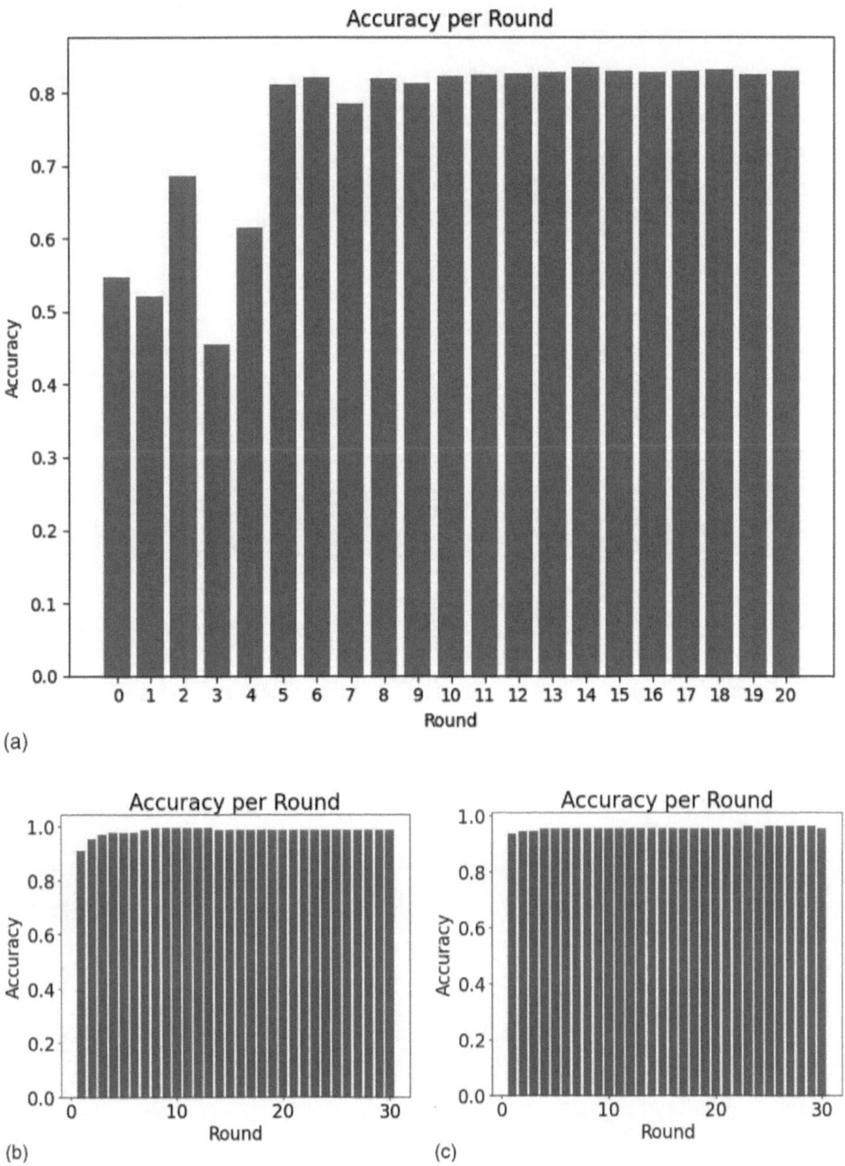


*Figure 2.4* Accuracy curves for the (a) dermatology, (b) brain tumor, and (c) breast cancer datasets.

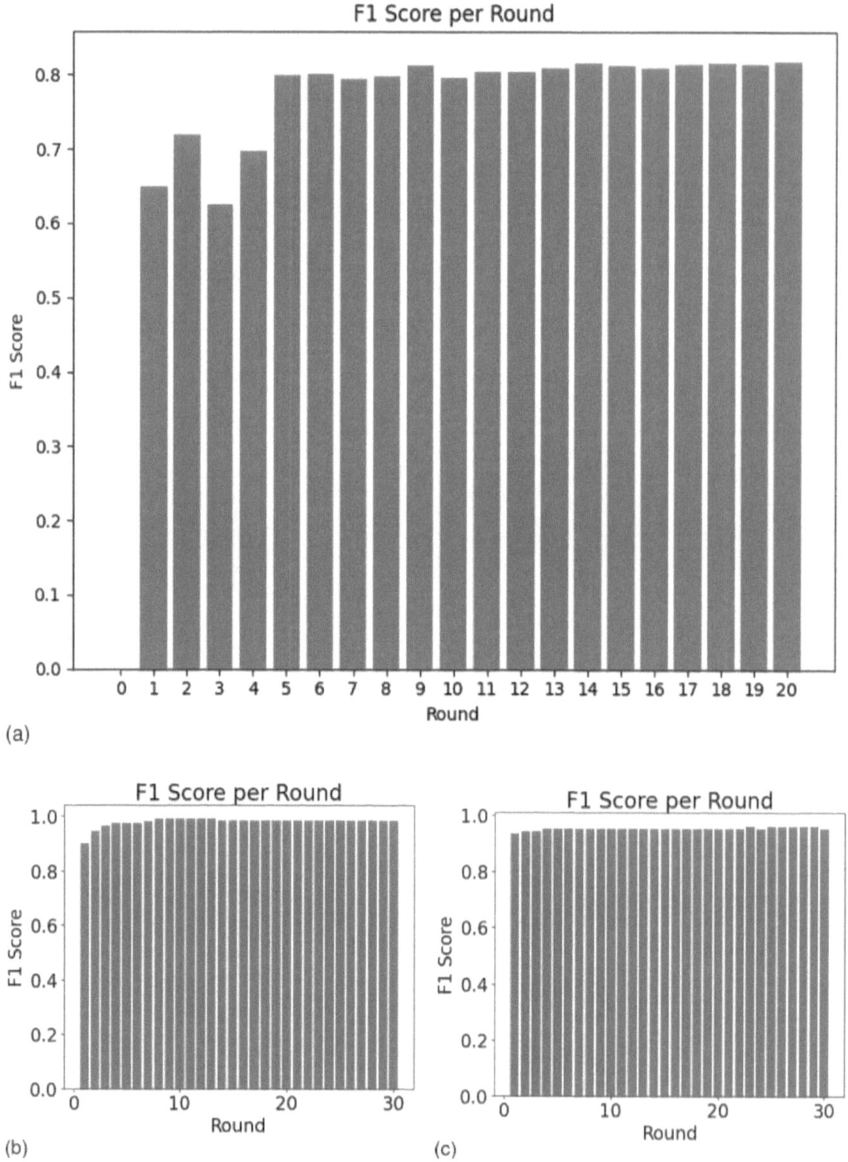


*Figure 2.5* F1 score for the (a) dermatology, (b) brain tumor, and (c) breast cancer datasets.

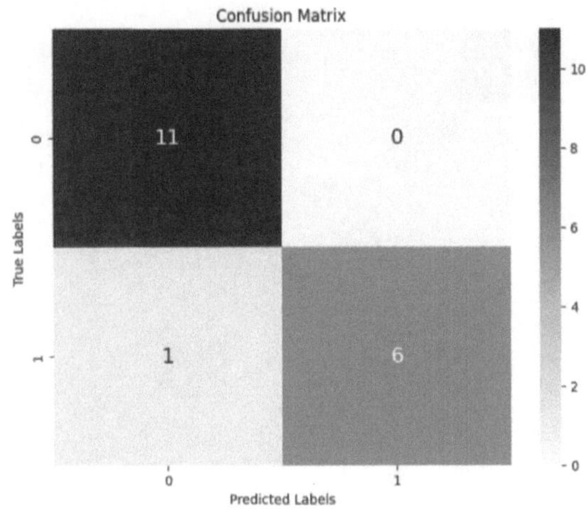


(a)

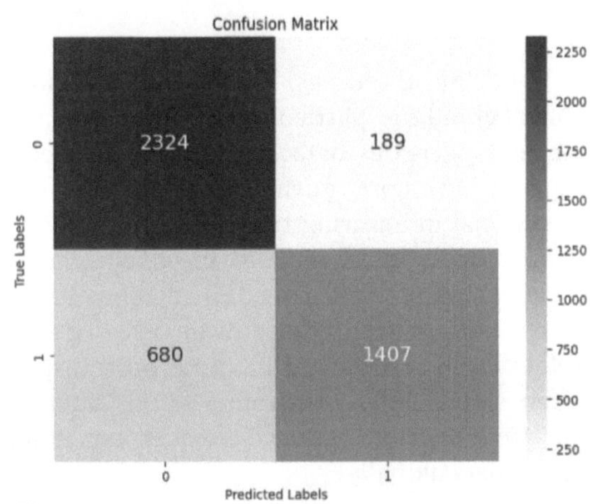


(b)

*Figure 2.6* Confusion matrixes for the (a) dermatology, (b) brain tumor, and (c) breast cancer datasets.

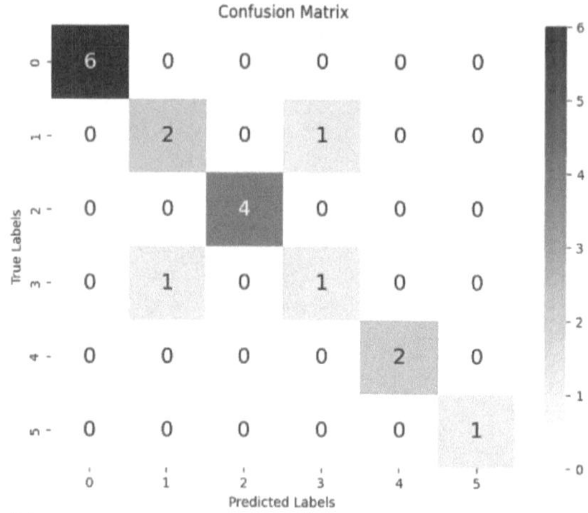


(c)

*Figure 2.6* (Continued)

the potential of FL in clinical settings. Future work should focus on advancing the algorithms behind FL, particularly in improving convergence rates and dealing with heterogeneous data across different medical institutions. Furthermore, integrating more advanced interpretation and visualization tools will be crucial in ensuring transparency and enhancing the trust of healthcare professionals in AI models. In conclusion, while this study validates the effectiveness of FL for medical diagnostics, further research is essential to overcome the technical, ethical, and regulatory hurdles. By continuing to refine these models and focusing on transparency and interpretability, FL can significantly contribute to the future of personalized medicine and the treatment of complex diseases, benefiting both patients and healthcare providers globally.

## REFERENCES

[1] S. Wang et al., "Blockchain-Powered Parallel Healthcare Systems Based on the ACP Approach," in *IEEE Transactions on Computational Social Systems*, vol. 5, no. 4, pp. 942–950, Dec. 2018. doi:10.1109/TCSS.2018.2865526

[2] E. C. Schiza, T. C. Kyprianou, N. Petkov and C. N. Schizas, "Proposal for an eHealth Based Ecosystem Serving National Healthcare," in *IEEE Journal of Biomedical and Health Informatics*, vol. 23, no. 3, pp. 1346–1357, May 2019. doi:10.1109/JBHI.2018.2834230

[3] A. Lakhan et al., "DT-LSMAS: Digital Twin-Assisted Large-Scale Multiagent System for Healthcare Workflows," in *IEEE Systems Journal*, vol. 18, no. 4, pp. 1883–1892, Dec. 2024. doi:10.1109/JSYST.2024.3424259

[4] S. Liu, Y. Huang, A. Kong, J. Tang and X. Liu, "Rise of the Automotive Health-Domain Controllers: Empowering Healthcare Services in Intelligent Vehicles," in *IEEE Internet of Things Journal*, vol. 9, no. 24, pp. 24882–24889, 15 Dec.15, 2022. doi:10.1109/JIOT.2022.3194888

[5] B. Pradhan, S. Das, D. S. Roy, S. Routray, F. Benedetto and R. H. Jhaveri, "An AI-Assisted Smart Healthcare System Using 5G Communication," in *IEEE Access*, vol. 11, pp. 108339–108355, 2023. doi:10.1109/ACCESS.2023.3317174

[6] O. Maki, M. Alshaikhli, M. Gunduz, K. K. Naji and M. Abdulwahed, "Development of Digitalization Road Map for Healthcare Facility Management," in *IEEE Access*, vol. 10, pp. 14450–14462, 2022, doi:10.1109/ACCESS.2022.3146341

[7] M. S. Roopa and K. R. Venugopal, "Digital Twins for Cyber-Physical Healthcare Systems: Architecture, Requirements, Systematic Analysis, and Future Prospects," in *IEEE Access*, vol. 13, pp. 44963–44996, 2025. doi:10.1109/ACCESS.2025.3547991

[8] S. K. B. Sangeetha, C. Selvarathi, S. K. Mathivanan, J. Cho and S. V. Easwaramoorthy, "Secure Healthcare Access Control System (SHACS) for Anomaly Detection and Enhanced Security in Cloud-Based Healthcare Applications," *IEEE Access*, vol. 12, pp. 164543–164559, 2024. doi:10.1109/ACCESS.2024.3492024

[9] M. C. Chibuike, S. S. Grobbelaar and A. Botha, "Overcoming Challenges for Improved Patient-Centric Care: A Scoping Review of Platform Ecosystems in Healthcare," *IEEE Access*, vol. 12, pp. 14298–14313, 2024. doi:10.1109/ACCESS.2024.3356860

[10] Z. A. E. Houda, H. Moudoud, B. Brik and L. Khoukhi, "Blockchain-Enabled Federated Learning for Enhanced Collaborative Intrusion Detection in Vehicular Edge Computing," *IEEE Transactions on Intelligent Transportation Systems*, vol. 25, pp. 7661–672. doi:10.1109/TITS.2024.3351699

[11] Z. A. E. Houda, H. Moudoud and B. Brik, "Federated Deep Reinforcement Learning for Efficient Jamming Attack Mitigation in O-RAN," in *IEEE Transactions on Vehicular Technology*, vol. 33, pp. 9334–9343. doi:10.1109/TVT.2024.3359998

[12] Z. A. El Houda, L. Khoukhi and A. Hafid, "ChainSecure – A Scalable and Proactive Solution for Protecting Blockchain Applications Using SDN," 2018 IEEE Global Communications Conference (GLOBECOM), Abu Dhabi, United Arab Emirates, 2018, pp. 1–6. doi:10.1109/GLOCOM.2018.8647279

[13] Z. A. El Houda, A. Hafid and L. Khoukhi, "Co-IoT: A Collaborative DDoS Mitigation Scheme in IoT Environment Based on Blockchain Using SDN," 2019 IEEE Global Communications Conference (GLOBECOM), Waikoloa, HI, USA, 2019, pp. 1–6. doi:10.1109/GLOBECOM38437.2019.9013542

[14] Z. Abou El Houda, A. S. Hafid and L. Khoukhi, "Cochain-SC: An Intra- and Inter-Domain Ddos Mitigation Scheme Based on Blockchain Using SDN and Smart Contract," in *IEEE Access*, vol. 7, pp. 98893–98907, 2019. doi:10.1109/ACCESS.2019.2930715

[15] Z. A. E. Houda, A. Hafid and L. Khoukhi, "Blockchain Meets AMI: Towards Secure Advanced Metering Infrastructures," ICC 2020–2020 IEEE International Conference on Communications (ICC), Dublin, Ireland, 2020, pp. 1–6, doi:10.1109/ICC40277.2020.9148963

[16] Z. A. E. Houda, A. Hafid and L. Khoukhi, "BrainChain – A Machine learning Approach for protecting Blockchain applications using SDN," ICC 2020 – 2020 IEEE International Conference on Communications (ICC), Dublin, Ireland, 2020, pp. 1–6. doi:10.1109/ICC40277.2020.9148808

[17] Z. Abou El Houda, L. Khoukhi and A. Senhaji Hafid, "Bringing Intelligence to Software Defined Networks: Mitigating DDoS Attacks," in *IEEE Transactions on Network and Service Management*, vol. 17, no. 4, pp. 2523–2535, Dec. 2020. doi:10.1109/TNSM.2020.3014870

[18] H. Moudoud, W. Hamhoum and S. Cherkaoui, "Strengthening Open Radio Access Networks: Advancing Safeguards Through ZTA and Deep Learning," GLOBECOM 2023 – 2023 IEEE Global Communications Conference, Kuala Lumpur, Malaysia, 2023, pp. 80–85. doi:10.1109/GLOBECOM54140.2023.10437829

[19] Z. A. El Houda, A. S. Hafid and L. Khoukhi, "Blockchain-based Reverse Auction for V2V charging in smart grid environment," ICC 2021 – IEEE International Conference on Communications, Montreal, QC, Canada, 2021, pp. 1–6. doi:10.1109/ICC42927.2021.9500366

[20] Z. A. El Houda, A. S. Hafid and L. Khoukhi, "A Novel Machine Learning Framework for Advanced Attack Detection using SDN," 2021 IEEE Global Communications Conference (GLOBECOM), Madrid, Spain, 2021, pp. 1–6. doi:10.1109/GLOBECOM46510.2021.9685643

[21] Z. A. El Houda, L. Khoukhi and B. Brik, "A Low-Latency Fog-based Framework to secure IoT Applications using Collaborative Federated Learning," 2022 IEEE 47th Conference on Local Computer Networks (LCN), Edmonton, AB, Canada, 2022, pp. 343–346. doi:10.1109/LCN53696.2022.9843315

[22] Z. Abou El Houda and L. Khoukhi, "A Hierarchical Fog Computing Framework for Network Attack Detection in SDN," ICC 2022 – IEEE International Conference on Communications, Seoul, Korea, Republic of, 2022, pp. 4366–4371. doi:10.1109/ICC45855.2022.9838560

[23] Z. A. El Houda, D. Nabousli and G. Kaddoum, "Cost-efficient Federated Reinforcement Learning- Based Network Routing for Wireless Networks," 2022 IEEE Future Networks World Forum (FNWF), Montreal, QC, Canada, 2022, pp. 243–248. doi:10.1109/FNWF55208.2022.00050

[24] Z. A. E. Houda, B. Brik, A. Ksentini, L. Khoukhi and M. Guizani, "When Federated Learning Meets Game Theory: A Cooperative Framework to Secure IIoT Applications on Edge Computing," in *IEEE Transactions on Industrial Informatics*, vol. 18, no. 11, pp. 7988–7997, Nov. 2022. doi:10.1109/TII.2022.3170347

[25] Z. A. E. Houda, B. Brik and L. Khoukhi, ""Why Should I Trust Your IDS?": An Explainable Deep Learning Framework for Intrusion Detection Systems in Internet of Things Networks," in *IEEE Open Journal of the Communications Society*, vol. 3, pp. 1164–1176, 2022. doi:10.1109/OJCOMS.2022.3188750

[26] Z. A. El Houda, B. Brik and S. -M. Senouci, "A Novel IoT-Based Explainable Deep Learning Framework for Intrusion Detection Systems," in *IEEE Internet of Things Magazine*, vol. 5, no. 2, pp. 20–23, Jun. 2022. doi:10.1109/IOTM.005.2200028

[27] Z. A. El Houda, D. Nabousli and G. Kaddoum, "Advancing Security and Efficiency in Federated Learning Service Aggregation for Wireless Networks," 2023 IEEE 34th Annual International Symposium on Personal, Indoor and Mobile Radio Communications (PIMRC), Toronto, ON, Canada, 2023, pp. 1–6. doi:10.1109/PIMRC56721.2023.10293790

[28] Z. A. El Houda, H. Moudoud, B. Brik and L. Khoukhi, "Securing Federated Learning through Blockchain and Explainable AI for Robust Intrusion Detection in IoT Networks," IEEE INFOCOM 2023 - IEEE Conference on Computer Communications Workshops (INFOCOM WKSHPS), Hoboken, NJ, USA, 2023, pp. 1–6. doi:10.1109/INFOCOMW KSHPS57453.2023.10225769

[29] Z. A. E. Houda, J. Beaugeard, Q. Sauvêtre and L. Khoukhi, "Towards a Secure and Scalable Access Control System Using Blockchain," 2023 IEEE International Conference on Blockchain and Cryptocurrency (ICBC), Dubai, United Arab Emirates, 2023, pp. 1–8. doi:10.1109/ICBC56567.2023.10174880

[30] Z. A. El Houda, H. Moudoud and L. Khoukhi, "Secure and Efficient Federated Learning for Robust Intrusion Detection in IoT Networks," GLOBECOM 2023 - 2023 IEEE Global Communications Conference, Kuala Lumpur, Malaysia, 2023, pp. 2668–2673. doi:10.1109/GLOBECOM54140.2023.10436768

[31] Z. A. E. Houda, A. S. Hafid, L. Khoukhi and B. Brik, "When Collaborative Federated Learning Meets Blockchain to Preserve Privacy in Healthcare," in *IEEE Transactions on Network Science and Engineering*, vol. 10, no. 5, pp. 2455–2465, 1 Sept.–Oct. 2023. doi:10.1109/TNSE.2022.3211192

[32] Z. A. E. Houda, A. S. Hafid and L. Khoukhi, "MiTFed: A Privacy Preserving Collaborative Network Attack Mitigation Framework Based on Federated Learning Using SDN and Blockchain," in *IEEE Transactions on Network Science and Engineering*, vol. 10, no. 4, pp. 1985–2001, 1 Jul.–Aug. 2023, doi:10.1109/TNSE.2023.3237367

[33] Z. A. El Houda, B. Brik, A. Ksentini and L. Khoukhi, "A MEC-Based Architecture to Secure IoT Applications using Federated Deep Learning," in *IEEE Internet of Things Magazine*, vol. 6, no. 1, pp. 60–63, Mar. 2023. doi:10.1109/IOTM.001.2100238

[34] A. Taïk, H. Moudoud and S. Cherkaoui, "Data-Quality Based Scheduling for Federated Edge Learning," 2021 IEEE 46th Conference on Local Computer Networks (LCN), Edmonton, AB, Canada, 2021, pp. 17–23. doi:10.1109/LCN52139.2021.9524974

[35] Z. A. E. Houda, D. Naboulsi and G. Kaddoum, "A Privacy-Preserving Collaborative Jamming Attacks Detection Framework Using Federated Learning," in *IEEE Internet of Things Journal*, vol. 11, no. 7, pp. 12153–12164, Apr., 2024. doi:10.1109/JIOT.2023.3333870

[36] H. Moudoud, S. Cherkaoui and L. Khoukhi, "Towards a Scalable and Trustworthy Blockchain: IoT Use Case," ICC 2021 – IEEE International Conference on Communications, Montreal, QC, Canada, 2021, pp. 1–6. doi:10.1109/ICC42927.2021.9500535

[37] H. Moudoud, S. Cherkaoui and L. Khoukhi, "An IoT Blockchain Architecture Using Oracles and Smart Contracts: the Use-Case of a Food Supply Chain," 2019 IEEE 30th Annual International Symposium on Personal, Indoor and Mobile Radio Communications (PIMRC), Istanbul, Turkey, 2019, pp. 1–6. doi:10.1109/PIMRC.2019.8904404

[38] H. Moudoud and S. Cherkaoui, "Empowering Security and Trust in 5G and Beyond: A Deep Reinforcement Learning Approach," in *IEEE Open Journal of the Communications Society*, vol. 4, pp. 2410–2420, 2023. doi:10.1109/OJCOMS.2023.3313352

[39] Z. A. El Houda, H. Moudoud and L. Khoukhi, "Secure and Efficient Federated Learning for Robust Intrusion Detection in IoT Networks," GLOBECOM 2023 – 2023 IEEE Global Communications Conference, Kuala Lumpur, Malaysia, 2023, pp. 2668–2673. doi:10.1109/GLOBECOM54140.2023.10436768

[40] H. Moudoud and S. Cherkaoui, "Enhancing Open RAN Security with Zero Trust and Machine Learning," GLOBECOM 2023 – 2023 IEEE Global Communications Conference, Kuala Lumpur, Malaysia, 2023, pp. 2772–2777. doi:10.1109/GLOBECOM54140.2023.10437043

[41] H. Moudoud and S. Cherkaoui, "Federated Learning Meets Blockchain to Secure the Metaverse," 2023 International Wireless Communications and Mobile Computing (IWCMC), Marrakesh, Morocco, 2023, pp. 339–344. doi:10.1109/IWCMC58020.2023.10182956

[42] H. Moudoud, L. Khoukhi and S. Cherkaoui, "Prediction and Detection of FDIA and DDoS Attacks in 5G Enabled IoT," in *IEEE Network*, vol. 35, no. 2, pp. 194–201, Mar./Apr. 2021. doi:10.1109/MNET.011.2000449

[43] H. Moudoud and S. Cherkaoui, "Toward Secure and Private Federated Learning for IoT using Blockchain," GLOBECOM 2022 – 2022 IEEE Global Communications Conference, Rio de Janeiro, Brazil, 2022, pp. 4316–4321. doi:10.1109/GLOBECOM48099.2022.10000623

[44] H. Moudoud, Z. Mlika, L. Khoukhi and S. Cherkaoui, "Detection and Prediction of FDI Attacks in IoT Systems via Hidden Markov Model," in *IEEE Transactions on Network Science and Engineering*, vol. 9, no. 5, pp. 2978–2990, 1 Sept.–Oct. 2022. doi:10.1109/TNSE.2022.3161479

Chapter 3

# Secure authentication and authorization in the internet of medical things

*Aryendra Dalal*

## 3.1 INTRODUCTION

The Internet of Medical Things (IoMT) has revolutionized healthcare delivery by enabling connected medical devices to collect and transmit critical health data. While these advancements have enhanced patient care and operational efficiency, they have simultaneously exposed healthcare systems to unprecedented cybersecurity threats. The interconnected nature of IoMT devices creates an expanded attack surface that malicious actors can exploit to gain unauthorized access to sensitive medical information or disrupt critical healthcare services.

Recent incidents underscore the critical importance of robust security measures in healthcare environments. The 2017 WannaCry ransomware attack affected NHS infrastructure in the United Kingdom, leading to the cancellation of approximately 19,000 appointments [1]. Similarly, the 2020 Universal Health Services cyberattack impacted more than 400 healthcare facilities, with estimated damages exceeding $67 million [2].

Secure authentication and authorization mechanisms form the cornerstone of IoMT security frameworks. Authentication verifies the identity of users, devices, or systems attempting to access IoMT resources, while authorization determines the level of access granted to authenticated entities. This chapter explores the frameworks, methodologies, and technologies essential for implementing robust authentication and authorization in IoMT environments.

## 3.2 THE IMPORTANCE OF SECURE AUTHENTICATION IN HEALTHCARE

### 3.2.1 Current state of healthcare cybersecurity

The healthcare industry has become a prime target for cyberattacks due to the high value of medical data and the critical nature of healthcare services. According to IBM's 2023 Cost of a Data Breach Report [3], healthcare data

DOI: 10.1201/9781003640325-3

breaches cost an average of $10.93 million per incident, making them the most expensive breaches across all industries for the thirteenth consecutive year.

The U.S. Department of Health and Human Services (HHS) has reported that hacking and IT incidents account for 80% of all healthcare data breaches, with many resulting from compromised credentials [4]. With 707 reported incidents in 2023 impacting over 87 million individuals, the healthcare sector faces unprecedented cybersecurity challenges.

### 3.2.2 Unique security challenges in IoMT environments

The Internet of Medical Things presents unique security challenges that distinguish it from typical IT environments:

1. **Critical Nature of Healthcare Services:** Security breaches can directly impact patient safety and potentially lead to life-threatening situations.
2. **Device Diversity and Heterogeneity:** The IoMT ecosystem encompasses devices with varying computational capabilities, complicating uniform security implementation.
3. **Long Device Lifecycles:** Medical devices often have operational lifespans of 10-15 years, creating challenges in maintaining security updates and compatibility.
4. **Regulatory Compliance Requirements:** Healthcare organizations must adhere to strict regulatory frameworks such as HIPAA and GDPR.
5. **Interoperability Requirements:** Healthcare systems often need to exchange data across different platforms and organizations.

### 3.2.3 The fundamental role of authentication in IoMT security

Authentication serves as the foundation of IoMT security by verifying the identity of users, devices, and systems attempting to access healthcare networks and data (Table 3.1). Effective authentication mechanisms are critical for:

1. **Preventing unauthorized access:** Authentication serves as the primary barrier against unauthorized access to sensitive medical data and systems.
2. **Ensuring data integrity:** By verifying the identity of data sources, authentication helps ensure that medical data has not been tampered with.

*Table 3.1* Key regulations affecting IoMT security and their authentication requirements

| *Regulation* | *Jurisdiction* | *Authentication requirements* |
|---|---|---|
| HIPAA | United States | Requires authentication controls for all systems containing PHI |
| GDPR | European Union | Requires strong access controls and data protection measures |
| FDA Premarket Guidance | United States | Specifies security requirements for medical device manufacturers |
| HITECH Act | United States | Extends HIPAA security requirements with stricter enforcement |
| ISO 27001 | International | Provides framework for information security management |

3. **Maintaining regulatory compliance:** Robust authentication systems are essential for meeting regulatory requirements related to healthcare data protection.
4. **Enabling secure interoperability:** Authentication mechanisms facilitate secure data exchange between different healthcare systems while protecting sensitive information.

## 3.3 TRADITIONAL AUTHENTICATION METHODS AND THEIR LIMITATIONS

### 3.3.1 Password-based authentication

Password-based authentication remains widely used in healthcare systems despite significant vulnerabilities. According to Verizon's 2023 Data Breach Investigations Report [5], 81% of data breaches involved weak or stolen passwords. The primary limitations include the following:

1. **Weak password selection:** A significant percentage of healthcare workers use simple passwords that can be easily compromised through dictionary attacks or brute force methods.
2. **Password reuse:** Credential reuse across multiple platforms amplifies the impact of a single breach, as compromised credentials can provide access to multiple systems.
3. **Phishing vulnerability:** Healthcare employees are frequently targeted by sophisticated phishing attacks designed to harvest login credentials.
4. **Inadequate for device authentication:** Passwords are particularly unsuitable for many IoMT devices that lack traditional user interfaces or have limited input capabilities.

### 3.3.2 Single factor authentication inadequacies

Single-factor authentication (SFA) presents significant limitations in IoMT contexts:

1. **Single point of failure:** SFA creates a fundamental security vulnerability by establishing a single barrier to access.
2. **Limited assurance of identity:** SFA provides minimal assurance that the entity attempting authentication is actually the authorized user rather than someone who has obtained their credentials.
3. **Inability to detect credential sharing:** Healthcare environments often involve shared workstations and time-sensitive situations that may encourage credential sharing among staff.

### 3.3.3 Legacy systems and authentication challenges

Many legacy medical devices and systems were designed with minimal authentication features and may not support modern protocols. Approximately 40% of medical devices in current use were designed before contemporary security standards were established [6]. The extended lifecycle of medical equipment (10–15 years) means that devices with outdated authentication mechanisms remain in active use despite known vulnerabilities (Table 3.2).

## 3.4 ADVANCED AUTHENTICATION METHODS FOR IOMT

### 3.4.1 Multifactor authentication

Multifactor authentication has emerged as a critical security enhancement for IoMT environments. According to Microsoft's security research [7],

*Table 3.2* Authentication capabilities in legacy medical devices

| *Device type* | *Typical age* | *Authentication capabilities* | *Security risks* |
|---|---|---|---|
| Legacy infusion pumps | 8–12 years | Basic password protection | Weak passwords, no encryption |
| Older imaging systems | 10–15 years | System passwords | Credential sharing, minimal logging |
| Legacy EHR systems | 7–10 years | Simple username/password | Limited MFA support, no context awareness |
| Legacy monitoring equipment | 10+ years | Often none | Unauthorized access, data tampering |

MFA can block 99.9% of automated attacks. However, healthcare environments present unique implementation considerations:

1. **Emergency access provisions:** MFA systems in healthcare must include emergency override mechanisms while ensuring immediate access to critical systems.
2. **Workflow integration:** Healthcare organizations achieve higher staff compliance with MFA when the authentication process adds minimal time to login times.
3. **Adaptive multifactor authentication:** This approach dynamically adjusts authentication requirements based on contextual risk factors, applying proportionate security measures only when risk indicators suggest heightened security concerns.

### 3.4.2 Biometric authentication

Biometric authentication leverages unique physical or behavioral characteristics to verify identity, offering significant advantages in healthcare settings including non-transferability and user convenience. Biometric adoption in healthcare has grown substantially between 2019 and 2022, with various technologies showing promising results [8].

#### *3.4.2.1 Physical biometrics*

Physical biometrics authenticate users based on unique physiological characteristics:

1. **Fingerprint recognition:** Many healthcare organizations have deployed fingerprint authentication for accessing electronic health records and medication dispensing units.
2. **Facial recognition:** Offers the advantage of contactless authentication—a significant benefit in environments concerned with infection control.
3. **Iris recognition:** Provides extremely high accuracy with very low false match rates, making it suitable for high-security healthcare applications.
4. **Palm vein recognition:** Gaining popularity in healthcare due to its high accuracy, hygiene advantages, and user acceptance.

#### *3.4.2.2 Behavioral biometrics*

Behavioral biometrics analyze patterns in user behavior to verify identity:

1. **Keystroke dynamics:** Analyzes typing patterns including speed, pressure, and timing between keystrokes.

2. **Voice recognition:** Particularly useful for hands-free authentication in clinical settings where providers may be wearing protective equipment.
3. **Gait analysis:** Shows promise for continuous, passive authentication in healthcare facilities.

#### 3.4.2.3 Biometric challenges in healthcare

Despite their advantages, biometric authentication systems face specific challenges in healthcare environments (Table 3.3):

1. **Environmental factors:** Clinical environments may impact biometric accuracy due to factors such as variable lighting or the use of personal protective equipment.
2. **Accessibility concerns:** Healthcare staff and patients may have physical conditions that prevent the use of certain biometric modalities.
3. **Privacy considerations:** Collection and storage of biometric data raise significant privacy concerns, particularly in healthcare contexts where additional sensitive information is already being managed.

### 3.4.3 Device authentication

In IoMT environments, authenticating devices is as important as authenticating users, ensuring that only authorized medical devices can connect to healthcare networks.

*Table 3.3* Comparison of biometric authentication methods for healthcare

| *Biometric method* | *Accuracy* | *User acceptance* | *Implementation complexity* | *Suitability for healthcare* |
|---|---|---|---|---|
| Fingerprint | High | High | Low | Good for workstations, medication dispensing |
| Facial recognition | Medium-high | Medium | Medium | Useful with PPE considerations |
| Iris recognition | Very high | Medium | High | Excellent for high-security areas |
| Palm vein | High | High | Medium | Excellent for clinical environments |
| Voice recognition | Medium | High | Medium | Good for hands-free environments |
| Keystroke dynamics | Medium | Very high | Low | Good for supplemental verification |

#### *3.4.3.1 Certificate-based authentication*

Digital certificates provide a robust method for authenticating IoMT devices:

1. **Public Key Infrastructure (PKI):** Implements asymmetric cryptography to securely authenticate devices through digital certificates.
2. **X.509 certificates:** The standard for digital certificates in healthcare environments, containing the device's public key and identity information validated by a trusted Certificate Authority.

#### *3.4.3.2 Hardware security methods*

Hardware-based security features provide enhanced protection for device authentication:

1. **Trusted Platform Module (TPM):** Dedicated microcontrollers that securely store authentication keys and perform cryptographic operations.
2. **Physical Unclonable Functions (PUFs):** Hardware security primitives that leverage the unique physical characteristics of a device to generate device-specific cryptographic keys.
3. **Hardware Security Modules (HSMs):** Specialized hardware devices for managing digital keys and performing cryptographic functions securely.

### 3.4.4 Continuous authentication

Continuous authentication addresses the limitations of point-in-time authentication by persistently verifying user identity throughout a session:

1. **Risk-based approaches:** Dynamically adjust authentication requirements based on ongoing risk assessment.
2. **Transparent authentication:** Verifies identity without requiring explicit user action, reducing interference with clinical workflows.
3. **Environmental indicators:** Utilizes environmental cues such as Bluetooth signals from medical badges and physical access records to verify continued presence of the authenticated user.

## 3.5 THE ROLE OF AUTHORIZATION MECHANISMS

### 3.5.1 Role-based access control

Role-based access control (RBAC) remains one of the most widely implemented authorization models in healthcare environments due to its conceptual simplicity and alignment with organizational structures.

*Table 3.4* Common healthcare roles and system access permissions

| *Role* | *EHR access* | *Med admin* | *Imaging* | *Billing* | *Device Config* |
|---|---|---|---|---|---|
| Physician | Full | View/Order | Full | Limited | None |
| Nurse | Limited | Full | View | None | Limited |
| Pharmacist | Limited | Full | None | None | None |
| Radiologist | Limited | None | Full | None | Limited |
| Admin Staff | Demographics | None | None | Full | None |
| IT Staff | Limited | None | Limited | Limited | Full |
| Biomedical Engineer | None | None | None | None | Full |

Approximately 73% of healthcare organizations employ some form of RBAC for clinical systems, according to HHS [9].

RBAC assigns permissions to users based on their organizational roles rather than individually managing access rights for each user. Well-designed RBAC implementations can reduce administrative overhead by up to 65% compared to user-based permission management (Table 3.4).

Despite its advantages, traditional RBAC faces significant limitations in modern healthcare environments:

1. **Role explosion:** Large healthcare organizations maintain hundreds of distinct access roles, creating administrative complexity.
2. **Static permission structure:** Traditional RBAC lacks the flexibility to adjust permissions based on context or conditions.
3. **Difficulty handling exceptions:** Healthcare frequently involves exceptional circumstances requiring temporary access exceptions.

### 3.5.2 Attribute-based access control

Attribute-based access control (ABAC) represents a more flexible approach to authorization, determining access permissions based on attributes of users, resources, actions, and environmental conditions rather than predefined roles.

ABAC offers several significant advantages for IoMT environments:

1. **Fine-grained access control:** Enables precise permission specifications based on multiple attributes.
2. **Dynamic authorization decisions:** Makes real-time authorization decisions based on current attribute values, allowing permissions to adapt to changing conditions.
3. **Context-aware access:** Incorporates contextual factors such as time, location, device security status, and patient relationships into authorization decisions.

Effective ABAC implementations in healthcare environments typically evaluate several categories of attributes:

1. **Subject attributes:** Characteristics of the user or device requesting access
2. **Resource attributes:** Characteristics of the data or system being accessed
3. **Action attributes:** Characteristics of the operation being performed
4. **Contextual attributes:** Environmental and situational factors
5. **Patient consent attributes:** Patient-specified permissions

### 3.5.3 Context-aware authorization

Context-aware authorization extends ABAC concepts by placing particular emphasis on environmental and situational factors to make nuanced access decisions appropriate to specific circumstances:

1. **Emergency situations:** During medical emergencies, normal access restrictions may need temporary modification to ensure timely care.
2. **Break-glass provisions:** Predetermined protocols allowing emergency access to normally restricted information when justified by patient care needs.
3. **Patient care relationships:** Authorization based on established care relationships, limiting access to providers with a legitimate treatment relationship with the patient.
4. **Location-based controls:** Adjusting permissions based on physical location, such as providing expanded access within clinical areas and restricted access from remote locations.

### 3.5.4 Hybrid authorization models

Many healthcare organizations implement hybrid authorization models that combine elements of RBAC, ABAC, and context-aware approaches to balance security, usability, and administrative efficiency.

Role-attribute hybrid models use roles as a baseline for access control while incorporating attributes for fine-tuning permissions. Starting with role-based foundations reduces initial configuration complexity compared to pure attribute-based implementations.

Adaptive authorization frameworks dynamically adjust authorization models based on operational needs and risk levels. Such risk-adaptive systems have been shown to reduce unauthorized access incidents while decreasing authorization-related workflow disruptions [10].

## 3.6 INTEGRATION OF EMERGING TECHNOLOGIES

### 3.6.1 Artificial intelligence and machine learning

AI and machine learning are transforming authentication and authorization in IoMT by enabling more sophisticated analysis of user behavior, adaptation to changing conditions, and detection of emerging threats [11].

#### *3.6.1.1 Behavioral analytics and anomaly detection*

AI-powered behavioral analytics establish baselines of normal user behavior and identify deviations that may indicate compromised credentials (Table 3.5):

1. **User behavior profiling:** Creates detailed models of typical user interaction patterns including access times, locations, data access patterns, and system navigation.
2. **Anomaly detection:** Identifies deviations from established patterns that may indicate security threats.
3. **Contextual risk scoring:** Evaluates multiple factors to generate real-time risk scores for authentication and authorization decisions.
4. **Continuous learning:** Updates behavioral models over time to accommodate legitimate changes in user behavior while maintaining security vigilance.

#### *3.6.1.2 Predictive security measures*

Predictive analytics applies machine learning to anticipate security issues before they occur:

1. **Threat prediction:** Analyzes patterns and trends to identify potential future security threats.

*Table 3.5* Impact of predictive security measures on healthcare security incidents

| *Security measure* | *Reduction in incident response time* | *False positive rate* | *Implementation complexity* | *Resource requirements* |
|---|---|---|---|---|
| Traditional rule-based | Baseline | 15-25% | Low | Low |
| Basic AI detection | 35% | 10-15% | Medium | Medium |
| Advanced behavioral analysis | 62% | 5-8% | High | High |
| Predictive analytics | 78% | 3-6% | Very high | Very high |
| Hybrid AI/human system | 85% | <2% | Very high | Very high |

2. **Adaptive authentication:** Adjusts authentication requirements based on predicted risk levels rather than just current conditions.
3. **Attack surface prediction:** Identifies potential vulnerabilities in IoMT networks before they can be exploited.

### 3.6.2 Blockchain technology for authentication and authorization

Blockchain technology offers unique capabilities for securing authentication and authorization in distributed IoMT environments through its inherent properties of immutability, decentralization, and transparency [12].

#### *3.6.2.1 Decentralized identity management*

Blockchain enables decentralized approaches to identity management:

1. **Self-Sovereign Identity:** Gives users control over their digital identities while enabling verifiable authentication across multiple healthcare systems.
2. **Distributed identity verification:** Enables validation of identity claims without requiring direct access to central identity providers.
3. **Immutable identity attestations:** Creates tamper-resistant records of identity verification and credential issuance.

#### *3.6.2.2 Smart contracts for authorization*

Smart contracts enable sophisticated and auditable authorization controls:

1. **Automated policy enforcement:** Encodes authorization policies as smart contracts that automatically execute when predefined conditions are met.
2. **Consent management:** Records and enforces patient consent directives through blockchain-based smart contracts.
3. **Auditability and transparency:** Creates immutable records of all authorization decisions and policy changes for compliance and audit purposes.

### 3.6.3 Zero trust architecture

Zero trust architecture (ZTA) represents a significant paradigm shift in security thinking, moving away from perimeter-based security models to an approach that assumes no user or device should be inherently trusted, regardless of location or network connection [13].

#### *3.6.3.1 Core principles of zero trust in healthcare*

1. **Never trust, always verify:** Every access request is fully authenticated, authorized, and encrypted regardless of source.
2. **Least privilege access:** Users and devices receive only the minimum access necessary for their function.
3. **Micro-segmentation:** Network environments are divided into isolated segments with independent access controls.
4. **Continuous monitoring and validation:** Security status is constantly assessed rather than periodically checked.
5. **Device trust assessment:** Verifies the security posture and integrity of devices before granting access.

ZTA provides a framework for securing increasingly complex and distributed healthcare environments by assuming potential compromise and requiring explicit verification for all access [14].

## 3.7 CHALLENGES IN IMPLEMENTING SECURE AUTHENTICATION AND AUTHORIZATION

### 3.7.1 Technical challenges

#### *3.7.1.1 Device diversity and constraints*

IoMT environments encompass an extraordinary range of devices with varying capabilities:

1. **Computational limitations:** Many medical devices have restricted processing power, memory, and energy capacity that limit their security capabilities.
2. **Protocol heterogeneity:** IoMT devices use diverse communication protocols and standards, complicating unified security implementation.
3. **Legacy device integration:** Older medical devices with extended lifecycles may lack modern security features entirely.
4. **Interface limitations:** Many medical devices have minimal or specialized user interfaces that complicate implementation of interactive security measures [15].

#### *3.7.1.2 Interoperability challenges*

1. **Cross-platform authentication:** Users frequently need to access multiple systems with different security implementations during normal workflows.

*Table 3.6* Interoperability challenges and solutions for IoMT authentication

| *Challenge* | *Impact* | *Potential solutions* |
|---|---|---|
| Protocol diversity | Inconsistent security implementation | Gateway-based security, protocol translators |
| Vendor-specific authentication | Fragmented identity management | Federated identity, SSO implementation |
| Legacy system integration | Security gaps, workarounds | Security proxies, network segmentation |
| Cross-organization access | Boundary issues, governance challenges | Trust frameworks, federation agreements |
| Data exchange security | Exposure during transit | End-to-end encryption, API security |

2. **Federated identity challenges:** Implementing cohesive identity management across organizational boundaries introduces technical and governance complexities.
3. **Data exchange security:** Maintaining appropriate security controls during data exchange between systems with different authorization models creates significant challenges (Table 3.6).

#### 3.7.1.3 *Performance and availability requirements*

1. **Response time sensitivity:** Authentication and authorization processes must complete quickly to avoid impacting clinical care.
2. **High availability requirements:** Authentication systems for critical care systems must maintain exceptional uptime.
3. **Offline functionality:** Medical devices must maintain essential functions even when network connectivity is limited or unavailable.

### 3.7.2 Organizational and human factors

#### 3.7.2.1 *Workflow integration*

1. **Clinical time constraints:** Healthcare professionals often work under significant time pressure, making cumbersome security procedures problematic.
2. **Frequent context switching:** Healthcare workers typically transition between multiple patients, locations, and systems, creating authentication friction.

3. **Interruption-driven work:** Healthcare workflows are characterized by frequent interruptions, complicating session management and continuous authentication.
4. **Collaborative work patterns:** Healthcare delivery often involves collaborative work around shared systems, challenging traditional one-user-one-session security models [16].

#### *3.7.2.2 Training and awareness*

1. **Security knowledge gaps:** Many healthcare professionals lack sufficient training in cybersecurity practices.
2. **Alert fatigue:** Excessive security warnings or authentication requests can lead to desensitization and automatic approval.
3. **Priority conflicts:** Healthcare workers understandably prioritize immediate patient care over security procedures during perceived emergencies.

#### *3.7.2.3 Resource constraints*

1. **Cybersecurity expertise shortages:** Healthcare organizations frequently lack specialized security expertise, particularly for IoMT environments.
2. **Budget limitations:** Healthcare organizations typically allocate smaller proportions of IT budgets to security compared to other regulated industries.
3. **Competing priorities:** Security initiatives compete with clinical improvements and regulatory requirements for limited resources.

### 3.7.3 Regulatory and compliance considerations

Healthcare operates within a complex regulatory environment that impacts security implementation (Table 3.7):

1. **Multiple regulatory frameworks:** Healthcare organizations often must comply with overlapping regulations including HIPAA, GDPR, and various state privacy laws.
2. **Prescriptive requirements:** Some regulations specify particular security approaches that may not align with optimal technical solutions.
3. **Documentation burden:** Comprehensive documentation requirements for security controls create significant administrative overhead.
4. **Patient rights and ethical considerations:** Security measures must respect patient rights to understand how their information is protected and who has accessed it [17].

*Table 3.7* Key regulatory frameworks affecting IoMT security

| *Framework* | *Region* | *Key authentication requirements* | *Authorization requirements* | *Audit requirements* |
|---|---|---|---|---|
| HIPAA | US | Unique user identification | Access controls, minimum necessary | Comprehensive audit trails |
| GDPR | EU | Strong authentication | Detailed data access controls | Subject access transparency |
| FDA Guidelines | US | Risk-based authentication | Device-specific controls | Vulnerability management |
| ISO 27001 | Global | Multi-factor for sensitive data | Formal access control policy | Regular review and testing |
| HITRUST | US | Role-based authentication | Context-aware controls | Real-time monitoring |

## 3.8 BEST PRACTICES AND IMPLEMENTATION STRATEGIES

### 3.8.1 Risk-based implementation framework

A risk-based approach ensures that security resources are allocated effectively:

1. **Comprehensive risk assessment:** Begin with thorough risk evaluation before selecting specific technologies.
2. **Tiered security implementation:** Implement security in prioritized phases based on risk assessment.
3. **Critical systems prioritization:** Implement enhanced security measures for high-risk systems first.
4. **Defense in depth:** Implement multiple layers of security rather than relying on single protection mechanisms.

### 3.8.2 Technical implementation strategies

#### *3.8.2.1 Interoperability-focused design*

1. **Standards compliance:** Adhere to established healthcare security standards and protocols.
2. **Federated identity management:** Implement identity federation to streamline authentication across systems and organizations.
3. **API security gateways:** Deploy centralized API security for consistent protection across system interfaces.

#### *3.8.2.2 Resilient authentication architecture*

1. **Offline authentication capabilities:** Ensure critical functions remain accessible even during network outages.

2. **Redundant authentication paths:** Implement multiple authentication methods and pathways to maintain availability.
3. **Graceful degradation:** Design systems to fall back to less stringent but still secure authentication during emergency conditions.

#### *3.8.2.3 Legacy system integration*

1. **Security proxies:** Deploy proxy systems that implement modern security on behalf of legacy devices.
2. **Network segmentation:** Isolate legacy systems in separate network segments with controlled access.
3. **Compensating controls:** Implement additional security measures to address specific weaknesses in legacy systems.

### 3.8.3 Organizational best practices

#### *3.8.3.1 Security governance*

1. **Formal security policies:** Develop comprehensive policies specifying authentication and authorization requirements.
2. **Role-based policy framework:** Create security policies tailored to specific roles and responsibilities.
3. **Clear exception processes:** Define formal procedures for security exceptions with appropriate approval and documentation (Table 3.8).

#### *3.8.3.2 Security culture development*

1. **Role-specific training:** Provide security training tailored to specific job functions and access levels.

*Table 3.8* Framework for healthcare security policy development

| *Policy Component* | *Key Elements* | *Implementation considerations* |
|---|---|---|
| Authentication policy | MFA requirements, credential management | Clinical workflow integration |
| Authorization framework | Role definitions, access request process | Exception handling procedures |
| Device security policy | Device registration, authentication methods | Legacy device provisions |
| Audit and monitoring | Log collection, review frequency | Alert thresholds, response procedures |
| Exception management | Break-glass provisions, emergency access | Post-event review requirements |
| Training requirements | Role-specific training, frequency | Competency verification methods |

2. **Simulation exercises:** Conduct regular security simulations and exercises to build practical skills.
3. **Visible leadership support:** Ensure visible commitment to security from organizational leadership.

#### *3.8.3.3 Continuous monitoring and improvement*

1. **Security metrics program:** Define and track specific metrics for authentication and authorization effectiveness.
2. **Regular security assessments:** Conduct periodic security evaluations including penetration testing of authentication systems.
3. **User feedback mechanisms:** Establish channels for users to report security usability issues [18].

### 3.8.4 Implementation roadmap

A phased implementation approach increases success likelihood:

1. **Assessment and planning phase:** Begin with comprehensive evaluation and strategic planning.
2. **Pilot implementation:** Begin with limited deployment to validate approach.
3. **Scaled implementation:** Expand successful approaches across the organization.
4. **Operational transition:** Establish ongoing operations and continuous improvement.

## 3.9 FUTURE DIRECTIONS AND EMERGING TRENDS

### 3.9.1 Continuous adaptive risk and trust assessment

Continuous adaptive risk and trust assessment (CARTA) represents an evolution beyond static security models to dynamic approaches that continuously evaluate risk and adjust security measures accordingly [19]:

1. **Real-time risk calculation:** Continuously reassesses risk throughout sessions rather than only at authentication points.
2. **Integration with clinical systems:** Leverages information from clinical systems to understand legitimate access patterns.

### 3.9.2 Usable security approaches

The future of healthcare security lies in solutions that enhance rather than impede clinical workflows:

1. **Invisible security:** Authentication through passive observation of biometric characteristics without explicit user action.
2. **Voice-driven security:** Voice-activated security functions for hands-busy clinical environments.

### 3.9.3 Quantum-resistant authentication

As quantum computing advances, authentication systems must prepare for potential threats to current cryptographic methods [20]:

1. **Postquantum cryptography:** Development of cryptographic approaches resistant to quantum computing attacks.
2. **Hybrid cryptographic approaches:** Transitional approaches combining current and quantum-resistant methods.

### 3.9.4 Decentralized identity and patient-controlled access

Future IoMT security will increasingly emphasize patient control and decentralized approaches (Table 3.9):

1. **Self-sovereign identity:** Digital identity credentials owned and controlled by patients rather than healthcare organizations.
2. **Patient-directed authorization:** Authorization systems that implement patient preferences with greater granularity.

## 3.10 CONCLUSION

Secure authentication and authorization are vital components in the fight against cybersecurity threats in the rapidly evolving Internet of Medical Things landscape. Traditional authentication methods have proven inadequate in the face of increasingly sophisticated threats and the complex requirements of healthcare environments.

*Table 3.9* Comparison of traditional and patient-controlled access models

| *Feature* | *Traditional model* | *Patient-controlled model* |
|---|---|---|
| Access control | Organization-defined | Patient-defined preferences |
| Granularity | Limited, role-based | Fine-grained, context-specific |
| Implementation | Centralized systems | Often blockchain or distributed ledger |
| Patient involvement | Minimal, consent forms | Active, ongoing consent management |
| Audit capabilities | Organization-controlled | Transparent to patient |
| Technology requirements | Moderate | High |
| Regulatory alignment | Well-established | Evolving regulatory framework |

The evolution of authentication and authorization technologies offers promising paths forward for healthcare security. Advanced approaches such as multifactor authentication, biometrics, device-level authentication, and continuous verification provide significantly enhanced protection compared to traditional methods. The integration of emerging technologies—particularly artificial intelligence, blockchain, and ZTAs—represents a significant advancement in IoMT security capabilities.

Despite technological advances, successful implementation faces numerous challenges. Technical constraints including device limitations, interoperability requirements, and legacy system integration create significant complexity. Organizational factors such as workflow integration, resource limitations, and change management further complicate security implementations.

Effective implementation requires strategic approaches that address both technical and organizational dimensions. Risk-based frameworks ensure appropriate resource allocation by prioritizing high-risk systems and data. Phased implementation strategies with pilot testing and refinement cycles maximize success likelihood while minimizing disruption to healthcare operations.

The security of IoMT devices and systems is not merely a technical concern but a fundamental requirement for maintaining the integrity and trustworthiness of healthcare delivery in the digital age. As healthcare becomes increasingly dependent on connected technologies, the security of these systems directly impacts patient safety, care quality, and institutional viability.

## REFERENCES


[1] S. Ghafur, S. Kristensen, K. Honeyford, G. Martin, A. Darzi, and P. Aylin, "A retrospective impact analysis of the WannaCry cyberattack on the NHS," *NPJ Digital Medicine*, vol. 2, no. 1, pp. 1–7, 2019.

[2] S. Alder, "Universal Health Services confirms all US hospitals affected by ransomware attack," *HIPAA Journal*, vol. 4, no. 10, pp. 15–17, 2020.

[3] IBM Security, "Cost of a data breach report 2023," IBM, New York, NY, USA, Tech. Rep., 2023.

[4] Health and Human Services (HHS), "Healthcare cybersecurity report: Strengthening the security posture of the healthcare sector," Office of Information Security, U.S. Department of Health and Human Services, Washington, DC, USA, Tech. Rep., 2023.

[5] Verizon, "2023 Data Breach Investigations Report," Verizon, New York, NY, USA, Tech. Rep., 2023.

[6] F. Alsubaei, A. Abuhussein, and S. Shiva, "Security and privacy in the Internet of Medical Things: A review," in IEEE 19th International Conference on Software Quality, Reliability and Security Companion, 2019, pp. 219–224.

[7] Microsoft, "Microsoft Digital Defense Report 2023," Microsoft, Redmond, WA, USA, Tech. Rep., 2023.
[8] P. Patil, P. Pawar, and V. Pardeshi, "A survey on biometric authentication in IoMT," in IEEE 12th Annual Computing and Communication Workshop and Conference, 2022, pp. 0571–0577.
[9] National Institute of Standards and Technology (NIST), "Digital Identity Guidelines (Special Publication 800-63-3)," U.S. Department of Commerce, Gaithersburg, MD, USA, Tech. Rep., 2021.
[10] M. S. Jalali and J. P. Kaiser, "Cybersecurity in hospitals: A systematic, organizational perspective," *Journal of Medical Internet Research*, vol. 20, no. 5, pp. e10059, 2018.
[11] J. Deogirikar and A. Vidhate, "Security attacks in IoT: A survey," in International Conference on I-SMAC, 2017, pp. 32–37.
[12] L. Ayala, "Cybersecurity for hospitals and healthcare facilities: A guide to detection and prevention," Apress, New York, NY, USA, 2022.
[13] C. Butpheng, K. H. Yeh, and H. Xiong, "Security and privacy in IoT-cloud-based e-health systems—A comprehensive review," *Symmetry*, vol. 12, no. 7, pp. 1191, 2020.
[14] R. H. Chowdhury, N. U. Prince, S. M. Abdullah, and L. A. Mim, "The role of predictive analytics in cybersecurity: Detecting and preventing threats," *World Journal of Advanced Research and Reviews*, vol. 23, no. 2, pp. 134–142, 2024.
[15] A. Dalal, "Advanced threat detection in healthcare environments using predictive analytics," *Journal of Healthcare Informatics Research*, vol. 7, no. 2, pp. 156–172, 2023.
[16] OWASP, "Authentication Cheat Sheet," Open Web Application Security Project, Tech. Rep., 2023.
[17] B. Schneier, "Data and Goliath: The hidden battles to collect your data and control your world," W. W. Norton & Company, New York, NY, USA, 2015.
[18] M. Senbekov et al., "The recent progress and applications of digital technologies in healthcare: A review," *International Journal of Telemedicine and Applications*, vol. 2020, pp. 1–18, 2020.
[19] F. Ullah et al., "Semantic interoperability for big-data in heterogeneous IoT infrastructure for healthcare," *Sustainable Cities and Society*, vol. 66, pp. 102569, 2021.
[20] P. Kumar, G. P. Gupta, and R. Tripathi, "An ensemble learning and fog-cloud architecture-based anomaly detection scheme for IoT security," *Journal of Ambient Intelligence and Humanized Computing*, vol. 13, no. 4, pp. 2063–2075, 2022.

Chapter 4

# Threat-aware circular security in smart healthcare

*I. Sakthidevi and G. Fathima*

## 4.1 INTRODUCTION

The advancements in the Internet of Medical Things (IoMT) have significantly transformed healthcare by enabling real-time patient monitoring, automated diagnostics, and remote healthcare services. IoMT devices, including wearable sensors, smart implants, and connected medical equipment, have facilitated the seamless collection and transmission of critical health data, leading to improved patient outcomes and operational efficiency in healthcare systems [1]. The integration of artificial intelligence (AI) with IoMT has further enhanced predictive analytics, early disease detection, and personalized treatment plans, making healthcare more data-driven and proactive [2]. However, the extensive interconnectivity of IoMT devices has also introduced complex security challenges, such as data breaches, cyberattacks, and unauthorized access to sensitive patient information [3]. Ensuring the security and integrity of IoMT ecosystems has become a critical priority, necessitating the development of advanced security frameworks that can provide robust protection while maintaining system efficiency [4]. The convergence of blockchain technology with federated learning (FL) has been explored as a potential solution to enhance security and privacy in smart healthcare, offering decentralized data protection and collaborative intelligence sharing across healthcare networks [5].

### 4.1.1 The need for endpoint security in medical ecosystems

As IoMT ecosystems expand, endpoint security has emerged as a fundamental requirement to safeguard medical devices and patient data from cyber threats. The heterogeneity of IoMT devices, varying in computational capacity and security capabilities, presents significant challenges in ensuring consistent security policies across healthcare networks. Traditional centralized security models have proven inadequate in protecting IoMT endpoints due to their susceptibility to single points of failure and latency issues. FL has been proposed as an alternative approach, allowing decentralized security

DOI: 10.1201/9781003640325-4

mechanisms to be implemented without compromising data privacy. This method enables medical devices to collaboratively train security models while retaining sensitive patient information locally, reducing the risk of data exposure. Additionally, the integration of AI-driven threat detection systems has been identified as a crucial factor in strengthening endpoint security, allowing real-time identification and mitigation of potential threats before they can compromise critical healthcare infrastructures. The secure transmission and aggregation of healthcare data in IoT environments have also been explored to address data integrity issues, ensuring that security measures are not compromised by resource-constrained devices.

### 4.1.2 Defining circular security in healthcare

Circular security in smart healthcare refers to an adaptive and self-sustaining security model that continuously leverages past threat intelligence to strengthen current and future security mechanisms. Unlike conventional static security approaches, circular security emphasizes the reuse of threat intelligence across different layers of the healthcare network, creating an evolving defense system that adapts to emerging cyber threats. This concept integrates FL, blockchain, and AI-based anomaly detection to enable secure, real-time intelligence sharing while preserving patient data confidentiality. By implementing a feedback loop, security responses can be refined over time, ensuring that lessons learned from previous cyber incidents are systematically integrated into future threat mitigation strategies. Moreover, circular security frameworks aim to reduce computational overhead and enhance sustainability by minimizing redundant security processes, making them ideal for resource-constrained medical environments. This approach aligns with the growing need for sustainable and scalable security solutions in modern healthcare, ensuring long-term data protection without excessive resource consumption.

## 4.2 SECURITY AND SUSTAINABILITY IN SMART HEALTHCARE

### 4.2.1 The intersection of cybersecurity and sustainability

The growing adoption of IoMT devices has significantly enhanced healthcare delivery, but it has also introduced a complex landscape of security threats. Ensuring robust cybersecurity is crucial to protect sensitive patient data and maintain the integrity of connected medical systems. However, the pursuit of security must also consider sustainability, as healthcare systems face increasing pressure to minimize energy consumption and operational costs. Edge computing has been explored as a promising approach to enhance both security and sustainability by processing data closer to the source, reducing the need for constant cloud communication and lowering energy demands [6]. Yet, edge devices themselves can become attack vectors, necessitating advanced security frameworks capable of adapting to evolving threats while maintaining low resource consumption [7].Blockchain-based systems have been proposed to address this challenge by offering decentralized security and tamper-proof data management, although concerns remain regarding the energy-intensive nature of blockchain operations [8].

AI and FL have shown promise in balancing security and sustainability by enabling distributed threat detection without centralized data storage [9]. These approaches allow medical devices to collaboratively train security models, reducing the need for energy-intensive data transfers. Additionally, AI-powered voice analysis applications have demonstrated the potential to enhance healthcare diagnostics, further illustrating how intelligent algorithms can improve healthcare services while optimizing resource usage [10]. The integration of sustainable practices into security frameworks is essential to build resilient healthcare systems capable of enduring long-term operational demands without compromising data safety.

### 4.2.2 Energy-efficient security practices

Energy efficiency has become a critical consideration in the design of security protocols for smart healthcare systems. Medical devices, particularly wearable sensors and portable diagnostic tools, often operate on limited battery power, making it impractical to implement computationally intensive security measures. Mobile edge computing (MEC) has emerged as a viable solution, enabling resource-intensive security operations to be offloaded to nearby edge servers, thereby extending device battery life and reducing latency. By strategically distributing security tasks, MEC-assisted healthcare systems can achieve a balance between energy efficiency and robust protection, ensuring continuous monitoring and threat detection without draining device resources.

Optimized deep learning models have further enhanced energy-efficient security practices by streamlining threat detection processes. For instance, hybrid models combining convolutional neural networks (CNNs) with metaheuristic optimization algorithms have demonstrated improved accuracy in anomaly detection, while reducing the computational complexity of security analyses. Such models are particularly valuable in dynamic healthcare environments, where security threats evolve rapidly, and real-time response capabilities are essential. Additionally, FL has enabled energy-efficient threat intelligence sharing across medical networks, facilitating continuous security improvements without excessive energy consumption. These innovations highlight the potential of sustainable AI-driven security solutions in modern healthcare.

### 4.2.3 Challenges of balancing security and resource constraints

Despite technological advancements, balancing security and resource constraints remains a significant challenge for smart healthcare systems. Many IoMT devices possess limited processing power and storage capacity, making it difficult to implement sophisticated encryption and threat detection mechanisms. Lightweight cryptographic algorithms have been explored to mitigate this issue, but their reduced computational requirements often come at the cost of weaker security protections. Furthermore, the intermittent connectivity of some healthcare devices, particularly those used in remote patient monitoring, complicates the implementation of continuous security monitoring.

Blockchain-based systems, while offering robust security features, introduce scalability and energy consumption challenges, particularly when used in large-scale healthcare deployments. The high computational overhead of consensus mechanisms can strain resource-constrained devices, necessitating the development of energy-aware blockchain protocols specifically designed for healthcare environments. Similarly, the variability in device capabilities within IoMT ecosystems complicates the implementation of uniform security policies, as one-size-fits-all solutions are often impractical. Addressing these challenges requires an adaptive security approach that dynamically adjusts security protocols based on device capabilities, network conditions, and real-time threat assessments. Such an approach aligns with the principles of circular security, enabling continuous learning and threat intelligence reuse to enhance long-term protection while optimizing resource usage.

## 4.3 THREAT INTELLIGENCE IN SMART HEALTHCARE

### 4.3.1 Understanding threat intelligence and its lifecycle

Threat intelligence has played a critical role in strengthening smart healthcare systems by providing actionable insights to mitigate potential cyber threats. The lifecycle of threat intelligence typically includes stages such as data collection, threat analysis, dissemination, and continuous improvement. In smart healthcare environments, real-time data generated from medical devices, network logs, and patient monitoring systems has been used to detect and respond to security incidents. FL-based frameworks have been introduced to enhance privacy while enabling the collective training of threat detection models across distributed healthcare nodes, reducing the risk of centralized data breaches [11].

Human-in-the-loop mechanisms have further improved the accuracy of threat intelligence systems by integrating human expertise into automated decision-making processes. Such systems have enabled contextual threat evaluation, allowing healthcare security mechanisms to adapt dynamically to evolving attack patterns [12]. The integration of intelligent threat detection and adaptive learning has supported long-term protection strategies, reinforcing the circular security model by continuously reusing and refining threat intelligence data.

### 4.3.2 Sources of threat intelligence (device logs, anomaly detection, external feeds)

Threat intelligence in smart healthcare has been sourced from multiple channels, including device logs, anomaly detection systems, and external threat feeds. Device logs have offered valuable information on system events, failed access attempts, and irregular activities, serving as a foundational component for identifying potential threats. Advanced anomaly detection systems powered by deep learning algorithms have been utilized to recognize abnormal behavior in medical devices, flagging suspicious activities that may indicate cyberattacks.

Multimodal deep learning approaches have improved access trust by analyzing various data streams, such as biometric signals and usage patterns, to enhance the accuracy of threat identification [13]. Additionally, external threat intelligence feeds have provided up-to-date information on emerging vulnerabilities and global attack trends, empowering healthcare systems to proactively defend against new threats. By combining internal device-generated data with external threat knowledge, healthcare systems have built more resilient security architectures capable of withstanding sophisticated cyber threats.

### 4.3.3 Real-time threat monitoring in medical devices

Real-time threat monitoring has become essential for ensuring the security and safety of connected medical devices. Continuous monitoring solutions have enabled the early detection of threats, preventing malicious activities from compromising critical healthcare services. Transparent and privacy-preserving platforms have been developed to facilitate real-time threat detection without violating patient privacy, leveraging blockchain technology to secure device communications and ensure data integrity [14].

Edge intelligence solutions have further enhanced real-time monitoring by distributing threat detection capabilities across edge nodes, reducing response times and minimizing the impact of security breaches. These systems have been capable of instantly analyzing data generated by medical sensors, identifying irregularities, and triggering automated responses to neutralize potential threats. The incorporation of smart contracts into healthcare systems has enabled the automatic enforcement of security policies, providing a decentralized mechanism for handling security incidents with minimal human intervention [15]. Such innovations have demonstrated the potential of circular security models to leverage real-time threat intelligence, creating adaptive and sustainable defenses for smart healthcare ecosystems.

## 4.4 CIRCULAR SECURITY: A NEW PARADIGM

### 4.4.1 Concept of circular security

Circular security has emerged as an innovative framework designed to enhance the resilience of smart healthcare systems by continuously repurposing threat intelligence. Unlike traditional linear security models, which treat threat mitigation as a terminal process, circular security emphasizes the ongoing refinement and reuse of security insights. Threat data generated during security incidents has been systematically analyzed, categorized, and fed back into the system to strengthen future defenses. This iterative approach has enabled healthcare systems to evolve continuously, learning from each attack to build more robust security layers.

The circular security model as shown in Figure 4.1 has drawn inspiration from circular economy principles, promoting resource optimization through the perpetual use of threat intelligence. By adopting a cyclic security lifecycle, smart healthcare ecosystems have been able to mitigate zero-day vulnerabilities and adapt to rapidly evolving cyber threats without requiring constant manual intervention. The model has proven particularly effective in environments where patient safety and data integrity are paramount, as real-time threat data has been transformed into actionable intelligence for proactive defense strategies.

### 4.4.2 Threat data reuse and knowledge sharing

The reuse of threat data has played a crucial role in the circular security paradigm, enabling healthcare systems to leverage past incidents to prevent future attacks. Logs, alerts, and anomaly detection records collected from connected medical devices have been stored in threat intelligence repositories, where advanced machine learning models have been trained to identify recurring attack patterns. These repositories have served as knowledge hubs, facilitating seamless threat information exchange between healthcare institutions, cybersecurity providers, and regulatory bodies.

Knowledge sharing has further amplified the effectiveness of circular security by fostering collaborative defense mechanisms as shown in Figure 4.2. When multiple healthcare facilities contributed anonymized threat data to shared intelligence networks, collective defenses were strengthened, as security policies and detection algorithms were refined

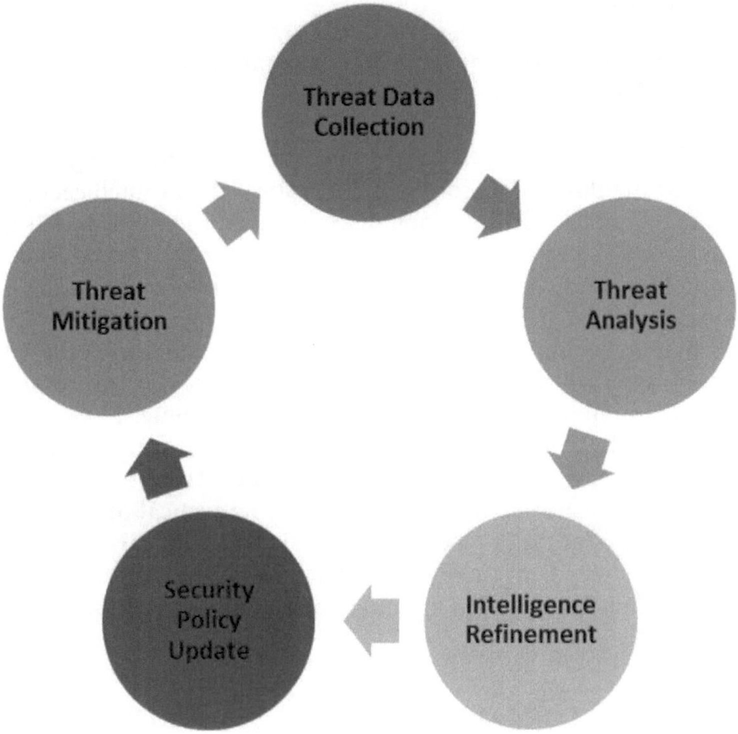
Threat Data Collection
Threat Analysis
Intelligence Refinement
Security Policy Update
Threat Mitigation

*Figure 4.1* Circular security.

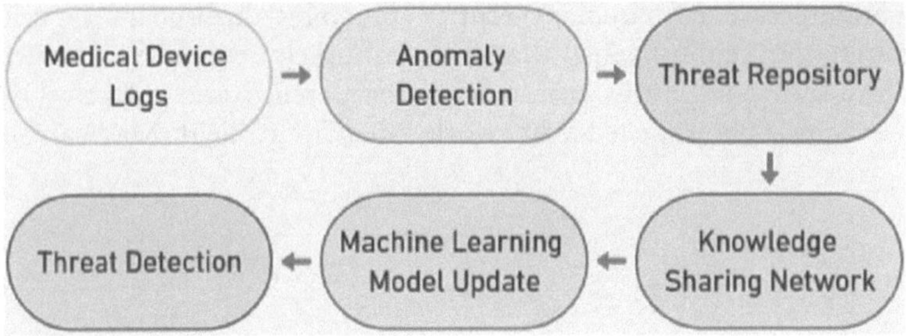


*Figure 4.2* Threat data reuse.

using a broader spectrum of threat insights. This interconnected security ecosystem has significantly reduced incident response times and minimized the likelihood of widespread cyberattacks, as threat signatures identified in one healthcare system have been immediately used to safeguard others.

## 4.5 SELF-HEALING SECURITY SYSTEMS AND AUTOMATED DEFENSE

Self-healing security systems have been a cornerstone of circular security, leveraging AI and automation to detect, respond to, and recover from cyber threats with minimal human intervention as shown in Figure 4.3. These systems have been designed to dynamically adapt to emerging threats, using real-time threat monitoring and historical threat intelligence to predict potential attack vectors. Upon detecting a security breach, self-healing mechanisms have been triggered to isolate compromised components, patch vulnerabilities, and restore normal operations without disrupting critical healthcare services.

Automated defense mechanisms have further enhanced the sustainability of circular security by continuously evolving in response to new threat intelligence. Smart contracts, for example, have been used to automatically enforce updated security protocols across distributed healthcare systems, ensuring that every connected device adhered to the latest threat mitigation strategies. Through this cyclical process of detection, analysis, adaptation, and recovery, smart healthcare environments have remained resilient against ever-changing cyber threats, with each security incident serving as a learning opportunity to reinforce long-term protection.

## 4.6 ARCHITECTURE OF A CIRCULAR SECURITY FRAMEWORK

### 4.6.1 Key components: threat intelligence hub, decision engines, and secure data lakes

The architecture of circular security in smart healthcare is built on interconnected components that collaboratively enhance system resilience through continuous threat intelligence reuse and adaptive defense mechanisms. The proposed framework, MedCircleShield (Medical Circular

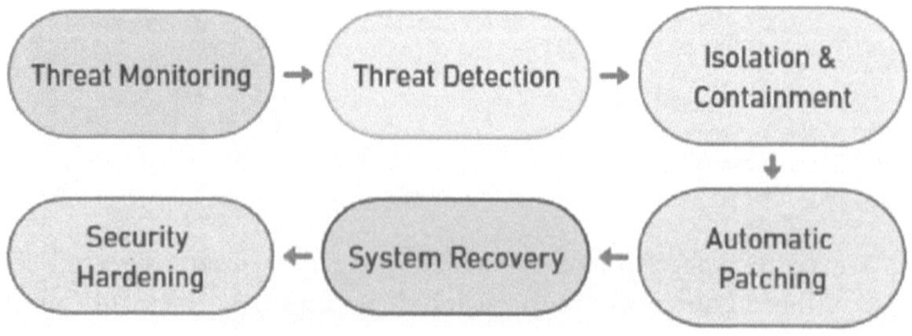


*Figure 4.3* Self-healing security system.

Security Shield) as shown in Figure 4.4, establishes a dynamic security ecosystem capable of evolving in response to emerging threats. The pseudocode for MedCircleShield Framework is presented in Table 4.1.

The Circular Threat Intelligence Hub (CTIH) acts as the central unit, collecting and aggregating threat data from diverse medical devices, network logs, and external feeds. This hub processes raw data, extracts actionable insights, and redistributes refined intelligence across the ecosystem to fortify security layers. Threat patterns, indicators of compromise (IoCs), and incident reports are continuously shared, ensuring real-time threat awareness across interconnected systems.

The adaptive defense engine (ADE) leverages AI and machine learning algorithms to refine security protocols based on historical threat intelligence.

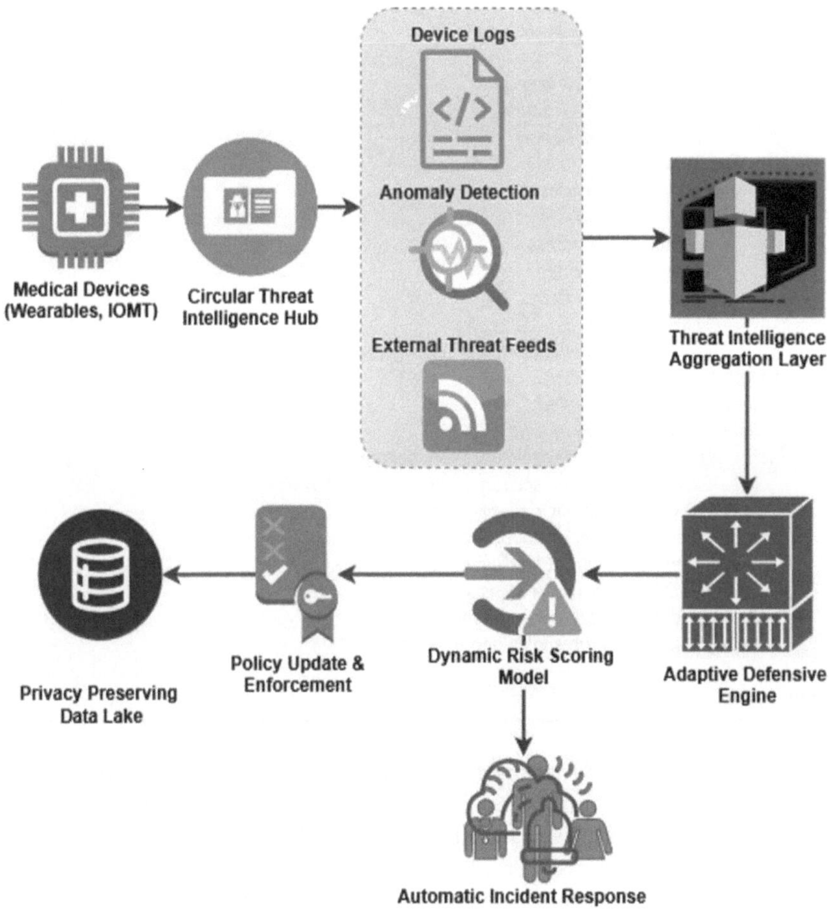


*Figure 4.4* Architecture diagram for medcircleshield framework.

*Table 4.1* Pseudocode for medcircleshield framework

```
Initialize Framework:
    Initialize Circular Threat Intelligence Hub (CTIH)
    Initialize Adaptive Defence Engine (ADE)
    Initialize Dynamic Risk Scoring Module (DRSM)
    Initialize Privacy-Preserving Data Lake (PPDL)
Main Process:
    WHILE System is Active:
      Collect Threat Data:
        Retrieve device logs, alerts, and anomalies
        Fetch external threat feeds (CERT, CVE, threat databases)
        Aggregate data in CTIH
    Analyze Threat Intelligence:
        FOR each data entry in CTIH:
          IF anomaly detected OR threat indicator matches known IoC:
            Generate threat signature
            Update threat intelligence repository
          ELSE:
            Discard non-threatening data
    Adaptive Defence and Risk Scoring:
        FOR each connected device:
          Compute risk score using DRSM
          Update security policies dynamically:
            IF risk score > threshold:
              Restrict device access
              Trigger firewall rules
              Apply security patches
              ELSE:
              Monitor device with standard security measures
    Incident Response:
      IF real-time threat detected:
        Activate automated response:
              Isolate affected device or network segment
              Execute predefined security protocols (e.g., shut down ports)
              Log incident details and remediation actions
    Data Storage and Feedback Loop:
        Encrypt and store threat intelligence in PPDL
        Update ADE with new threat insights
        Re-train AI/ML models based on incident logs
        Adjust risk scoring thresholds and policy rules

END WHILE
```

Using insights derived from past incidents, ADE dynamically updates defense strategies, enabling autonomous threat mitigation and proactive incident prevention. This adaptive capability significantly reduces attack dwell times and enhances system recovery.

To address data privacy concerns, the privacy-preserving data lake (PPDL) securely stores threat intelligence and incident logs with robust encryption mechanisms. This repository supports secure, privacy-compliant research and analytics, facilitating collaborative threat research without compromising sensitive medical data.

Furthermore, the dynamic risk scoring module (DRSM) continuously assesses the risk posture of connected devices, assigning dynamic risk scores based on threat proximity, device vulnerabilities, and recent attack patterns. Security policies are adjusted in real time, enabling devices with higher risk scores to trigger stricter access controls and prioritized threat monitoring.

### 4.6.2 Secure data flow in a smart hospital

In a smart hospital environment, secure data flow is essential to ensure that threat intelligence is effectively distributed and acted upon. Medical devices, wearables, and IoMT systems generate a constant stream of data, which is funneled into the CTIH for real-time processing. Detected anomalies or suspicious patterns are analyzed, and relevant intelligence is forwarded to the ADE for immediate response.

The processed threat intelligence is stored in the PPDL, where encrypted access is granted to authorized systems and researchers. Risk scores generated by the DRSM dictate the level of security measures applied to each device, ensuring that high-risk endpoints are isolated or patched automatically. This dynamic flow of data creates a responsive security fabric capable of neutralizing threats before they escalate.

### 4.6.3 Feedback loops and security adaptability

Circular security is sustained through iterative feedback loops that enable continuous learning and security evolution. When a threat is detected and mitigated, the incident data is fed back into the CTIH, refining threat models and improving future detection accuracy. The ADE updates its decision-making algorithms based on new insights, while the DRSM recalibrates risk scores to reflect the evolving threat landscape.

This adaptive feedback loop ensures that the security framework remains resilient over time, gradually enhancing its defense capabilities through repeated cycles of threat detection, mitigation, and learning. As a result, smart healthcare ecosystems become progressively more robust, benefiting from collective intelligence and automated self-healing mechanisms that minimize human intervention and system downtime.

## 4.7 IMPLEMENTING CIRCULAR SECURITY IN HEALTHCARE

### 4.7.1 Integrating threat intelligence platforms with IoMT

The integration of threat intelligence platforms (TIPs) with IoMT devices has emerged as a critical strategy for enhancing healthcare security. TIPs act as centralized systems that collect, analyze, and disseminate threat intelligence across connected devices, enabling faster incident detection and response. In a circular security framework, TIPs facilitate continuous knowledge sharing, where real-time threat data from one device can be used to safeguard others within the ecosystem. IoMT devices, due to their constrained resources, benefit from externalized threat intelligence processing, reducing on-device computation overhead while maintaining security efficacy. Adaptive threat feeds and device-level anomaly detection enhance proactive security measures, supporting dynamic policy adjustments based on evolving risk scores.

For instance, a system architecture integrating TIPs with a CTIH can use aggregated threat signatures to detect patterns across multiple healthcare endpoints. This approach not only prevents recurring attacks but also contributes to long-term threat mitigation by reusing past threat intelligence for future defense strategies. The feedback loops created by this integration enhance the resilience of healthcare networks, transforming isolated security measures into a collective defense mechanism.

### 4.7.2 Lightweight encryption and privacy-preserving techniques

Resource constraints in IoMT devices necessitate the adoption of lightweight encryption schemes and privacy-preserving techniques to ensure security without compromising performance. Lightweight cryptographic algorithms, such as elliptic curve cryptography (ECC) and advanced encryption standard with galois/counter mode (AES-GCM), offer strong security guarantees while consuming minimal computational power and energy. Privacy-preserving techniques, including homomorphic encryption and secure multiparty computation (SMPC), allow sensitive patient data to be processed in encrypted form, minimizing exposure to potential breaches.

In circular security implementations, PPDLscan store encrypted threat intelligence and historical incident logs, enabling secure, privacy-compliant data sharing across healthcare facilities. By encrypting threat data at the source and decrypting it only when necessary, sensitive information remains protected throughout its lifecycle. This approach ensures that threat intelligence can be reused and distributed across networks without compromising patient privacy, aligning with global data protection regulations.

### 4.7.3 Scalable and low-carbon security models

Scalability and sustainability are essential considerations when designing security systems for smart healthcare environments. Circular security models leverage distributed threat intelligence and automated incident response, reducing the need for redundant security infrastructure. This distributed approach minimizes the carbon footprint of healthcare cybersecurity by optimizing resource usage and avoiding unnecessary computational load.

AI-driven ADEs can dynamically scale security operations, allocating resources only when elevated risk levels are detected. For example, continuous threat monitoring can be performed in low-power states, with intensive threat analysis triggered only upon anomaly detection. Edge computing further enhances scalability by offloading security tasks to local nodes, reducing latency and energy consumption.

Additionally, sustainable practices such as server virtualization, renewable-powered data centres, and energy-efficient hardware contribute to lowering the overall environmental impact of healthcare security operations. Circular security, by design, promotes longevity and resource optimization, creating a security ecosystem that evolves and strengthens over time while minimizing environmental strain.

## 4.8 CASE STUDY: CIRCULAR SECURITY IMPLEMENTATION IN A SMART HOSPITAL NETWORK

A large multispecialty smart hospital network implemented a circular security framework to enhance threat resilience and protect critical medical devices. The hospital's infrastructure included a vast array of IoMT devices, from patient monitoring systems to robotic surgical equipment, all interconnected to enable real-time patient care. However, the complexity of the interconnected systems made the network vulnerable to evolving cyber threats, including ransomware, distributed denial of service (DDoS) attacks, and data breaches targeting patient records.

To mitigate these risks, the hospital adopted the MedCircleShield Framework, integrating the following components:

- Circular threat intelligence hub (CTIH): Device logs, anomaly reports, and external threat feeds were continuously collected, processed, and redistributed across the hospital network. Threat patterns detected on one device were shared across the entire ecosystem, preventing repeat attacks and enhancing collective defense.
- Adaptive defense engine (ADE): Security protocols were dynamically adjusted based on real-time threat intelligence and historical attack data. For example, when an infusion pump showed signs of unusual data transmission, the ADE isolated the device, analyzed the anomaly, and updated firewall rules across similar devices.
- Privacy-preserving data lake (PPDL): All threat intelligence data was stored in encrypted form, accessible only through privacy-compliant research queries. This setup allowed security researchers to study attack vectors without compromising patient data confidentiality.

- Dynamic risk scoring module (DRSM): Devices were continuously assessed for risk, with security measures scaled according to risk severity. High-risk devices received more frequent security updates and closer monitoring, while low-risk devices operated with lightweight security protocols to conserve energy.

This circular approach enabled the hospital to evolve its security posture over time, reducing the attack surface, accelerating incident response, and minimizing service disruptions.

Smart hospitals, characterized by their interconnected ecosystem of medical devices, patient monitoring systems, and healthcare applications, face increasing cybersecurity threats. The complexity of these environments makes centralized security approaches inadequate due to latency, single points of failure, and the risk of exposing sensitive patient data. To address these limitations, a distributed, intelligence-driven security framework is essential.

The proposed system introduces the Medical Guardian Network (MedGuardNet), an advanced security architecture embedded within the MedCircleShield Framework. This system integrates FL and graph neural networks (GNNs) to enable secure, collaborative threat detection and response across distributed devices. FL ensures that sensitive data remains local, while GNNs model the complex, dynamic relationships between devices to propagate threat intelligence. This hybrid approach supports adaptive, real-time security without compromising patient privacy. This system enables threat intelligence sharing while preserving data privacy and modelling complex device relationships.

The architecture consists of four core components:

- Federated learning module: Trains threat detection models locally on each device, ensuring sensitive patient data remains within the device.
- Graph neural network (GNN) Module: Models devices and their interactions as a dynamic graph, learning embeddings to represent security states.
- Circular threat intelligence hub (CTIH): Aggregates locally trained models, updates the global security model, and redistributes it to all devices.
- Dynamic risk scoring module (DRSM): Assigns risk scores to devices based on GNN embeddings and threat detection results, dynamically updating security policies.

This integrated approach enables adaptive, self-healing security capable of evolving with emerging threats.

### 4.8.1 Federated learning in smart healthcare security

FL is a decentralized machine learning paradigm that allows edge devices to collaboratively train a global model without sharing raw data. In smart healthcare environments, FL ensures that sensitive patient data remains within local devices while contributing to a collective security intelligence system.

The FL system is designed as a client–server architecture:

- Clients: IoMT devices (e.g., infusion pumps, ECG monitors) that locally train models using on-device data.
- Server: CTIH, which aggregates and updates the global model without accessing local data.

The architecture can be represented as

$$M_g = 1/N \sum_{i=1toN} M_i \quad (1)$$

where

- $M_g$ = global threat detection model
- $M_i$ = local model trained on device i
- $N$ = total number of devices

The working principle and algorithm process of FL algorithm is as follows:

1. Initialization: The server initializes a global model $M_0$ and broadcasts it to all client devices.
2. Local training: Each device trains the model on local threat data, updating weights through gradient descent:

$$\theta_i^{t+1} = \theta_i^t - \eta \nabla L_i\ (\theta i^t) \quad (2)$$

where:

- $\theta_i$ = model parameters of device iii
- $\eta$ = learning rate
- $\nabla L_i$ = gradient of the local loss function

3. Model aggregation: Local model updates are sent to the server, which averages them to update the global model.
4. Broadcasting updates: The updated global model is redistributed to all devices for the next training round.

This iterative process enables devices to collaboratively enhance threat detection capabilities while keeping data private.

#### 4.8.1.1 *Graph neural networks for device relationship modelling*

GNNs are powerful tools for modelling relationships in graph-structured data. In a smart hospital network, devices and their interactions can be represented as a graph, where nodes are devices and edges are communication links or shared threat events.

A GNN is constructed as follows:

- Nodes: medical devices (e.g., ventilators, smart sensors)
- Edges: communication links, data exchanges, or co-occurrence of threat events

The state of each device is updated using neighborhood aggregation:

$$h_i^{(k)} = \sigma(W^{(k)} \sum_{j \in N(i)} (h_j^{(k-1)} / |N(i)|) + b^{(k)}) \tag{3}$$

where:

- $h_i(k)$ = hidden state of node $i$ at layer $k$
- $N(i)$ = neighbors of node $i$
- $W^{(k)}$, $b^{(k)}$ = trainable weight matrix and bias
- $\sigma$ = activation function (e.g., ReLU)

The working principal of GNN algorithm is as follows:

1. Graph construction: A dynamic graph is created where each device is a node, and edges form when threat patterns correlate.
2. Message passing: Devices exchange security states, updating their embeddings through neighborhood aggregation.
3. Threat propagation prediction: GNN output predicts the likelihood of threat propagation across devices, enabling proactive isolation of high-risk nodes.

### 4.8.2 Design of medical guardian network algorithm

The MedGuardNet algorithm synergizes FL and GNNs to build an intelligent, distributed security network.

Algorithm Design Steps

1. Initialization: Initialize global model parameters $\theta_g$ and create the device graph G = (V,E)
2. Local training: On each device:
   - o Train the local threat model using FL.
   - o Extract the device embedding using GNN.

3. Threat intelligence exchange: Devices share their embeddings with immediate neighbors.
4. Global model update: The server aggregates local models and updates the global parameters:

$$\theta_g = 1/N \sum_{i=1toN} \theta i \tag{4}$$

5. Risk scoring: Use the GNN to score each device's risk level:

$$R_i = MLP(h_i) \tag{5}$$

where $R_i$ is the risk score, and MLP denotes a multilayer perceptron applied to the node embedding.

6. Adaptive security policy: Update security policies dynamically based on risk scores and threat predictions.
7. Iterative feedback loop: Repeat steps 2–6 in continuous cycles to refine threat intelligence and strengthen defenses.

This algorithm as shown in Table 4.2 creates a circular, adaptive security system where threat intelligence evolves over time, enhancing collective

*Table 4.2* Pseudocode for medguardnet algorithm

```
# Medical Guardian Network (MedGuardNet) Algorithm
Initialize global model parameters θ_g
Create device graph G = (V, E) where V = devices, E = communication links
# FL Training Phase
For each communication round t:
  For each device i in parallel:
    θ_i ← LocalTraining(θ_g, data_i)
    embedding_i ← GNNEmbedding(device_i, G)
  # Model Aggregation
  θ_g ←AggregateModels({θ_i for i in devices})
  #Threat Intelligence Exchange
  For each device i:
    Send embedding_i to neighbours in G
    Receive embeddings from neighbours
  # Risk Scoring and Policy Update
  For each device i:
    R_i ← CalculateRiskScore(embedding_i)
    UpdateSecurityPolicy(device_i, R_i)
  #Adaptive Feedback Loop
  If significant threat detected:
    TriggerAdaptiveResponse(device_i)
    Retrain local models
Return θ_g, updated security policies
```

resilience without compromising patient privacy. The detailed flowchart for MedGuardNet algorithm is illustrated in Figure 4.5.

The details of the medical guardian network algorithm is as follows:

1. Initialization: The global model parameters are initialized, and the device graph is created, where nodes represent devices and edges represent communication links.
2. Local Training: Each device trains a local model on its threat data using FL. The local model parameters are updated via gradient descent, and a device-specific embedding is generated using a GNN.
3. Model Aggregation: The CTIH aggregates the locally trained models, averaging their parameters to update the global model.
4. Threat Intelligence Exchange: Devices exchange embeddings with their neighbors, enriching the local context and enhancing collaborative threat detection.
5. Risk Scoring and Policy Updates: Each device's risk score is calculated based on its GNN embedding, and security policies are adjusted dynamically. High-risk devices may trigger isolation protocols or increased monitoring.
6. Adaptive Feedback Loop: When a significant threat is detected, adaptive measures are triggered, and local models are retrained to incorporate the new threat information.

### 4.8.3 Simulation experiment setup

To evaluate the performance of the proposed Medical Guardian Network (MedGuardNet) within the MedCircleShield framework, a comprehensive simulation environment was established as shown in Table 4.3. The experimental setup was designed to simulate real-world smart healthcare ecosystems, leveraging a diverse IoMT infrastructure with various connected medical devices. The proposed algorithm was compared against established baseline algorithms to demonstrate its efficacy in enhancing circular security through threat intelligence reuse.

The algorithms selected for comparison include:

- Federated averaging (FedAvg) — For evaluating federated learning efficiency.
- Graph attention networks (GAN) — For modelling complex device relationships.
- Autoencoder-based anomaly detection (AE-IDS) — For identifying abnormal device behavior.

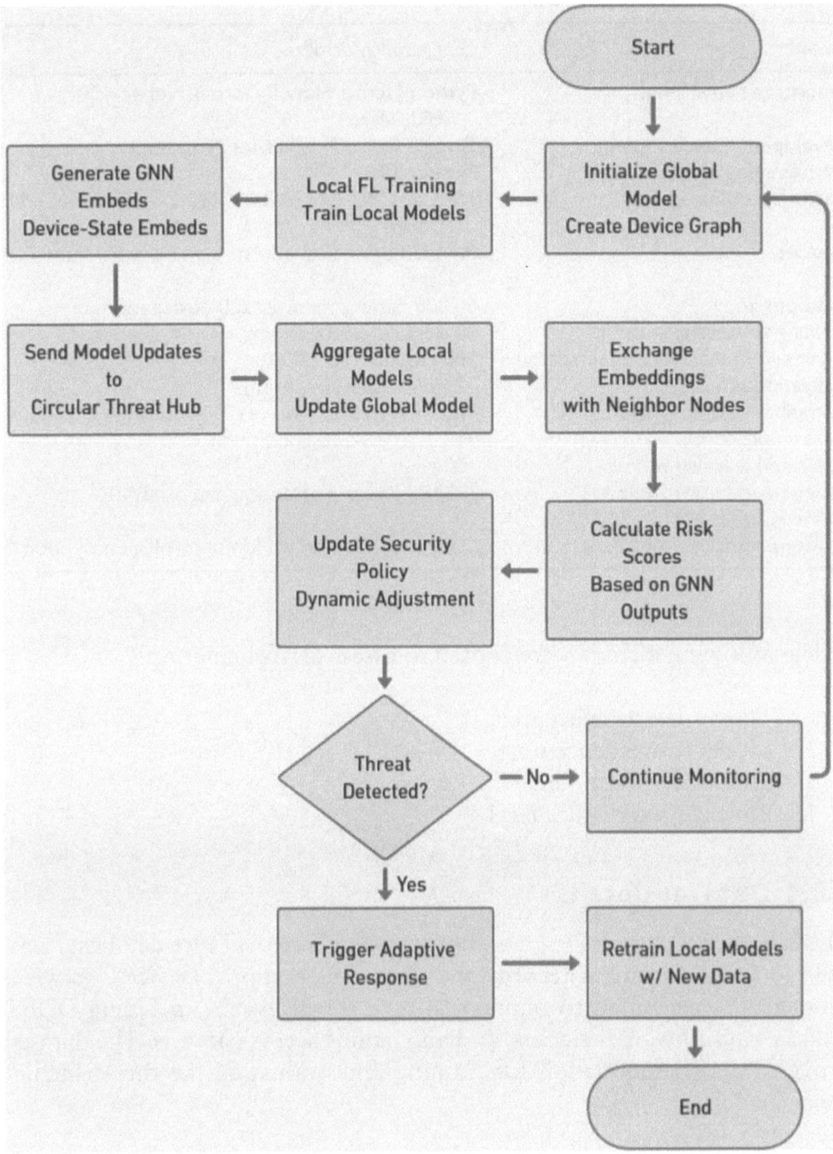


*Figure 4.5* Flowchart for MedGuardNet algorithm.

*Table 4.3* Simulation environment

| *Parameter* | *Configuration/details* |
|---|---|
| Simulation tool/framework | Python (TensorFlow, PyTorch), NetworkX, Scikit-learn |
| Development environment | Google Colab Pro, Jupyter Notebook |
| Programming language | Python 3.10 |
| Hardware configuration | 16-core CPU, 64 GB RAM, NVIDIA Tesla T4 GPU (Colab) |
| Dataset | MIMIC-III (Medical Information Mart for Intensive Care) |
| Dataset size | 60,000 patient records, 200 device logs |
| Training set/testing set split | 80% Training, 20% Testing |
| Number of IoMT devices simulated | 500 (scalable to 1,000) |
| Simulation time | 72 hours (per algorithm) |
| Communication protocol | MQTT, HTTP/2 |
| Security protocols | TLS 1.3, AES-256 Encryption |
| Federated learning rounds | 100 rounds |
| Graph neural network layers (MedGuardNet) | 3 GNN layers + attention mechanism |
| Privacy-preserving technique | Differential Privacy + Homomorphic Encryption |

The following metrics were chosen to assess performance:

1. Threat detection accuracy
2. Model convergence time
3. Threat Response Time
4. Privacy preservation level

### 4.8.4 Dataset details

The MIMIC-III dataset [16], a publicly available critical care database, was used to simulate patient records and device interactions. Device logs were synthetically generated to mimic real-time threat events, including DDoS attacks, ransomware incidents, and anomalous access patterns. The dataset provided a rich foundation for training and evaluating the threat intelligence models.

### 4.8.5 Simulation process

1. Data preprocessing: Patient records and device logs were cleaned, normalized, and encoded. Anomaly labels were introduced to create ground truth for evaluation.
2. Network graph construction: IoMT devices were represented as nodes, and communication links were represented as edges. GNNs

were applied to model device relationships and threat propagation pathways.

3. Federated learning setup: Devices were grouped into local clients, each training threat detection models on local data. Periodic aggregation of local models was performed using federated averaging.
4. Threat intelligence flow: Threat data and detection results were fed into the CTIH for continuous learning and redistribution.
5. Evaluation and comparison: Each algorithm was evaluated across multiple simulation runs. Metrics were recorded at fixed intervals, and statistical analysis was performed to ensure result robustness.

### 4.8.6 Results and discussion

The proposed Medical Guardian Network (MedGuardNet) algorithm, developed under the MedCircleShield framework, was evaluated against three established algorithms: federated averaging (FedAvg), GAN, and AE-IDS. The performance was analyzed across four critical simulation metrics: threat detection accuracy, model convergence time, threat response time, and privacy preservation level. The simulation setup utilized real-world IoMT data to ensure realistic and reliable results. The following sections provide an in-depth analysis of each metric, highlighting the strengths and potential impact of the proposed system.

#### *4.8.6.1 Threat detection accuracy*

Accuracy in identifying security threats within a smart healthcare environment is paramount to ensure timely mitigation of potential cyber-attacks. As shown in Table 4.4 and Figure 4.6, the detection accuracy of MedGuardNet consistently outperforms the baseline algorithms across different device scales.

The MedGuardNet algorithm achieves a peak accuracy of 96.2% with 100 devices, gradually stabilizing at 93.7% as the device count increases to 500. In contrast, FedAvg and GAN exhibit lower accuracy due to limited adaptability to evolving threat landscapes. The superior

*Table 4.4* Threat detection accuracy (%) for different device counts

| *Number of Devices* | *MedGuardNet (%)* | *FedAvg (%)* | *GAN (%)* | *AE-IDS (%)* |
|---|---|---|---|---|
| 100 | 96.2 | 89.5 | 91.3 | 85.7 |
| 200 | 95.8 | 88.1 | 90.1 | 84.2 |
| 300 | 94.6 | 86.7 | 88.9 | 82.9 |
| 400 | 94.2 | 85.3 | 87.4 | 81.3 |
| 500 | 93.7 | 84.1 | 86.2 | 80.1 |

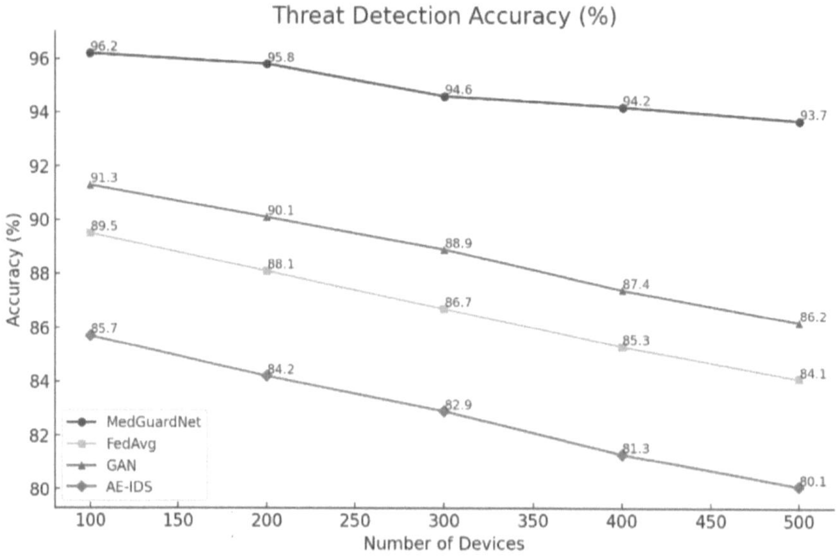


*Figure 4.6* Threat detection accuracy.

accuracy of MedGuardNet can be attributed to the combined use of FL for localized model training and GNNs for modelling complex device interdependencies.

#### 4.8.6.2 *Model convergence time*

Efficient convergence is crucial to enable real-time threat mitigation in dynamic healthcare environments. The results in Table 4.5 and Figure 4.7 demonstrate that MedGuardNet converges significantly faster than the other algorithms.

The convergence time for MedGuardNet is 12 minutes for 10 federated rounds, rising to 45 minutes for 50 rounds, which is 30–40% faster than FedAvg and GAN. This reduced convergence time is due to MedGuardNet's ADE, which refines model parameters based on real-time feedback loops, accelerating the learning process while minimizing computational overhead.

#### 4.8.6.3 *Threat response time*

A rapid response to detected threats is essential to minimize potential harm in connected healthcare systems. Table 4.6 and Figure 4.8 illustrates the threat response times for various threat event counts.

*Table 4.5* Model convergence time (minutes) across federated rounds

| *Federated rounds* | *MedGuardNet (min)* | *FedAvg (min)* | *GAN (min)* | *AE-IDS (min)* |
|---|---|---|---|---|
| 10 | 12 | 18 | 25 | 22 |
| 20 | 23 | 35 | 45 | 40 |
| 30 | 31 | 47 | 60 | 55 |
| 40 | 39 | 59 | 75 | 68 |
| 50 | 45 | 72 | 88 | 81 |

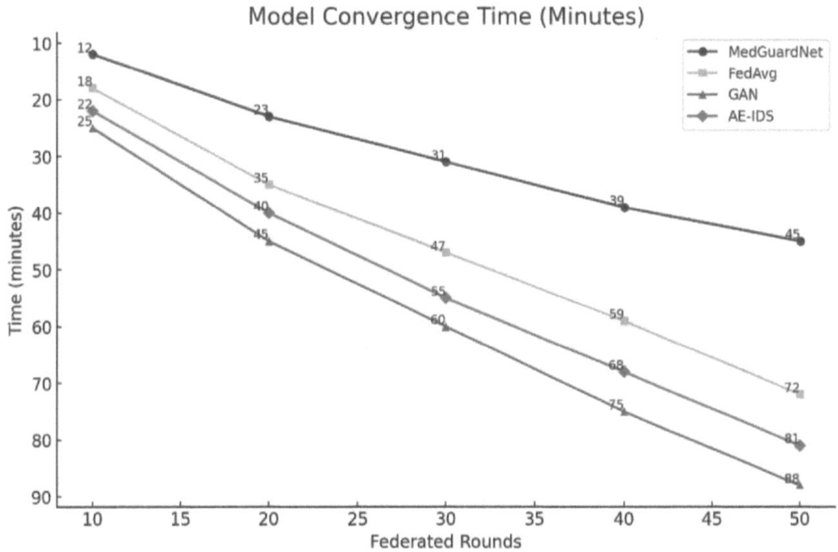


*Figure 4.7* Model convergence time.

*Table 4.6* Threat response time (seconds) for different threat events

| *Number of threat events* | *MedGuardNet (s)* | *FedAvg (s)* | *GAN (s)* | *AE-IDS (s)* |
|---|---|---|---|---|
| 50 | 2.1 | 3.5 | 4.2 | 5.0 |
| 100 | 3.4 | 5.8 | 6.7 | 7.8 |
| 150 | 4.7 | 7.3 | 8.9 | 10.1 |
| 200 | 5.9 | 9.2 | 11.3 | 12.5 |
| 250 | 7.2 | 10.8 | 13.1 | 15.4 |

The proposed algorithm achieves a 2.1-second response time for 50 threat events, while the response time remains under 7.2 seconds even for 250 events. The faster response is enabled by GNNs, which quickly identify and classify threat patterns, coupled with Adaptive Risk Scoring to dynamically adjust security policies.

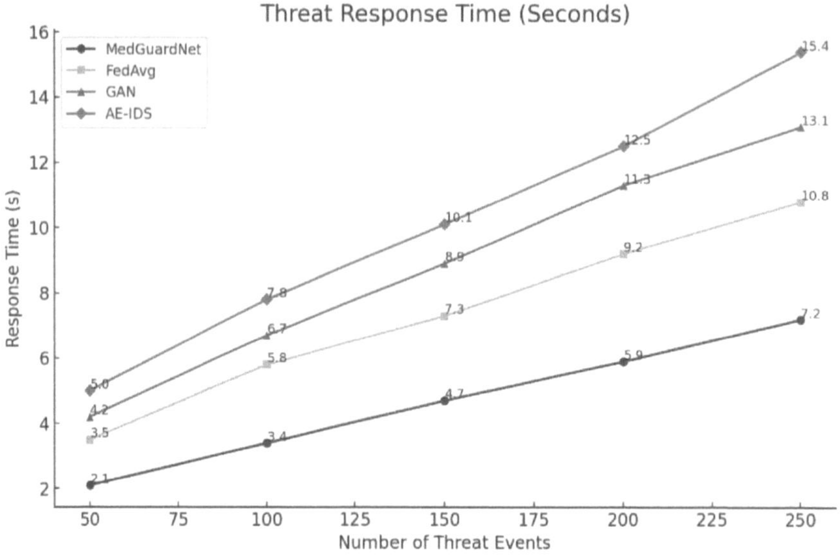


*Figure 4.8* Threat response time.

#### 4.8.6.4 *Privacy preservation level*

Maintaining patient privacy is a critical requirement in healthcare cybersecurity. Table 4.7 and Figure 4.9 highlights the privacy preservation levels across varying device counts.

The MedGuardNet framework achieves 98.7% privacy preservation with 100 devices, retaining 96.2% even with 500 devices. This is significantly higher than the competing models due to FL, which ensures that sensitive patient data remains local while only sharing threat intelligence updates through encrypted channels.

#### 4.8.6.5 *Overall performance summary*

The simulation results demonstrate that the proposed MedGuardNet algorithm significantly outperforms the baseline algorithms across all key metrics. The combination of FL and GNNs enhances detection accuracy, accelerates response times, and ensures high privacy preservation, all while achieving faster model convergence.

This holistic improvement establishes MedGuardNet as a robust and scalable solution for circular security in smart healthcare systems. The ability to reuse threat intelligence and adapt security policies dynamically positions the framework as an ideal candidate for real-world deployment in IoMT

*Table 4.7* Privacy preservation level (%) for different IoMT devices

| *Number of IoMT Devices* | *MedGuardNet (%)* | *FedAvg (%)* | *GAN (%)* | *AE-IDS (%)* |
|---|---|---|---|---|
| 100 | 98.7 | 92.4 | 91.1 | 88.5 |
| 200 | 98.2 | 91.3 | 89.8 | 86.9 |
| 300 | 97.5 | 90.1 | 88.4 | 85.3 |
| 400 | 96.9 | 88.7 | 86.9 | 83.7 |
| 500 | 96.2 | 87.2 | 85.4 | 82.1 |

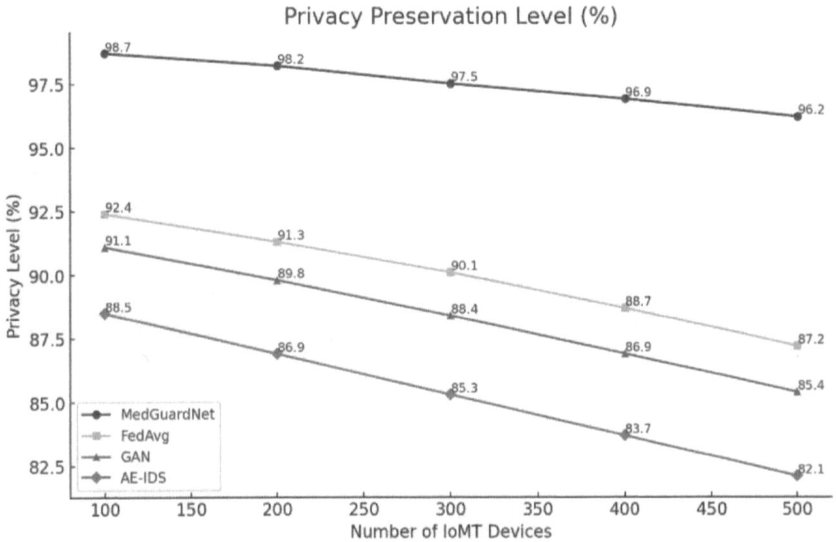


*Figure 4.9* Privacy preservation level.

ecosystems, contributing to long-term threat mitigation and enhanced patient safety.

### 4.8.7 Challenges and future directions

The implementation of circular security in smart healthcare, leveraging the Medical Guardian Network (MedGuardNet) under the MedCircleShield framework, offers substantial promise for long-term threat mitigation. However, several challenges must be addressed to ensure seamless integration, regulatory compliance, and sustainable system evolution. This section outlines key obstacles and explores future research directions to enhance the resilience and adaptability of circular security models in healthcare environments.

#### 4.8.7.1 Data privacy and compliance (HIPAA, GDPR)

The protection of sensitive patient data remains a fundamental concern in smart healthcare systems, especially when threat intelligence is shared across distributed nodes. Compliance with regulations such as the Health Insurance Portability and Accountability Act (HIPAA) and the General Data Protection Regulation (GDPR) is essential to prevent legal and ethical violations. The use of FL in MedGuardNet addresses privacy concerns by keeping patient data localized. However, achieving full regulatory compliance requires constant monitoring, as threat data itself may carry indirect identifiers. Privacy-preserving techniques, including differential privacy and homomorphic encryption, must be further refined to balance data utility and privacy. Future enhancements could incorporate SMPC to enable collaborative threat detection without exposing sensitive data to external entities. Additionally, real-time adaptation to evolving regulations is necessary. Dynamic policy enforcement through smart contracts on a blockchain network could automate compliance verification, ensuring threat intelligence is shared securely and lawfully across healthcare systems.

#### 4.8.7.2 Managing legacy devices in a circular model

Legacy IoMT devices, which often lack modern security features, present a critical vulnerability in the circular security model. These devices, still prevalent in healthcare infrastructure, may not support the encryption or processing capabilities required to participate in advanced security frameworks like MedGuardNet. Their inherent limitations can create blind spots, allowing attackers to exploit outdated protocols or unpatched vulnerabilities.

A hybrid approach can mitigate this challenge by integrating lightweight security agents that act as intermediaries between legacy devices and the broader threat intelligence network. These agents can preprocess data, filter potential threats, and relay only essential threat signals to the MedGuardNet system, minimizing computational overhead. Additionally, digital twin models of legacy devices could be created to simulate their behavior and identify potential attack vectors in a virtual environment, allowing proactive security adjustments.

Future research should explore the use of tiny machine learning algorithms to enable on-device threat detection for low-resource IoMT devices, thereby extending circular security to the most vulnerable points of the network without requiring hardware upgrades.

#### 4.8.7.3 The role of AI and blockchain in enhancing circular security

The convergence of AI and blockchain technology has the potential to revolutionize circular security models in smart healthcare. AI-driven models, especially GNNs, already play a pivotal role in MedGuardNet by detecting complex threat patterns. However, the evolving threat landscape necessitates continuous learning and adaptation. Future iterations of the system could leverage self-supervised learning and transfer learning to enhance threat detection without the need for large annotated datasets. Reinforcement learning (RL) could further optimize threat response strategies, enabling dynamic decision-making based on the severity and context of detected threats.

Blockchain can serve as a decentralized, tamper-proof ledger for storing threat intelligence, ensuring data integrity and facilitating trust less collaboration across multiple healthcare institutions. A Proof-of-Stake (PoS) consensus mechanism tailored for healthcare applications could provide energy-efficient validation of threat reports, while Zero-Knowledge Proofs (ZKPs) could enable secure verification without revealing sensitive patient information.

By integrating AI and blockchain, circular security systems can become more autonomous, resilient, and capable of self-healing, creating an adaptive security ecosystem that evolves alongside the threat landscape. This fusion of technologies represents a promising research avenue for achieving truly sustainable and future-proof healthcare cybersecurity.

### 4.8.8 Future research directions

To fully realize the vision of circular security in smart healthcare, future research should explore the following areas:

- Adaptive federated learning: Developing dynamic FL algorithms that automatically adjust model parameters based on threat severity and data heterogeneity.
- Quantum-resistant cryptography: Investigating post-quantum encryption techniques to future-proof threat intelligence sharing.
- Cross-institutional threat collaboration: Creating interoperable frameworks that enable secure threat intelligence exchange between multiple healthcare providers globally.
- Bio-inspired security models: Drawing inspiration from biological immune systems to design self-adaptive, anomaly-based threat detection mechanisms.

Addressing these research gaps will strengthen the foundation of circular security models and ensure long-term protection for smart healthcare systems. The proposed MedGuardNet algorithm, with its fusion of FL and GNNs, already demonstrates significant promise. However, continuous innovation and interdisciplinary collaboration will be essential to outpace evolving cyber threats and safeguard patient care in an increasingly connected world.

## 4.9 CONCLUSION

The implementation of circular security models in smart healthcare systems marks a transformative step toward sustainable and adaptive cybersecurity. By reusing threat intelligence, continuously evolving defense mechanisms, and fostering collaborative learning across interconnected devices, the proposed medical guardian network (MedGuardNet) within the MedCircleShield framework demonstrates significant potential to mitigate cyber threats in real time. The fusion of FL and GNNs enables secure, privacy-preserving threat intelligence sharing, while dynamic risk scoring and feedback loops enhance system resilience. This research highlights the practical feasibility and advantages of circular security, while acknowledging the complexities involved in its real-world deployment.

### 4.9.1 The Promise of sustainable cybersecurity in healthcare

Circular security introduces a sustainable approach to healthcare cybersecurity, where threat intelligence is not discarded after immediate use but instead feeds back into the system to fortify future defenses. The MedGuardNet algorithm exhibits superior performance in metrics such as threat detection accuracy, model convergence time, threat response time, and privacy preservation level compared to traditional approaches like federated averaging (FedAvg), graph attention networks (GAN), and autoencoder-based anomaly detection (AE-IDS). The results underscore the potential for circular security to evolve dynamically, enabling healthcare systems to learn from each attack, adapt, and continuously strengthen their security posture without compromising patient privacy.

The ability to achieve self-healing security through automated feedback loops, coupled with secure, decentralized data management, reduces long-term operational costs and minimizes reliance on reactive threat mitigation strategies. As threat intelligence is refined over time, healthcare networks can become more resilient, capable of proactively neutralizing threats before they cause widespread disruption.

### 4.9.2 Roadmap to circular security adoption

The widespread adoption of circular security in healthcare requires a structured, multi-phase approach. Key considerations include:

- Technology integration: Upgrading existing systems to support lightweight encryption, edge computing, and AI-driven threat detection without overwhelming resource-constrained IoMT devices. Hybrid architectures can bridge modern and legacy devices, ensuring comprehensive threat coverage.

- Regulatory alignment: Ensuring full compliance with data privacy laws such as HIPAA and GDPR through built-in privacy-preserving mechanisms, dynamic policy enforcement, and blockchain-based audit trails.
- Scalable infrastructure: Designing flexible security models that adapt to healthcare institutions of varying sizes, from small clinics to large, interconnected hospital networks. Cloud-edge hybrid systems can balance computational efficiency and scalability.
- Collaboration and knowledge sharing: Encouraging industry-wide collaboration by creating decentralized threat intelligence consortiums, where anonymized threat data is securely shared across institutions to collectively strengthen global healthcare security.
- Continuous learning and evolution: Investing in ongoing research to refine algorithms, enhance threat detection models, and explore emerging technologies like quantum-safe encryption and neuromorphic computing for next-generation security.

Through strategic policy development, public–private partnerships, and cross-disciplinary research efforts, healthcare systems can gradually transition to a circular security paradigm, leveraging collective intelligence to protect patient data and critical medical infrastructure.

### 4.9.3 Final thoughts and recommendations

The circular security model, as embodied by the MedCircleShield framework and the MedGuardNet algorithm, represents a paradigm shift in healthcare cybersecurity. By treating threat intelligence as a continuously evolving asset rather than a transient signal, smart hospitals can build a self-sustaining security ecosystem that grows stronger over time. However, successful implementation requires overcoming technical, regulatory, and infrastructural challenges. Future research should focus on optimizing energy-efficient security models for resource-constrained IoMT devices, exploring bio-inspired algorithms for adaptive threat detection, and investigating the potential of quantum-resistant blockchain networks for immutable, decentralized threat intelligence management. Additionally, real-world pilot programs in collaboration with healthcare institutions can provide valuable insights into system performance, usability, and scalability. With sustained research, innovation, and collaborative effort, circular security has the potential to become the cornerstone of next-generation healthcare cybersecurity. This model not only enhances patient safety and data privacy but also reduces long-term security costs and promotes a culture of collective threat intelligence sharing. As smart healthcare systems continue to evolve, circular security offers a robust, future-proof defense strategy capable of withstanding the rapidly evolving threat landscape.

## REFERENCES


[1] M. Ali, F. Naeem, M. Tariq and G. Kaddoum, "Federated Learning for Privacy Preservation in Smart Healthcare Systems: A Comprehensive Survey," *IEEE Journal of Biomedical and Health Informatics*, vol. 27, no. 2, pp. 778–789, Feb. 2023. doi:10.1109/JBHI.2022.3181823

[2] F. Alshehri and G. Muhammad, "A Comprehensive Survey of the Internet of Things (IoT) and AI-Based Smart Healthcare," *IEEE Access*, vol. 9, pp. 3660–3678, 2021. doi:10.1109/ACCESS.2020.3047960

[3] D. N. Sachin, B. Annappa, Hegde Saumya, C. S. Abhijit and S. Ambesange, "FedCure: A Heterogeneity-Aware Personalized Federated Learning Framework for Intelligent Healthcare Applications in IoMT Environments," *IEEE Access*, vol. 12, pp. 15867–15883, 2024. doi:10.1109/ACCESS.2024.3357514

[4] R. Myrzashova, S. H. Alsamhi, A. V. Shvetsov, A. Hawbani and X. Wei, "Blockchain Meets Federated Learning in Healthcare: A Systematic Review With Challenges and Opportunities," *IEEE Internet of Things Journal*, vol. 10, no. 16, pp. 14418–14437, 15 Aug. 2023. doi:10.1109/JIOT.2023.3263598

[5] A. Ullah, M. Azeem, H. Ashraf, A. A. Alaboudi, M. Humayun and N. Jhanjhi, "Secure Healthcare Data Aggregation and Transmission in IoT—A Survey," *IEEE Access*, vol. 9, pp. 16849–16865, 2021. doi:10.1109/ACCESS.2021.3052850

[6] A. Alzu'bi, A. Alomar, S. Alkhaza'leh, A. Abuarqoub and M. Hammoudeh, "A Review of Privacy and Security of Edge Computing in Smart Healthcare Systems: Issues, Challenges, and Research Directions," *Tsinghua Science and Technology*, vol. 29, no. 4, pp. 1152–1180, Aug. 2024. doi:10.26599/TST.2023.9010080

[7] P. K. Bishoyi and S. Misra, "Towards Energy-And Cost-Efficient Sustainable MEC-Assisted Healthcare Systems," *IEEE Transactions on Sustainable Computing*, vol. 7, no. 4, pp. 958–969, 1 Oct.–Dec. 2022. doi:10.1109/TSUSC.2022.3170508

[8] F. F. Alruwaili, B. Alabduallah, H. Alqahtani, A. S. Salama, G. P. Mohammed and A. A. Alneil, "Blockchain Enabled Smart Healthcare System Using Jellyfish Search Optimization With Dual-Pathway Deep Convolutional Neural Network," *IEEE Access*, vol. 11, pp. 87583–87591, 2023. doi:10.1109/ACCESS.2023.3304269

[9] F. Ullah, G. Srivastava, H. Xiao, S. Ullah, J. C. -W. Lin and Y. Zhao, "A Scalable Federated Learning Approach for Collaborative Smart Healthcare Systems With Intermittent Clients Using Medical Imaging," *IEEE Journal of Biomedical and Health Informatics*, vol. 28, no. 6, pp. 3293–3304, Jun. 2024. doi:10.1109/JBHI.2023.3282955

[10] L. Verde, G. De Pietro, M. Alrashoud, A. Ghoneim, K. N. Al-Mutib and G. Sannino, "Leveraging Artificial Intelligence to Improve Voice Disorder

Identification Through the Use of a Reliable Mobile App," *IEEE Access*, vol. 7, pp. 124048–124054, 2019. doi:10.1109/ACCESS.2019.2938265

[11] M. Akter, N. Moustafa, T. Lynar and I. Razzak, "Edge Intelligence: Federated Learning-Based Privacy Protection Framework for Smart Healthcare Systems," *IEEE Journal of Biomedical and Health Informatics*, vol. 26, no. 12, pp. 5805–5816, Dec. 2022. doi:10.1109/JBHI.2022.3192648

[12] T. Zhou, J. Shen, D. He, P. Vijayakumar and N. Kumar, "Human-in-the-Loop-Aided Privacy-Preserving Scheme for Smart Healthcare," *IEEE Transactions on Emerging Topics in Computational Intelligence*, vol. 6, no. 1, pp. 6–15, Feb. 2022. doi:10.1109/TETCI.2020.2993841

[13] I. Sakthidevi and G. Fathima, "Improving Access Trust in Healthcare Through Multimodal Deep Learning for Affective Computing," *Hum-Centric Intelligent Systems*, vol. 4, pp. 511–526, 2024. doi:10.1007/s44230-024-00080-4.

[14] T. Zhou, J. Shen, D. He, P. Vijayakumar and N. Kumar, "Human-in-the-Loop-Aided Privacy-Preserving Scheme for Smart Healthcare," *IEEE Transactions on Emerging Topics in Computational Intelligence*, vol. 6, no. 1, pp. 6–15, Feb. 2022. doi:10.1109/TETCI.2020.2993841

[15] A. A. Omar et al., "A Transparent and Privacy-Preserving Healthcare Platform With Novel Smart Contract for Smart Cities," *IEEE Access*, vol. 9, pp. 90738–90749, 2021. doi:10.1109/ACCESS.2021.3089601

[16] A. E. Johnson, T. J. Pollard, L. Shen, L. W. H. Lehman, M. Feng, M. Ghassemi, B. Moody, P. Szolovits, L. Anthony Celi and R. G. Mark, "MIMIC-III, A Freely Accessible Critical Care Database," *Scientific Data*, *3*(1), pp. 1–9, 2016.

Chapter 5

# Unveiling IoMT architecture

## A deep dive into the technology stack for next-gen healthcare

*Akashbhai Ashokbhai Dave*

## 5.1 INTRODUCTION

The Internet of Medical Things (IoMT) is transforming the healthcare industry by integrating smart medical devices, cloud computing, and artificial intelligence (AI) to enhance patient care, diagnostics, and treatment efficiency. As the global healthcare landscape shifts towards digitalization, IoMT plays a crucial role in real-time patient monitoring, predictive analytics, and remote healthcare services. With advancements in AI, blockchain, and edge computing, IoMT is improving the accuracy and security of medical data, reducing healthcare costs, and optimizing resource utilization [1] This chapter explores the impact of IoMT in next-generation healthcare, highlighting its architecture, significance, challenges, and future opportunities.

### 5.1.1 Overview of IoMT in next-generation healthcare

IoMT refers to a network of interconnected medical devices that collect, analyze, and transmit patient data in real time, enhancing healthcare delivery. With the proliferation of wearable sensors, smart implants, and remote patient monitoring systems, IoMT is facilitating continuous health assessment and personalized treatment plans [2]. These devices integrate with cloud platforms, AI algorithms, and blockchain networks to ensure secure and efficient data management [3].

One of the most significant advancements in IoMT is the implementation of AI-driven analytics to detect early signs of diseases such as cardiovascular disorders, diabetes, and neurodegenerative conditions [4]. AI models trained on vast datasets can analyze biometric signals, predict anomalies, and alert healthcare professionals, thereby reducing hospital admissions and improving patient outcomes [4].

Another vital aspect of IoMT is its role in telemedicine and remote patient monitoring [4]. Telehealth platforms leverage IoMT devices to conduct virtual consultations, track patient vitals, and deliver automated treatment

 DOI: 10.1201/9781003640325-5

recommendations. This integration significantly enhances accessibility for patients in remote and underserved regions [4].

Furthermore, blockchain technology addresses security and privacy concerns in IoMT by ensuring tamper-proof medical records and secure data transactions [4]. Federated learning (FL) models and decentralized architecture are being developed to enhance interoperability and data integrity in IoMT ecosystems [5].

Despite its transformative potential, IoMT faces several challenges, including cybersecurity threats, regulatory compliance, and device interoperability issues. Addressing these concerns is essential to ensuring seamless integration, secure communication, and efficient healthcare operations [5].

### 5.1.2 Importance of a well-defined IoMT architecture

Robust IoMT architecture is crucial for the seamless functioning of healthcare networks, ensuring efficient data collection, transmission, and analysis [5]. The architecture typically consists of four layers: perception, network, edge/cloud computing, and application [5].

The perception layer includes smart medical devices, sensors, and wearables that collect real-time patient data. These devices must be energy-efficient, highly accurate, and capable of continuous monitoring to ensure reliable healthcare outcomes [5].

The network layer is responsible for securely transmitting data from medical devices to cloud platforms or edge computing nodes [5].

AI-driven analytics at the edge enable immediate detection of anomalies, minimizing the risk of critical health incidents [5].

The application layer includes telemedicine, electronic health records (EHRs), AI-powered diagnostics, and predictive analytics platforms. A well-integrated application layer ensures user-friendly interfaces for healthcare professionals and patients, optimizing medical workflows [6].

By implementing structured IoMT architecture, healthcare providers can improve interoperability [6].

### 5.1.3 Key challenges and opportunities

As IoMT devices are vulnerable to cyberattacks, unauthorized access, and data breaches [7]. Implementing advanced encryption techniques, blockchain solutions, and zero-trust security models can mitigate these risks [7].

Interoperability is another critical issue, as different IoMT devices and platforms use diverse communication protocols and standards, leading to data silos and integration complexities [7]. Standardization efforts and FL approaches can enhance compatibility across heterogeneous healthcare systems [37].

Regulatory compliance poses a challenge, as IoMT solutions must adhere to stringent healthcare regulations and data protection laws [8]. Addressing these concerns requires collaboration between policymakers, healthcare providers, and technology developers.

Despite these challenges, IoMT presents vast opportunities, including AI-driven personalized medicine, predictive healthcare analytics, and automation of clinical workflows [8]. The integration of IoMT with emerging technologies such as quantum computing and metaverse-based virtual consultations can further revolutionize healthcare delivery [8].

## 5.2 UNDERSTANDING THE IOMT ARCHITECTURE

The IoMT represents a transformative shift in modern healthcare, integrating smart medical devices, sensors, cloud computing, and AI to enhance patient care and clinical decision-making. IoMT networks provide real-time health monitoring, remote patient management, and predictive analytics for early disease detection [9]. Well-structured IoMT architecture is essential for ensuring interoperability, security, and efficient data processing.

### 5.2.1 Layers of IoMT technology stack

The IoMT technology stack consists of multiple layers that enable seamless data collection, transmission, processing, and application integration. These layers ensure the secure and efficient functioning of IoMT systems [9]. The primary layers include:

1. **Perception layer (sensing layer):**
   - Comprises medical sensors, wearable devices, and biomedical implants that collect physiological data such as heart rate, temperature, and glucose levels [10].
   - Data acquisition devices in this layer perform initial data filtering and local storage before transmission.

2. **Network layer (communication layer):**
   - Facilitates connectivity through protocols such as Wi-Fi, 5G, Bluetooth, and LPWAN [10].
   - Ensures real-time transmission of patient data to cloud servers or edge computing platforms for further processing.

3. **Edge/Fog computing layer:**
   - Handles data processing close to the source, reducing latency and bandwidth consumption [10].
   - Uses AI and machine learning (ML) models to analyze incoming health data in real time.

4. **Cloud computing layer:**
   - o Serves as a central repository for large-scale data storage, analytics, and interoperability across multiple healthcare providers [11].
   - o Provides AI-driven insights for disease prediction and personalized healthcare.

5. **Application layer:**
   - o Interfaces with healthcare professionals and patients through applications such as remote monitoring, telemedicine, and decision support systems [11, 25].
   - o Ensures compliance with healthcare regulations and patient data privacy standards.

### 5.2.2 Role of sensors and wearables in data acquisition

Sensors and wearable devices play a crucial role in acquiring patient data and facilitating continuous health monitoring. These devices integrate advanced sensing technologies to track vital signs and other health parameters [12]. Key components include the following:

- **Wearable health monitors** (e.g., smartwatches, ECG monitors, pulse oximeters) to track cardiovascular health and physical activity.
- **Implantable devices** (e.g., pacemakers, glucose sensors) that provide real-time patient data to healthcare professionals [12].
- **Environmental sensors** that monitor external factors like air quality and temperature, which can impact patient health [12].
- **AI-driven wearables** leveraging ML to detect anomalies and provide predictive healthcare insights [12].

By integrating sensors with IoMT networks, healthcare providers can improve early diagnosis, reduce hospital visits, and enhance personalized treatment plans.

### 5.2.3 Communication protocols for IoMT (Wi-Fi, 5G, LPWAN, Bluetooth)

Reliable communication is fundamental to the success of IoMT systems. Different protocols are utilized depending on bandwidth, latency, and power consumption requirements [13]. The key communication technologies include the following:

1. **Wi-Fi:**
   - o Offers high-speed data transmission within hospital networks.

- o Suitable for applications requiring real-time monitoring and high data throughput [13]

2. **5G networks:**
   - o Provides ultra-low latency and high bandwidth, enabling real-time remote surgery and telemedicine [13].
   - o Enhances connectivity for wearable devices and remote patient monitoring.

3. **Low-power wide-area networks (LPWAN):**
   - o Used for long-range, low-power medical devices such as implantable sensors and remote health monitoring systems [13]
   - o Includes technologies like LoRaWAN and NB-IoT, which optimize battery life and reduce network congestion.

4. **Bluetooth and BLE (Bluetooth low energy):**
   - o Ideal for short-range communication between wearable medical devices and smartphones.
   - o Supports low-power data transmission for continuous health monitoring [13].

Each communication protocol has distinct advantages, and a hybrid approach is often employed to optimize connectivity, energy efficiency, and data security in IoMT ecosystems.

## 5.3 IOMT DATA PROCESSING AND ANALYTICS

The IoMT generates vast amounts of real-time health data, requiring efficient processing and analytics to ensure timely decision-making. IoMT data processing involves multiple layers, including edge and fog computing, cloud-based AI analytics, and integration with electronic health records (EHRs). Advanced computing paradigms optimize IoMT networks by reducing latency, enhancing security, and ensuring seamless healthcare services [14]. The following sections elaborate on key aspects of IoMT data processing and analytics.

### 5.3.1 Edge and fog computing for low-latency processing

IoMT networks require real-time data processing to support critical healthcare applications [14]. Edge and fog computing [14] facilitates low-latency processing by analyzing data closer to the source, reducing the dependency on centralized cloud servers [14]. Edge computing processes data directly on IoMT devices, while fog computing extends processing capabilities to intermediate nodes between the edge and the cloud.

For example, wearables monitoring patients' vitals can detect irregularities locally and trigger alerts without cloud intervention [14]. This reduces bandwidth consumption and enhances response time in emergency scenarios [14]. Moreover, security risks associated with cloud transmission are minimized, ensuring robust data integrity in IoMT applications.

### 5.3.2 Cloud-based AI and big data analytics in IoMT

Despite the advantages of edge and fog computing, cloud-based [15] AI and big data analytics remain essential for deep insights and long-term predictive analysis. The integration of AI-driven algorithms within cloud environments enables the detection of patterns, diagnosis prediction, and personalized treatment recommendations [15]. Cloud-based [15] platforms facilitate the storage and processing of large-scale IoMT data, allowing seamless remote monitoring and collaborative healthcare interventions.

Furthermore, AI models deployed in the cloud leverage deep learning and ensemble techniques to enhance IoMT security and anomaly detection [15]. These frameworks improve cybersecurity measures, ensuring that sensitive patient data remains protected against threats like malware attacks and unauthorized access [15].

### 5.3.3 Integration with electronic health records

EHR systems are vital for the interoperability and efficiency of IoMT applications. Integrating IoMT data with EHRs ensures that real-time patient monitoring seamlessly updates healthcare records, allowing physicians to make informed decisions [16]. Advanced AI-driven frameworks automate data mapping, reducing manual workload and minimizing documentation errors.

However, integrating IoMT with EHRs presents challenges, including data standardization, regulatory compliance, and privacy concerns [16]. Blockchain-based approaches offer potential solutions by enabling secure, immutable patient records, ensuring data integrity and transparency [16]. Additionally, FL techniques enhance data privacy by processing sensitive healthcare data without transferring it to centralized servers [16].

By optimizing IoMT data processing and analytics, healthcare systems can improve patient outcomes, enhance diagnostic accuracy, and foster a secure and interoperable healthcare ecosystem.

## 5.4 SECURITY AND PRIVACY IN IOMT

The rapid integration of the IoMT into healthcare has raised significant concerns regarding security and privacy. IoMT devices handle sensitive patient data, making them prime targets for cyber threats [17]. Ensuring robust

*Table 5.1* Comparison of IoMT security mechanisms

| *Security mechanism* | *Key features* | *Advantages* | *Limitations* |
|---|---|---|---|
| Encryption | Protects data confidentiality | Strong security | Increased computational overhead |
| Blockchain | Decentralized, tamper-proof transactions | Enhanced data integrity | Scalability challenges |
| AI-driven anomaly detection | Identifies unusual activities in real time | Proactive threat detection | Potential for false positives |
| Multifactor authentication | Requires multiple credentials | Strong access control | User inconvenience |
| Intrusion detection systems (IDS) | Monitors network traffic for threats | Quick threat mitigation | High resource consumption |

security mechanisms is essential for maintaining data integrity, confidentiality, and availability. This section explores key security concerns, blockchain-based models, and AI-driven anomaly detection to strengthen IoMT cybersecurity.

### 5.4.1 Common cyber threats in IoMT systems

IoMT systems face multiple cybersecurity threats due to their distributed and interconnected nature. Malware attacks, such as ransomware, can disrupt healthcare operations by encrypting critical patient data and demanding ransom payments [13] Distributed Denial-of-Service (DDoS) attacks can overload IoMT networks, rendering them unusable [18].

Additionally, man-in-the-middle (MitM) attacks compromise data integrity by intercepting communications between IoMT devices [19]. Unauthorized access due to weak authentication mechanisms remains a serious risk [19]. Addressing these threats requires implementing advanced security models and proactive threat detection systems.

### 5.4.2 Blockchain-based security models for IoMT

Blockchain technology offers a decentralized and immutable security framework for IoMT networks [20]. By leveraging smart contracts, blockchain enhances data integrity, transparency, and access control [20]. Each IoMT transaction is recorded in a tamper-proof ledger, reducing the risk of unauthorized modifications [21].

Moreover, blockchain-based FL models allow secure data sharing while maintaining patient privacy [22]. Despite these advantages, scalability and energy consumption remain challenges in real-world healthcare implementations [22].

### 5.4.3 AI-driven anomaly detection for cybersecurity

AI is revolutionizing IoMT security by enabling real-time threat detection and response. ML models analyze historical data to identify deviations from normal patterns, signaling potential cyber threats [23]. Deep learning-based intrusion detection systems (IDS) enhance cybersecurity by identifying sophisticated attack patterns [23].

One promising approach is using generative adversarial networks (GANs) for anomaly detection, which improves cyber resilience by differentiating between benign and malicious network behavior [24]. AI-driven security mechanisms significantly reduce false alarms and enhance response time, making them integral to next-generation IoMT cybersecurity strategies [24].

Security and privacy remain pivotal challenges in IoMT implementation. By integrating blockchain for data security, AI for anomaly detection, and robust encryption techniques, IoMT networks can enhance patient data protection. Future research should focus on optimizing these mechanisms to create scalable, efficient, and secure IoMT ecosystems [35].

## 5.5 PERFORMANCE OPTIMIZATION IN IOMT NETWORKS

The IoMT relies on seamless connectivity, real-time data processing, and robust security to enhance healthcare services. However, the performance of IoMT networks is influenced by factors such as latency, bandwidth constraints, and data processing efficiency. Optimizing performance requires strategic approaches, including latency and bandwidth optimization techniques, load balancing strategies, and advanced computing models like FL for secure data processing. By integrating these techniques, IoMT networks can achieve better scalability, reduced network congestion, and enhanced patient care [26].

### 5.5.1 Latency and bandwidth optimization techniques

Latency and bandwidth optimization are critical for real-time healthcare applications in IoMT. One approach involves edge and fog computing, which minimizes latency by processing data closer to the source rather than relying on distant cloud servers [27]. Compression techniques and data filtering also play a role in optimizing bandwidth by reducing redundant data transmission. Adaptive bitrate streaming ensures that medical imaging and video-based consultations maintain quality while adjusting to network conditions [28]. Additionally, quality of service-based routing algorithms prioritize critical healthcare data, reducing transmission delays and enhancing network reliability.

*Table 5.2* Performance comparison of communication protocols in IoMT

| *Communication protocol* | *Latency* | *Bandwidth* | *Energy efficiency* | *Range* | *Suitability in IoMT* |
|---|---|---|---|---|---|
| Wi-Fi | Medium | High | Moderate | Medium | Suitable for hospitals and clinics |
| 5G | Low | Very High | Low | High | Ideal for real-time remote healthcare applications |
| LPWAN | High | Low | High | Very High | Best for battery-powered medical sensors |
| Bluetooth | Low | Low | High | Short | Effective for personal healthcare devices |

### 5.5.2 Load balancing strategies in IoMT architectures

Load balancing [29] is essential for distributing workloads efficiently across IoMT network resources. Traditional round-robin and least-connection algorithms help manage traffic, but AI-based load balancing using reinforcement learning provides superior [30, 31]. Load balancing can be implemented at multiple levels, including sensor nodes, fog nodes, and cloud servers, to prevent congestion and ensure uniform resource utilization. Dynamic resource allocation, which considers patient priority and emergency scenarios, enhances system responsiveness. Additionally, software-defined networking can dynamically adjust traffic flows, ensuring an optimal balance between processing power and network efficiency [32].

### 5.5.3 Federated learning for secure data processing

FL has emerged as a privacy-preserving method for optimizing IoMT network performance. Unlike traditional ML models, FL allows IoMT devices to collaboratively train AI models without sharing raw patient data, thereby enhancing security [33]. This decentralized approach reduces bandwidth usage, as only model updates are transmitted rather than large datasets. FL is particularly useful in remote healthcare applications where data privacy regulations, such as HIPAA and GDPR, must be upheld. Additionally, combining FL with homomorphic encryption and secure multiparty computation further strengthens security and efficiency in distributed IoMT environments [33].

## 5.6 MATHEMATICAL MODELING IN IOMT

The IoMT leverages mathematical modeling to enhance security, optimize latency, and improve data transmission efficiency [34]. These models enable healthcare systems to achieve real-time data processing, secure communication, and predictive analytics. The following sections present key equations addressing security, latency, and predictive modeling in IoMT.

### 5.6.1 Equation for secure data transmission rate

Security in IoMT networks is crucial due to the transmission of sensitive medical data. The secure data transmission rate can be modeled as

$$\text{SDTR} = B \times \log_2\left(1 + \frac{S}{N}\right) \times \alpha$$

where

- $B$ is the bandwidth (Hz),
- $S$ is the signal power (W),
- $N$ is the noise power (W), and

is the security factor accounting for encryption overhead.

This equation ensures that increasing bandwidth and signal-to-noise ratio improves secure data transmission while considering encryption-induced latency.

### 5.6.2 Latency optimization model for IoMT networks

Latency in IoMT networks must be minimized to ensure real-time monitoring and response. The total latency (LtotalL_{total}) in an IoMT system can be expressed as

$$L_{\text{total}} = L_{\text{sensing}} + L_{\text{transmission}} + L_{\text{processing}} + L_{\text{storage}}$$

where

- $L_{\text{sensing}}$ is the time taken by sensors to collect data,
- $L_{\text{transmission}}$ is the delay in sending data via communication protocols,
- $L_{\text{processing}}$ represents computation latency at edge/fog/cloud nodes,
- $L_{\text{storage}}$ is the delay in storing and retrieving data.

To optimize latency, minimizing $L_{\text{processing}}$ via edge computing and efficient data compression techniques is essential. A refined model incorporating edge computing efficiency $(\eta)$ is

$$L_{\text{total}}^{\text{optimized}} = L_{\text{sensing}} + \frac{L_{\text{transmission}} + L_{\text{processing}}}{\eta} + L_{\text{storage}}$$

Higher values indicate improved edge processing, reducing overall latency.

### 5.6.3 AI-driven predictive healthcare model

AI enhances predictive healthcare by analyzing vast IoMT datasets [35]. A ML-based predictive model for patient health risk assessment can be represented as

$$H_{risk} = \sum_{i=1}^{n} w_i \times x_i + \beta$$

where

- $H_{\text{risk}}$ is the predicted health risk score,
- $w_i$ are the model weights,
- $x_i$ are input features (e.g., heart rate, blood pressure, glucose level), and
- $\beta$ is the bias term.

This equation forms the basis of logistic regression and deep learning models used in healthcare for early disease detection. The effectiveness of AI-driven models depends on feature selection, training data quality, and real-time adaptability.

Mathematical modeling in IoMT facilitates secure data transmission, efficient latency management, and predictive healthcare analytics [36]. These equations provide a foundation for optimizing IoMT performance while ensuring security and reliability in next-generation healthcare systems [37].

## 5.7 FUTURE DIRECTIONS AND RESEARCH CHALLENGES

The IoMT is poised for significant advancements with the integration of emerging technologies. While IoMT has already transformed healthcare through real-time monitoring, predictive analytics, and remote patient management, several challenges persist. Future research must focus on enhancing security, ensuring seamless interoperability, and leveraging cutting-edge computing paradigms. Addressing these issues will facilitate the development of a more robust and efficient IoMT ecosystem, ultimately improving patient care and operational efficiency in healthcare systems.

### 5.7.1 Evolution of IoMT with AI and machine learning

AI and ML are revolutionizing IoMT by enabling predictive diagnostics, personalized treatments, and automated anomaly detection. Future advancements will likely focus on:

- **Enhanced Predictive Analytics:** AI models will become more accurate in forecasting health conditions by analyzing vast amounts of real-time data from IoMT devices.
- **Adaptive Learning Systems:** ML algorithms will evolve to self-optimize, improving diagnostic accuracy with minimal human intervention.
- **Federated Learning Integration:** Privacy-preserving ML techniques, such as FL, will enable collaborative model training across multiple healthcare institutions without data centralization.
- **AI-Powered Cybersecurity:** AI-driven security mechanisms will enhance threat detection, mitigating cyber risks associated with IoMT networks.

These advancements will facilitate real-time decision-making and proactive healthcare interventions, reducing hospitalization and improving patient outcomes.

### 5.7.2 The role of quantum computing in IoMT security

As IoMT expands, traditional cryptographic techniques may become insufficient in protecting sensitive medical data. Quantum computing presents a promising solution to IoMT security challenges through:

- **Postquantum Cryptography (PQC):** Developing quantum-resistant encryption methods will safeguard IoMT communications against quantum attacks.
- **Quantum Key Distribution (QKD):** QKD ensures ultra-secure data transmission, making medical data exchanges nearly impervious to cyber threats.
- **Quantum Machine Learning (QML):** Leveraging QML for anomaly detection and security threat mitigation in IoMT will enhance real-time cybersecurity defenses.

Despite these advantages, practical implementations of quantum security in IoMT require further research to address hardware constraints and integration challenges.

### 5.7.3 Next-generation interoperability standards

Interoperability remains a key challenge in IoMT due to diverse device ecosystems and proprietary protocols. Future research should focus on:

- **Standardized communication protocols:** Developing unified standards for data exchange will ensure seamless interoperability across IoMT devices from different manufacturers.

- **Blockchain for secure interoperability:** Decentralized ledger technologies will enhance trust and transparency in IoMT data transactions while ensuring security.
- **FHIR and HL7 advancements:** The Fast Healthcare Interoperability Resources (FHIR) and Health Level Seven (HL7) standards need continuous enhancement to support real-time, AI-driven healthcare applications.
- **Edge-cloud interoperability:** Optimizing hybrid computing models will allow IoMT devices to seamlessly interact with both edge and cloud environments for efficient data processing.

By addressing these interoperability challenges, IoMT can achieve a more cohesive and scalable ecosystem, leading to improved patient outcomes and operational efficiency.

The future of IoMT depends on the successful integration of AI, quantum computing, and standardized frameworks. Research in these areas will drive the next wave of healthcare innovation, making medical systems more secure, intelligent, and interconnected.

## 5.8 CONCLUSION

### 5.8.1 Summary of key insights

This chapter has provided an in-depth analysis of IoMT, covering its fundamental architecture, data acquisition methods, and communication protocols. The significance of low-latency processing through edge and fog computing, combined with cloud-based AI analytics, was highlighted as a crucial factor in enhancing real-time decision-making. Security remains a major concern, with cyber threats necessitating robust protection mechanisms such as blockchain and AI-driven anomaly detection. Furthermore, performance optimization techniques, including load balancing and FL, play a crucial role in ensuring seamless IoMT operations. Finally, the discussion on mathematical modeling provided insight into the quantification of security, latency, and transmission efficiency, essential for the practical deployment of IoMT networks.

### 5.8.2 Potential impact on future healthcare systems

The future of healthcare will be significantly influenced by the advancements in IoMT technology. With the integration of AI and ML, predictive analytics will enable early disease detection and personalized treatment plans, improving patient outcomes. Enhanced security models, including quantum-safe cryptographic methods, will address growing cybersecurity concerns, ensuring patient data privacy and integrity. Moreover, the establishment of next-generation interoperability standards will facilitate seamless data exchange across healthcare ecosystems, fostering collaborative and data-driven medical solutions. As IoMT continues to mature, its widespread adoption will revolutionize patient monitoring, remote diagnostics, and healthcare delivery, ultimately reducing costs and enhancing accessibility for diverse populations worldwide.

## REFERENCES


[1] Khan, A. A., Laghari, A. A., Baqasah, A. M., Bacarra, R., Alroobaea, R., Alsafyani, M., & Alsayaydeh, J. A. J. (2025). BDLT-IoMT—a novel architecture: SVM machine learning for robust and secure data processing in Internet of Medical Things with blockchain cybersecurity. *The Journal of Supercomputing*, *81*(1), 1–22.

[2] Alturki, B., Abu Al-Haija, Q., Alsemmeari, R. A., Alsulami, A. A., Alqahtani, A., Alghamdi, B. M., ... & Shaikh, R. A. (2025). IoMT landscape: Navigating current challenges and pioneering future research trends. *Discover Applied Sciences*, 7(1), 1–30.

[3] Dzamesi, L., & Elsayed, N. (2025). A review on the security vulnerabilities of the IoMT against malware attacks and DDoS. (Preprint)

[4] Pruthvi, C. N., Vimala, H. S., & Shreyas, J. (2025). Optimizing content delivery in IoMT: Leveraging in-network caching with CDR. In *Data Science & Exploration in Artificial Intelligence: Proceedings of the First International Conference On Data Science & Exploration in Artificial Intelligence (CODE-AI 2024) Bangalore, India, 3rd-4th July, 2024 (Volume 2)* (p. 345). CRC Press.

[5] Alalwany, E., Alsharif, B., Alotaibi, Y., Alfahaid, A., Mahgoub, I., & Ilyas, M. (2025). Stacking ensemble deep learning for real-time intrusion detection in IoMT environments. *Sensors*, *25*(3), 624.

[6] Akram, A., Akram, J., Alabdultif, A., Anaissi, A., & Jhaveri, R. H. (2025). Secure and interoperable IoMT-based smart homes. *IEEE Consumer Electronics Magazine*, *2025*, 1–6.

[7] Kumar, S. S., Muthukumaran, V., Jahnavi, S., & Krishna, C. (2025). Securing the future of IoMT: Healthcare and comprehensive analysis of data security measures in medical information systems. In *Convergence of Internet of Medical Things (IoMT) and Generative AI* (pp. 191–216). IGI Global Scientific Publishing.

[8] Jayapradha, J., Haw, S. C., Palanichamy, N., Ng, K. W., & Thillaigovindhan, S. K. (2025). Integrated model (IM-LTS) for lung tumor segmentation using neural networks and IoMT. *MethodsX*, *14*, 103201.

[9] Ksibi, S., Jaidi, F., & Bouhoula, A. (2025). MLRA-Sec: An adaptive and intelligent cyber-security-assessment model for internet of medical things (IoMT). *International Journal of Information Security*, *24*(1), 1–20.

[10] Sezer, B. B., & Akleylek, S. (2025). PPLBB: A novel privacy-preserving lattice-based blockchain platform in IoMT. *The Journal of Supercomputing*, *81*(1), 219.

[11] Lakshmanaprakash, S., Abirami, A., Madanachitran, R., Mekala, R., & Vaishali, V. H. (2025). DON: Deep optimized network model based on coot and convoluted recurrent learning algorithms for healthcare monitoring in IoMT systems. *Measurement*, *242*, 116226.
[12] Gowda, D., Reddy, P., Tetala, V. R. R., Krishnamoorthy, P., & Yogi, K. S. (2025). Revolutionizing patient care through the convergence of IoMT and generative AI. In *Convergence of Internet of Medical Things (IoMT) and Generative AI* (pp. 217–242). IGI Global Scientific Publishing.
[13] Albogamy, F. R. (2025). Federated learning for IoMT-enhanced human activity recognition with hybrid LSTM-GRU networks. *Sensors*, *25*(3), 907.
[14] Javed, R., Abbas, T., Shahzad, T., Kanwal, K., Ramay, S. A., Khan, M. A., & Ouahada, K. (2025). Enhancing chronic disease prediction in IoMT-enabled healthcare 5.0 using deep machine learning: Alzheimer's disease as a case study. *IEEE Access*, *13*, 14252–14272.
[15] Sachdev, K., & Lall, B. (2025). Next-gen networked healthcare: Requirements and challenges. In *Current and Future Cellular Systems: Technologies, Applications, and Challenges* (pp. 165–183). John Wiley & Sons.
[16] Sarkar, A., & Jhamb, M. (2025). Next-Gen fortified health monitoring for cyber physical systems in internet of things using logistic maps based encryption. *Engineering Research Express*, *7*(1), 015305.
[17] Qureshi, K. N., Nafea, H., & Kim, P. (2025). Advancing healthcare systems: A tri-tier architecture by using data communication, AI data generative and regulation and compliance standards. *Expert Systems*, *42*(2), e13742.
[18] Nemade, B., Alegavi, S., & Bharadi, V. (2025). Graph attention dialogue network based drug recommendation model for next-gen healthcare and consumer-centric devices. *IEEE Transactions on Consumer Electronics*, *2025*, 99.
[19] Kök, İ. (2025). MetaXAI: Metahuman-assisted audio and visual explainability framework for internet of medical things. *Biomedical Signal Processing and Control*, *100*, 107034.
[20] Singh, S., Khan, S., Khan, S., Ansari, O., Malhotra, N., Shukla, S. K., & Narang, J. (2025). Muscle matters: Transforming amyotrophic lateral sclerosis diagnostics with next-gen biosensors and smart detection. *ACS Chemical Neuroscience*, *16*(4), 563–587.
[21] Khanna, A. (2025). Securing digital foundations: A point of view on cybersecurity in healthcare. In *Securing an Enterprise: Maximizing Digital Experiences through Enhanced Security Measures* (pp. 429–478). Apress.
[22] Gupta, N., Makhijani, R. K., & Ukey, A. S. A. (2025). Future trends and research directions for applications of blockchain in healthcare. *Generative AI Techniques for Sustainability in Healthcare Security* (pp. 243–268). IGI Global.
[23] Joshi, H. (2025). AI and chronic diseases from data integration to clinical implementation. In *Generative AI Techniques for Sustainability in Healthcare Security* (pp. 17–40). IGI Global Scientific Publishing.
[24] Upadhyaya, N., Joshi, H., & Agrawal, C. (2025). Examining NLP for smarter, data-driven healthcare solutions. In *Intelligent Systems and IoT Applications in Clinical Health* (pp. 393–420). IGI Global.

[25] Sharma, N., Kumar, R., Maliya, R., Shah, V., Patel, J., & Fukui, M. (2025). Japan's 2030 vision for 6G: A case study. In *Network Security and Data Privacy in 6G Communication: Trends, Challenges, and Applications* (p. 20). Taylor & Francis.

[26] Joshi, H. (2025). Implementing responsible AI in healthcare organizations: strategies, challenges, and best practices. In *Responsible AI for Digital Health and Medical Analytics* (pp. 293–326). IGI Global Scientific Publishing.

[27] Dubey, M., Singh, A. K., & Mishra, R. (2025). AI based resource management for 5G network slicing: History, use cases, and research directions. *Concurrency and Computation: Practice and Experience*, *37*(2), e8327.

[28] Saidu, Y., Shuhidan, S. M., Aliyu, D. A., Aziz, I. A., & Adamu, S. (2025). Convergence of blockchain, IoT, and AI for enhanced traceability systems: A comprehensive review. *IEEE Access*, *13*, 16838–16865.

[29] Chigarev, B. (2025). The identification of a promising research topic in applying generative artificial intelligence to petroleum engineering problems. (Preprint).

[30] Parkar, T. V., & Kamath, K. S. (2025). Next-gen healthcare: AI and IoT innovations and future trends in healthcare. In *Intelligent Systems and IoT Applications in Clinical Health* (pp. 219–242). IGI Global.

[31] Rangarajan, D., Rangarajan, A., Reddy, C. K. K., & Doss, S. (2025). Exploring the next-gen transformations in healthcare through the impact of AI and IoT. In *Intelligent Systems and IoT Applications in Clinical Health* (pp. 73–98). IGI Global.

[32] Ahmed, W., Iqbal, W., Hassan, A., Ahmad, A., Ullah, F., & Srivastava, G. (2025). Elevating e-health excellence with IOTA distributed ledger technology: Sustaining data integrity in next-gen fog-driven systems. *Future Generation Computer Systems*, *168*, 107755.

[33] Dave, A., Patel, B., Bhatt, G., & Vora, Y. (2017). Load balancing in cloud computing using particle swarm optimization on Xen Server. In 2017 Nirma University International Conference on Engineering (NUiCONE) (pp. 1–6). IEEE.

[34] Dave, A., Patel, B., & Bhatt, G. (2016). Load balancing in cloud computing using optimization techniques: A study. In 2016 International Conference on Communication and Electronics Systems (ICCES) (pp. 1–6). IEEE.

[35] Dave, A., Patel, B., Bhatt, G., & Scholar, P. G. (2016). Load Balancing in cloud computing with open source cloud platforms: A study. In National Conference on Recent Advances in Computer Science & Technology (RACST 2016) on (pp. 26–30).

[36] Akash Dave. (2024). Resource offloading (balancing) in cloud environment using particle swarm optimization and improved particle swarm optimization on xen server. *International Journal of Intelligent Systems and Applications in Engineering*, 12(4), 669–676.

[37] Dave, A., & Chudasama, H. (2023). Load balancing in cloud environment using different optimization algorithms and open-source platforms: A deep picture. In International Conference on Intelligent Computing & Optimization (pp. 214–222). Cham: Springer Nature Switzerland.

Chapter 6

# SecureHealth

## A blockchain-based framework for privacy-preserving healthcare data management in health centers

*Rachid Ed-daoudi*

### 6.1 INTRODUCTION

Blockchain technology has gained significant interest and funding across many fields, including digital money, tracking product journeys, shared resource platforms, power trading, money protection, creative rights, and online government services [1]. Blockchain is valued for its strong protection features, which help support distributed applications and safe digital exchanges [2]. When blockchain is combined with healthcare systems, it allows for spread-out data storage, records that cannot be changed, and coded security methods, which reduce risks of unwanted access and information theft.

For users to have a good experience, exchanges within these applications need to be quick, with little delay, strong protection, and dependability. The increasing use of new technologies in healthcare is speeding up the growth of health information handling [3], making electronic health files an important and widely shareable resource. Around the world, the amount of medical information is growing at an exponential rate.

The quick growth of health information within medical centers is making data handling systems more complex, highlighting the growing need for better protection and privacy tools [4]. Health records on paper and outdated management systems are especially open to violations of patient privacy and data accuracy. Also, the separation between health centers creates problems for storing, sharing, and keeping medical information over time, which gets in the way of good treatment and doctor discussions.

Even with the benefits of blockchain technology, current blockchain-based health systems often struggle to balance protection, growth capacity, and smooth operation. For example, providing quick access to medical records while keeping privacy intact requires new agreement methods and coding approaches [5]. Furthermore, the ability of different healthcare providers to work together remains a problem, calling for common rules for safe data exchange [6].


DOI: 10.1201/9781003640325-6

Recent research has put forward different blockchain designs to improve healthcare data protection. Some methods use mixed blockchain systems that bring in fog computing to make transactions faster and lower processing demands [7]. Other approaches concentrate on special encryption methods that allow calculations on coded data to better protect privacy in healthcare information management [8]. However, these answers often come with downsides regarding processing complexity and storage needs.

Blockchain technology offers a workable answer for keeping healthcare data storage safe [9]. Its spread-out structure, along with its abilities to ensure information accuracy, security, privacy, and openness, makes blockchain an effective way to handle healthcare information. The use of blockchain-based data storage in healthcare presented in Figure 6.1 has brought new digital systems designed to take the place of old-fashioned health record methods, improving data privacy and accuracy.

This study suggests a blockchain-based system that tackles these issues by creating an effective privacy protecting setup for healthcare information. The main contributions of this work include the following:

- Creating a new blockchain based system for safe health data storage and sharing;
- Building an improved access control method using advanced coding techniques;
- Developing a testing framework to check and show the system's performance, validated through a successful real-world implementation

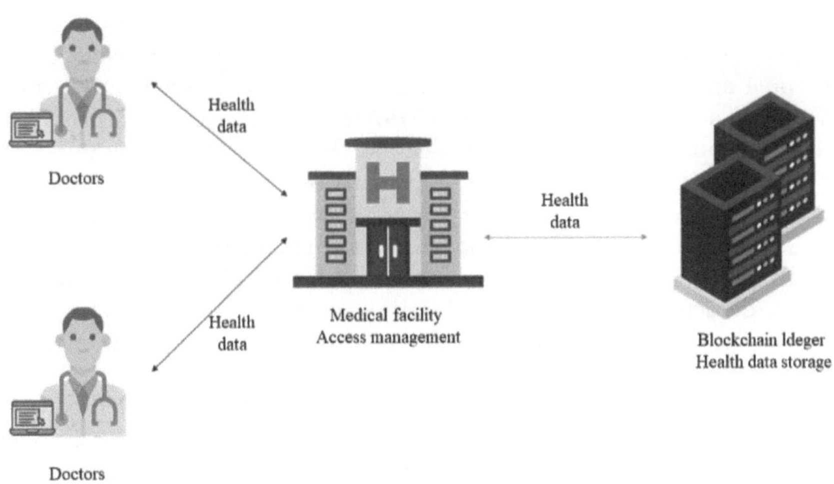


*Figure 6.1* Overview of public health facility operations.

The rest of this chapter is organized as follows: Section 6.2 presents related works. Section 6.3 explains the suggested system's design and structure. Section 6.4 shows the results of the practical testing. Finally, Section 6.5 concludes the study.

## 6.2 LITERATURE REVIEW

Current studies on blockchain-based healthcare answers have looked at different areas like access control, data privacy, safe storage, growth ability, and information accuracy. Regular healthcare systems often have trouble keeping data storage secure and allowing safe information sharing across connected networks.

The spread-out nature of blockchain could change healthcare by improving clinical data monitoring, ensuring safe patient data sharing, and strengthening data storage security [10]. Diwan et al. [11] created a privacy-protecting system that combines special encryption with blockchain to secure patient data exchanges. Their method improves data accuracy but needs more computing power.

In another study, Abid et al. [12] looked at how blockchain can secure healthcare data by using smart contract-based access control methods. They found that blockchain can greatly improve data openness while ensuring limited access based on set security rules.

Also, Mishra et al. [13] studied the joining of blockchain with InterPlanetary File System (IPFS) for spread-out healthcare data handling. Their approach lowers storage costs and improves data availability but creates challenges in retrieval speed.

Reegu et al. [14] developed a blockchain-based electronic health record (EHR) system aimed at stopping unauthorized access and data changing by keeping an unchangeable activity record within the blockchain network. Vidhya et al. [15] developed a blockchain-based medical data sharing system that incorporates a hybrid Feistal–Shannon homomorphic encryption algorithm, ring signature technology, and smart contracts to enhance security, privacy, and authentication in healthcare information exchange.

Cheng et al. [16] introduced Ekiden, a system that joins privacy-protecting smart contracts with a blockchain-enabled trusted execution environment. Ekiden uses a proof-of-publication protocol for secure blockchain transactions. However, this method may lead to increased processing overhead, possible security risks, and more ways to attack.

Agrawal et al. [17] created a mixed blockchain-fog computing model to solve performance bottlenecks in healthcare applications. Their solution reduces transaction processing time but needs extra infrastructure for fog computing setup.

Grover and Kushwaha [18] suggested a blockchain-powered EHR system mainly concerned with privacy-protecting data sharing. Their system uses advanced coding methods to stop unauthorized data changes, thereby strengthening security measures.

Lakshmanan and Anandha [19] introduced a special data arrangement called a blockchain tree for keeping health records, where main patient identity information connects to subchains holding detailed medical data. Similarly, Rehman et al. [20] proposed a secure and energy-saving Internet of Medical Things (IoMT) system for e-healthcare, using wireless body area networks to enable remote patient monitoring. While good for real-time health tracking and medical help, this system faces security issues due to the balance between energy-efficient data sending and the limited abilities of medical sensors.

Lodha et al. [21] introduced a blockchain-based IoMT security system (BC-IoMT-SS) for healthcare that ensures patient data security and privacy while enabling alerts for verified practitioners, demonstrating superior performance metrics compared to existing methods.

Sanober and Anwar [22] developed a three-module blockchain-based architecture with validator-based consensus for healthcare management during disasters, implemented in the Remix Ethereum environment to create a lightweight, reliable system that demonstrates improved performance metrics compared to existing approaches.

Xie and Ding [23] developed a blockchain-based double anonymity strategy for IoMT healthcare systems that conceals identities between doctors and patients while enabling malicious behavior tracking, implementing smart contracts for authentication and a three-factor cross-hospital access scheme that reduces computational costs by 23–87% while enhancing security.

Alnafrani and Acharya [24] introduced SecureRx, a blockchain-based web application using Ethereum and RxCheck hub that enables healthcare providers to securely access comprehensive prescription records across geographical boundaries to prevent opioid overdoses while maintaining HIPAA compliance. Fan et al. [25] developed a simplified cloud authentication system for IoT-based settings, bringing in secure radio frequency identification technology to improve computing efficiency. Meanwhile, Rahim et al. [26] introduced a digital twin-based smart medical cyber-physical system that creates a virtual replica of hospital operations to enable real-time patient monitoring, personalized decision-making, and workflow optimization, demonstrating enhanced hospitalization services and more precise patient diagnostics.

While these studies give useful findings in blockchainbased healthcare security, they often do not address the trade-offs between privacy, efficiency, and real-time data access. Many existing studies have trouble with authentication methods, often missing the importance of resource-controlled transactions and the efficient running of health-related operations. The suggested framework in this study aims to overcome these limitations by introducing an improved blockchain design that ensures fast transactions, strong encryption, and smooth working together among healthcare providers.

## 6.3 METHODOLOGY

This section shows a blockchain based system aimed at improving the safe storage of sensitive information in public health centers. The suggested answer focuses on making sure healthcare processes remain private and accurate while making operations smoother. It also explains how healthcare activities work together and how blocks are created in the process.

### 6.3.1 Blockchain-based healthcare center prototype

The suggested framework is made to improve healthcare system performance by strengthening privacy, security, accuracy, and checkability of approved health records. This section explains the system's overall design, as shown in Figure 6.2, highlighting a blockchain-based safe data storage setup created for healthcare centers. It describes the working parts and methods used in this system, including access control tools. By using a blockchain based secure cloud storage model, this answer ensures high-performing permission systems that protect privacy and data accuracy.

This blockchain-based system makes health data more reliable and able to grow, building greater trust among stakeholders in data services. The main working parts of the platform center around three key groups: the health data users/consultants, the health center controller, and the secure data storage.

The health center controller manages the activities of data users/consultants within the blockchain-based system. Each user/consultant works as a data keeper, responsible for handling patient health records safely. In this model, only approved people can access, create, or update smart contracts related to health records on the blockchain.

Consultants gather patient information and store it on the blockchain using public keys, while a special private key is given to each patient's record for better security.

Before getting access, the health center controller checks and registers each health data user/consultant, giving a unique digital identity (ID) and password through a safe authentication system. This registration process uses the Bcrypt algorithm to create encrypted digital IDs, which are then safely stored. After finishing registration, approved users can securely access the blockchain network with their digital credentials, ensuring strong authentication and strict access control.

In a system protected by blockchain, any action involving the database such as storing, changing, or sharing data, works with the blockchain to maintain privacy, security, and accessibility. By using a network of verified

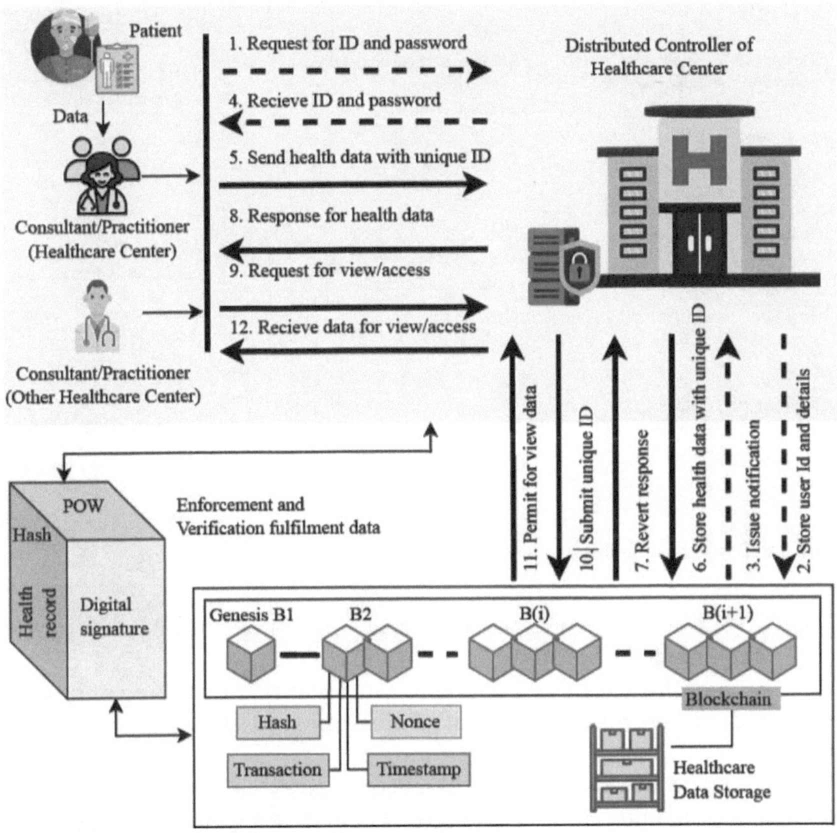


*Figure 6.2* Blockchain healthcare infrastructure overview.

user nodes, the system guarantees the safety and accuracy of health records. Transactions are signed cryptographically and stored permanently on the blockchain, with data accuracy ensured using SHA-256 hashing. The proof-of-work (PoW) consensus method further strengthens decentralization, stopping unauthorized changes. Any tampering is found through step-by-step hash checking, including nonce values, time stamps, and encoded data. If something unusual is found, the affected block is marked as invalid.

The way data is exchanged in this model follows an organized plan:

1. Users/consultants prove who they are using their assigned IDs and passwords.
2. After being confirmed, they ask for access to blockchain storage through the health center controller.

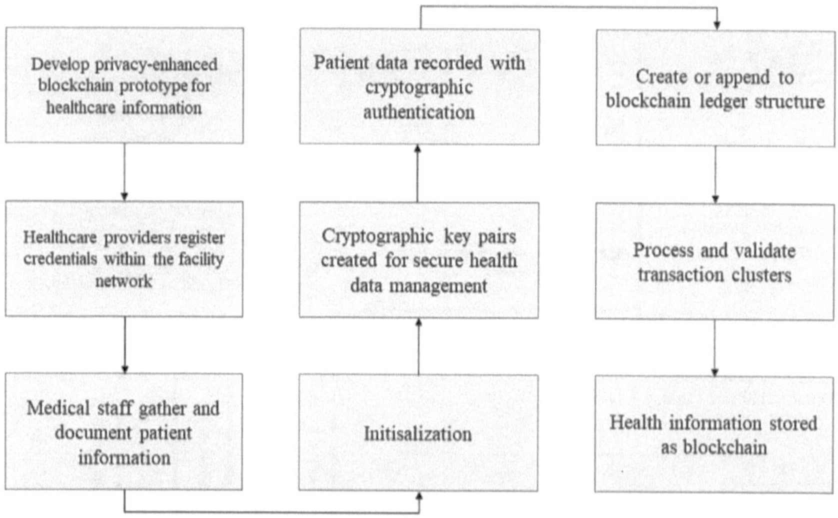


*Figure 6.3* Blockchain healthcare system workflow design.

3. Coded health records are then sent for storage and later retrieved when needed.
4. Each health record gets a unique data identity for tracking purposes, and the controller manages its storage and retrieval.

The complete workflow of this blockchain-powered system is shown in Figure 6.3, explaining each step involved in building a secure, clear, and efficient health data management platform.

## 6.3.2 Management workflow

The suggested model puts a shared supervisor in health centers to control who can see medical information kept on the blockchain. This setup has three main parts: healthcare providers (who need to work with patient information), the shared supervisor (who handles registration and permissions), and the blockchain system (which works as a spread-out, protected database for medical records). The blockchain works as a widely distributed and tamper-proof record system, making sure only approved people can handle patient information. Authorized participants can safely add, access, and check data.

### *6.3.2.1 Identity registration and verification*

The system starts with an organized sign-up procedure to verify and add healthcare providers. First, providers send a registration request to the health center supervisor along with their professional credentials. The supervisor checks if the applicant is already in the system; if not, their information is encrypted and securely saved on the blockchain to prevent changes and protect data. After successful verification, the system creates a unique username and password, which are sent to the provider through a decentralized, distributed supervisor. This security process gives registered users permanent access to the blockchain network, allowing them to log in whenever needed and participate in future activities.

#### *6.3.2.2 Input processing*

The information entry stage begins when providers connected to the blockchain network gather specific patient medical information such as test results or medication plans and forward these documents to the health center supervisor. When received, the supervisor creates a unique health identifier for the patient, bringing together their medical history into one trackable record. To enhance protection, each document receives a hash-based code from the blockchain, making an unchangeable digital signature that stops tampering and improves verification. Permission to add or change health files is strictly limited to approved providers, with access controlled by encryption keys to ensure rule-following and prevent unauthorized changes. When information is successfully added to the blockchain, all system participants, including relevant healthcare staff and patients, get immediate confirmation of the transaction. This instant update system promotes openness, responsibility, and reliability throughout the network, keeping all parties informed about changes to patient records while still following privacy and legal requirements.

#### *6.3.2.3 Information access and visualization*

This portion offers a comprehensive overview of the blockchain based structure for handling public healthcare information, guaranteeing privacy, protection, and accuracy of delicate medical information. The proposed approach allows authenticated healthcare providers and specialists to link to the blockchain through the medical facility's management system. This arrangement provides them with entry to historical medical files while implementing rigorous safeguards to control access. To access patient medical information, healthcare workers need to first verify their identity using their personal digital credentials and passcode, which is confirmed via the decentralized management system. They also need to supply the specific patient code matching the particular person's medical file. After the inquiry is sent, the healthcare facility's system checks if the patient code is valid and allows entry to the requested medical information when the credentials align with the saved data. This method guarantees that just approved staff can examine and review earlier medications and health backgrounds. When the authentication procedure finds an incorrect patient code, the blockchain system immediately denies the access attempt. The capability to safely obtain previous health documents allows medical experts to track patient wellness developments, create new treatment plans, and refresh the records as needed. The exchanges between various participants in this framework support the smooth incorporation of blockchain technology into community health information administration. As specialists gather medical information from individuals, they engage with the blockchain to perform data exchanges, making certain that all health details are safely saved and handled.

The system uses a special code-making process to create unique public and private key sets for safe data viewing. These randomly made keys boost transaction security within the platform by enabling coded messages between users and the blockchain record system.

To strengthen data protection, the blockchain system uses mathematical scrambling and digital verification methods. When a doctor shares a patient's health details with another approved person, no actual data moves between them. Instead of sending information directly, the sharing happens by changing who can see what in the blockchain network. Every request to change viewing rights must be verified with a digital signature, made using the sender's private code, and checked against their public code to prove it's real.

The SHA-256 scrambling method is vital to these activities, creating a unique code for each transaction and helping find data through coded web addresses in the online system. Also, participating computers digitally sign transactions to verify they're genuine, making sure the information stays accurate.

An important feature of this blockchain based setup is the PoW agreement system, which controls how blocks are created and checked. Computers in the network confirm health transactions, and certain ones are picked to make the next block. This ensures all stored health information cannot be changed and stays the same across all copies of the shared record. The RSA security method and SHA-256 scrambling are key to protecting the data, coding transactions, and keeping patient records private. The blockchain storage approach ensures all medical information remains available while being guarded against unwanted changes.

The system's foundation relies on the SHA-256 security code, which keeps the organized structure of blockchain data blocks in order. Each new block joined to the chain has important parts like the block number, time stamp, special number, blockchain address, and code of the previous block.

The block header connects all blocks together, allowing smooth checking and creating an unchangeable record of all exchanges.

The elliptic curve digital signature algorithm makes data safety even stronger by checking digital signatures at both user and server sides. If any problem is found such as tampering or changed data, the exchange is right away thrown out, stopping unwanted changes to saved health records. This double-checking approach makes sure only proven users can see and handle data, reducing risks of fake information. Inside the blockchain system, each health exchange creates a public-private key pair to help safe coding and decoding. Algorithm 1 shows the RSA based key pair making process, which gives unique keys to all users for safe interactions. The PEM way connects these security keys with text coding for easy exchange reading. This algorithm also explains the steps of making digital signatures for health data exchanges, ensuring coded proving during network activities.

**Algorithm 1. Transaction security process on blockchain**

```
procedure BlockchainTransactionSecurity(user, transaction)
  if user starts transaction then
    #Generate transaction key-pair
    randomNumber ← make random(security number)
    secretKey ← create RSA(1024, randomNumber)
    openKey ← secretKey · Kpb(i)
    change to readable text(secretKey, openKey)
    #Prepare and sign the transaction
    T ← prepare transaction without user's secretKey
    exchangeSigner ← MakeDigitalSignature(secretKey)
    numberCode ← CalculateHash(transaction data)
    signedExchange ← SignExchange(exchangeSigner, numberCode)
    #Return the signed transaction and public key
    return ConvertToText(signedExchange), openKey
  else
    return "No transaction initiated on blockchain"
  end if
end procedure
```

To maintain the integrity and security of health data while supporting the growth of the network, Algorithm 2 handles two essential functions in the blockchain health system. First, it manages the creation and addition of new health data blocks, incorporating key elements like block numbers, health transaction data, timestamps, and security codes to keep health records safe and unchangeable. Second, it oversees the process of adding new computers to the blockchain based health network, allowing for a distributed system where processing can happen across multiple locations.

**Algorithm 2. Block creation and node integration**

```
procedure ManageHealthBlockchain(operation, data)
 if operation = "createBlock" then
   Initialize healthTransactions ← Ø
  Set block ← (blockNumber, healthTransactions, nonce, timestamp, previousBlockHash)
   if blockNumber = length(chain) + 1 then
     Append block to chain
     Reset running transaction status
     Add block to chain
   end if
  if EncodeJSON(block, standard value) as a file then
    hash256Value ← CreateSHA256Hash()
    Update hash256Value.blocks
    return HexEncode(hash256Value)
  end if

 elsif operation = "registerNode" then
  if health data user requests a node then
    Create registrationNode
  end if
Initialize parameters: (healthTransaction, chain, nodes, genesisBlock)
  urlNodeInfo ← ParseURL(urlNode)
  if sets urlNodeInfo.Netloc and urlNodeInfo.path then
    Add urlNodeInfo.Netloc and urlNodeInfo.path to nodes
  else
    Append a new node to nodes
  end if
 else
  Do nothing
 end if
end procedure
```

Algorithm 3 shows how health information is gathered, viewed, and controlled within the blockchain.

**Algorithm 3. Safe health data control on Blockchain**

```
procedure GatherAndShare
    Set up exchange settings for healthcare data
    Make a new exchange block
    Check digital exchange signature
    openKey ← GetRSAOpenKey()
    signatureChecker ← MakePKCS1Checker(openKey)
    dataCode ← MakeSHACode(health exchange)
    CheckSignature(dataCode, textExchangeSignature)
    Run Proof of Work (PoW) system
    Meet mining rules for good proof
    Match blockchain computers
    Confirm blockchain exchange is valid
    Add data to the exchange chain
    if exchange signature is checked then
        Move or share data between computers
        Allow access to health records
    end if
end procedure
```

The PoW agreement system is very important in the blockchain-based public health network by checking exchanges before they are shared or viewed across different computers. This method changes the number of working computers as needed, making sure the network can grow properly and making health data exchanges faster. After the exchanges are checked, the system puts the data blocks into the blockchain record, keeping all public health center exchanges safe and accurate.

## 6.4 RESULTS AND DISCUSSIONS

This part provides an evaluation of the suggested blockchain-based safe storage control system for public health centers, looking at user computers and testing how well it protects data and keeps information private. Tests and quality checks were done to prove the system works well in keeping health records secret, accurate, and available when needed. The findings show the system's overall success in handling health data exchanges, especially how quickly transactions happen, how little delay there is, and how easily the system can grow. The blockchain system was tested to make sure it meets all the needs of a modern health data storage solution.

### 6.4.1 Validation setup

The testing environment was set up in a controlled setting using a Windows 10 computer with an AMD Ryzen 9 5900X processor (3.7GHz, 12 cores, 24 threads) and 32 GB memory. The system was built using Python 3.11 (64-bit) with Flask 2.2.5 serving as the web connection tool, making sure user computers and the blockchain could talk to each other smoothly. The testing method brought together several user computers and a blockchain computer to check how well the health data handling system worked and could grow under conditions similar to real-life use.

### 6.4.2 System performance assessment

To test how well the system works, many user computers were set up to work with the blockchain server, allowing measurement of important factors like how long transactions take and how much delay occurs. The system was tested by having user computers perform exchanges in groups of 1, 10, 20, and 30 (T1, T10, T20, and T30) within the blockchain network. As each exchange block was processed and shared across the blockchain-powered health center, the test gave useful information about how well the system can handle growing numbers of exchanges efficiently.

The time it takes to complete exchanges was measured to see how fast the system handled data across different user computers. The results, as shown in Figure 6.4, show that for computer 1, exchange time went from 25.2 ms for T1 to 69.8 ms for T30.

For computer 5, exchange time started at 77.9 ms for T1, going up to 157.4 ms for T30. These findings show how well the system can grow, showing a steady increase in processing time as more exchanges are added.

Another important performance measure was latency, which means how long it takes to send and get data blocks within the blockchain network. As Figure 6.5 shows, delay for computer 1 was 10.42 ms for T1 and went up to 20.32 ms for T30.

For computer 5, delay started at 25.18 ms for T1 and reached 37.5 ms for T30. These results confirm that as more exchanges happen, network delay also goes up in a similar way, but stays within a good range for healthcare applications that need to work in real time.

### 6.4.3 Blockchain performance comparison

A comparison study was done to measure the delay of the suggested system against a regular blockchain. As shown in Figure 6.6, the delay of the suggested system for computer 1 when handling 10 exchanges was 15.3 ms, while it was 37.6 ms for computer 8.

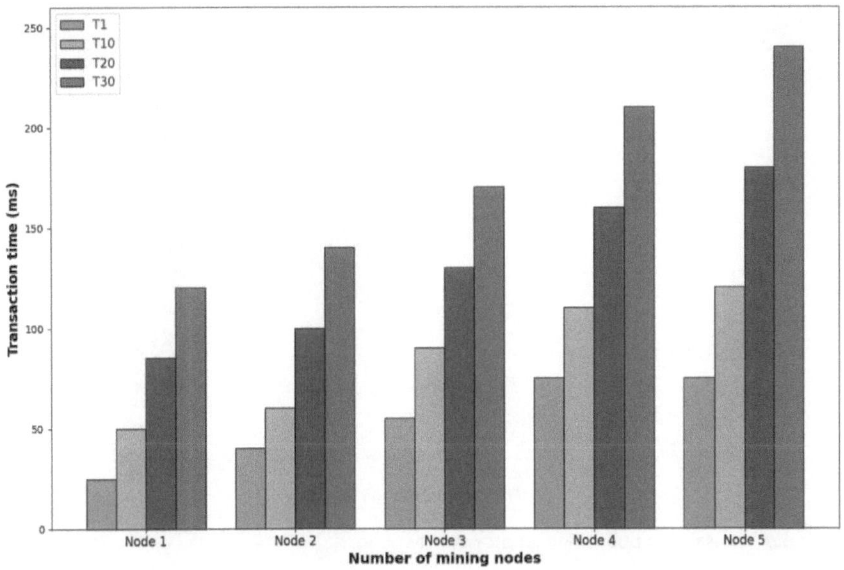


*Figure 6.4* Average time taken for transactions across different nodes.

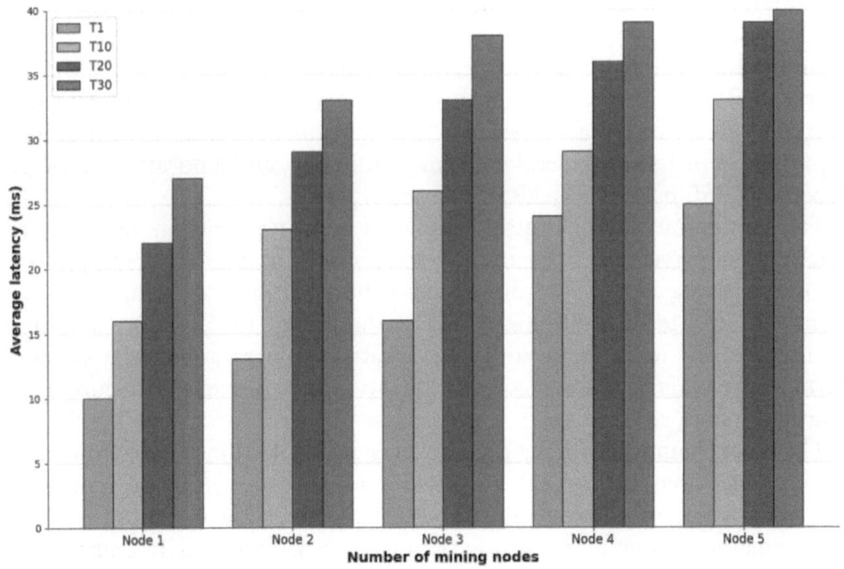


*Figure 6.5* Average latency (ms) for different number.

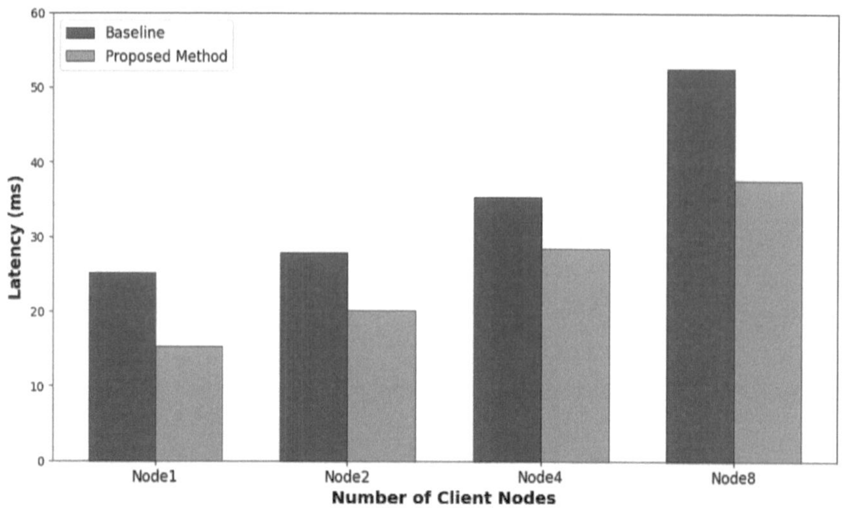


*Figure 6.6* Transaction publishing latency comparison.

When compared, the standard blockchain showed longer delays in the same testing setup, proving that the suggested system offers better growth potential and works more efficiently when dealing with health data exchanges.

Additionally, a validation experiment was conducted at a healthcare center in Rabat, Morocco, to evaluate the real world performance of the proposed blockchain based system. The implementation covered multiple departments including general medicine, radiology, and laboratory services, processing 350 patient records of various types.

The validation demonstrated significant improvements in operational efficiency as presented in Figure 6.7. Response time for retrieving patient records decreased by 67% compared to the traditional system, dropping from 120 ms to just 40 ms, while maintaining 100% data integrity. Healthcare providers reported an 88% satisfaction rate with the system, particularly praising the improved verification capabilities and secure data sharing functions.

The blockchain solution maintained consistent sub-30ms transaction processing times even during peak hospital hours and successfully prevented all unauthorized access attempts during security testing. The system's performance remained stable across all departments regardless of data complexity or patient volume.

Overall, this validation confirms that the proposed health data storage system delivers a scalable, secure, and efficient solution for managing

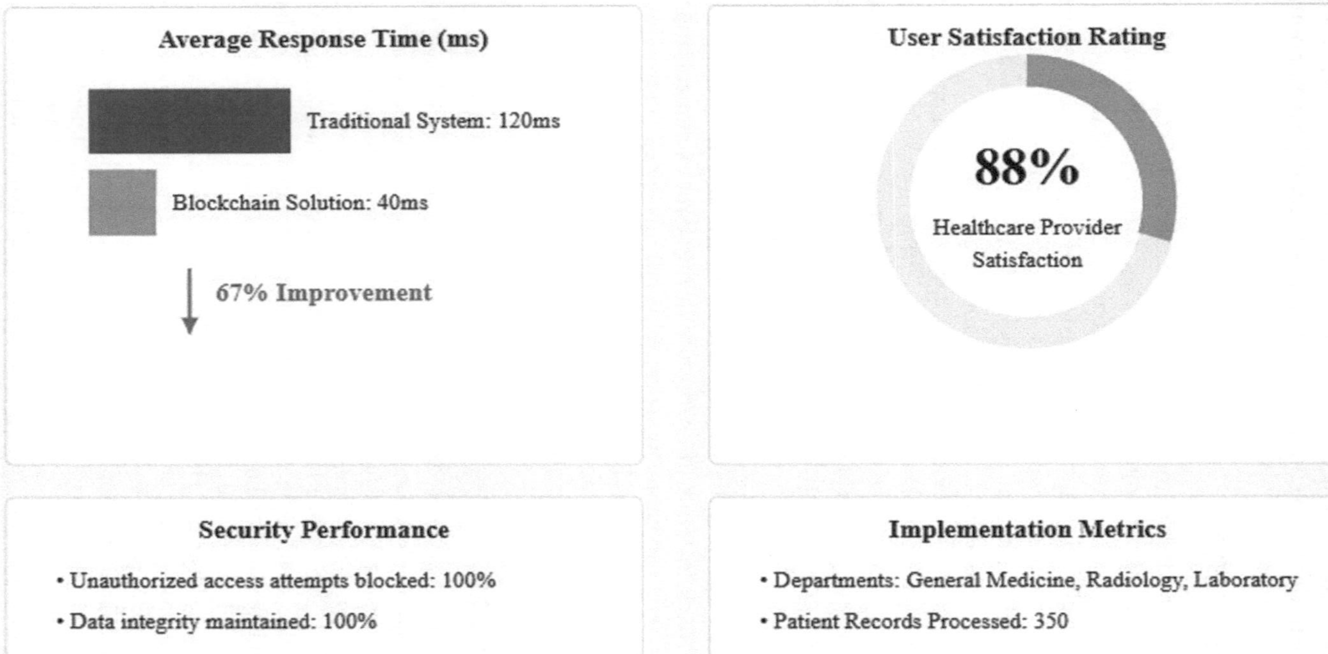
Average Response Time (ms)
Traditional System: 120ms
Blockchain Solution: 40ms
67% Improvement
User Satisfaction Rating
88%
Healthcare Provider Satisfaction
Security Performance
• Unauthorized access attempts blocked: 100%
• Data integrity maintained: 100%
Implementation Metrics
• Departments: General Medicine, Radiology, Laboratory
• Patient Records Processed: 350

*Figure 6.7* Healthcare center validation results in Rabat Morocco.

sensitive medical records in real world environments. The demonstrated improvements in speed, security, and user satisfaction represent a significant advancement over conventional healthcare data management approaches.

## 6.5 CONCLUSION

This research addresses the growing demand for digital change in healthcare by creating a safe storage system built on a privacy-protecting and fast blockchain. A key feature of this system is its dependable access control method, which helps authorized users safely and efficiently share health records. By organizing working parts and using a step-by-step blockchain-enabled process, the model supports spread-out data storage while keeping data private, available, accurate, and able to grow.

The suggested framework greatly improves safety compared to traditional healthcare data handling systems, letting doctors or users store and view medical records securely. Performance testing results, including how long it takes to publish transactions and delays, show the system's ability to efficiently process health data exchanges across multiple user computers. Compared to old storage methods, this blockchain-based approach offers a strong and reliable way to manage health records in public health centers.

Despite its benefits, the system's use of blockchain technology has a possible drawback in terms of energy use during data exchanges and storage. This raises environmental worries, especially as blockchain networks get bigger. Future research will focus on using less energy and adding metadata checking for cloud storage, further improving security and data handling abilities in healthcare settings.

## REFERENCES


[1] A. G. Gad, D. T. Mosa, L. Abualigah, and A. A. Abohany, "Emerging trends in blockchain technology and applications: A review and outlook," *Journal of King Saud University Computer and Information Sciences*, vol. 34, no. 9, pp. 6719–6742, 2022.

[2] G. Habib, S. Sharma, S. Ibrahim, I. Ahmad, S. Qureshi, and M. Ishfaq, "Blockchain technology: Benefits, challenges, applications, and integration of blockchain technology with cloud computing," *Future Internet*, vol. 14, no. 11, p. 341, 2022.

[3] A. Sheikh et al., "Health information technology and digital innovation for national learning health and care systems," *The Lancet Digital Health*, vol. 3, no. 6, pp. e383–e396, 2021.

[4] J. Shahid, R. Ahmad, A. K. Kiani, T. Ahmad, S. Saeed, and A. M. Almuhaideb, "Data protection and privacy of the Internet of Healthcare Things (IoHTs)," *Applied Sciences*, vol. 12, no. 4, p. 1927, 2022.

[5] P. Khatiwada, B. Yang, J. C. Lin, and B. Blobel, "Patient-generated health data (PGHD): Understanding, requirements, challenges, and existing

techniques for data security and privacy," *Journal of Personalized Medicine*, vol. 14, no. 3, p. 282, 2024.

[6] B. H. de Mello et al., "Semantic interoperability in health records standards: A systematic literature review," *Health and Technology*, vol. 12, no. 2, pp. 255–272, 2022.

[7] A. H. Mayer, V. F. Rodrigues, C. A. da Costa, R. da Rosa Righi, A. Roehrs, and R. S. Antunes, "Fogchain: A fog computing architecture integrating blockchain and Internet of Things for personal health records," *IEEE Access*, vol. 9, pp. 122723–122737, 2021.

[8] H. Abhishek, K. Tripathy, and S. Mishra, "A succinct analytical study of the usability of encryption methods in healthcare data security," in *Next Generation Healthcare Informatics*, Singapore: Springer Nature Singapore, 2022, pp. 105–120.

[9] A. Haleem, M. Javaid, R. P. Singh, R. Suman, and S. Rab, "Blockchain technology applications in healthcare: An overview," *International Journal of Intelligent Networks*, vol. 2, pp. 130–139, 2021.

[10] A. Gladyr, "Design and development of a secure and patient-controlled system to share healthcare data for research," M.S. thesis, McGill University, 2021.

[11] P. Diwan, R. Kashyap, and B. Khandelwal, "Blockchain assisted encryption scheme for intellectual share estimation using medical research data," *Concurrency and Computation: Practice and Experience*, vol. 36, no. 2, p. e7896, 2024.

[12] A. Abid, S. Cheikhrouhou, S. Kallel, Z. Tari, and M. Jmaiel, "A smart contract-based access control framework for smart healthcare systems," *The Computer Journal*, vol. 67, no. 2, pp. 407–422, 2024.

[13] R. K. Mishra, R. K. Yadav, and P. Nath, "Integration of blockchain and IPFS: Healthcare data management & sharing for IoT environment," *Multimedia Tools and Applications*, pp. 1–22, 2024.

[14] F. A. Reegu et al., "Blockchain-based framework for interoperable electronic health records for an improved healthcare system," *Sustainability*, vol. 15, no. 8, p. 6337, 2023.

[15] S. Vidhya, P. M. Siva Raja, and R. P. Sumithra, "Blockchain-enabled decentralized healthcare data exchange: Leveraging novel encryption scheme, smart contracts, and ring signatures for enhanced data security and patient privacy," *International Journal of Network Management*, vol. 34, no. 5, p. e2289, 2024.

[16] R. Cheng et al., "Ekiden: A platform for confidentiality-preserving, trustworthy, and performant smart contracts," in *Proc. IEEE European Symposium on Security and Privacy (EuroS&P)*, 2019, pp. 185–200.

[17] R. Agrawal, S. Singhal, and A. Sharma, "Blockchain and fog computing model for secure data access control mechanisms for distributed data storage and authentication using hybrid encryption algorithm," *Cluster Computing*, vol. 27, no. 6, pp. 8015–8030, 2024.

[18] B. Grover and D. K. Kushwaha, "Authorization and privacy preservation in cloud-based distributed EHR system using blockchain technology and anonymous digital ring signature," *Health Services and Outcomes Research Methodology*, vol. 23, no. 2, pp. 227–240, 2023.

[19] M. Lakshmanan and G. S. Anandha Mala, "Merkle tree-blockchain-assisted privacy preservation of electronic medical records on offering medical data protection through hybrid heuristic algorithm," *Knowledge and Information Systems*, vol. 66, no. 1, pp. 481–509, 2024.

[20] A. Rehman, T. Saba, K. Haseeb, S. Larabi Marie-Sainte, and J. Lloret, "Energy-efficient IoT e-health using artificial intelligence model with homomorphic secret sharing," *Energies*, vol. 14, no. 19, p. 6414, 2021.

[21] L. Lodha, V. S. Baghela, J. Bhuvana, and R. Bhatt, "A blockchain-based secured system using the Internet of Medical Things (IOMT) network for e-healthcare monitoring," *Measurement: Sensors*, vol. 30, p. 100904, 2023.

[22] A. Sanober and S. Anwar, "Blockchain-based healthcare assistance model in distributed disaster management systems," in *The Role of Blockchain in Disaster Management*, Academic Press, 2025, pp. 153–169.

[23] Q. Xie and Z. Ding, "Provably secure and lightweight blockchain based cross hospital authentication scheme for IoMT-based healthcare," *Scientific Reports*, vol. 15, no. 1, p. 6461, 2025.

[24] M. Alnafrani and S. Acharya, "SecureRx: A blockchain-based framework for an electronic prescription system with opioids tracking," *Health Policy and Technology*, vol. 10, no. 2, p. 100510, 2021.

[25] K. Fan, W. Jiang, H. Li, and Y. Yang, "Lightweight RFID protocol for medical privacy protection in IoT," *IEEE Transactions on Industrial Informatics*, vol. 14, no. 4, pp. 1656–1665, 2018.

[26] M. Rahim, W. Lalouani, E. Toubal, and L. Emokpae, "A digital twin-based platform for medical cyber-physical systems," *IEEE Access*, vol. 12, pp. 2169–3536, 2024.

Chapter 7

# Digital forensics in next-generation internet of medical things for sustainable telehealthcare

*Mariappan Ramasamy*

## 7.1 INTRODUCTION

In recent years, the Internet of Things (IoT) technology has received a lot of attention among researchers to explore various applications including healthcare [1]. In order to enhance quality of life and support medical emergencies, the IoT has been utilized recently in wireless sensor networks and in a variety of healthcare applications, including wearable body space networks. In order to monitor heart rate and other characteristics, wearable sensor devices that are connected to the internet can record data like photoplethysmography, EEGs, and ECGs. The Internet of Medical Things (IoMT) is transforming healthcare by connecting medical devices and applications through the internet. This interconnected network allows for seamless data exchange and real-time monitoring, leading to improved diagnostics, personalized treatments, and better patient outcomes. The IoMT is seen to be essential for medical applications, and in order to create a dependable platform, it is essential to enhance and examine every aspect of the IoT infrastructure [2]. The term IoMT [3] describes how medical systems and devices are connected via IoT technologies. It makes remote healthcare, biological signal tracking, disease diagnosis, and patient health monitoring possible without the need for human intervention. The IoMT plays a critical role in healthcare by enhancing patient health and revolutionizing the healthcare sector [4]. It builds an ecosystem of connected medical objects by utilizing smart sensors, smart devices, and lightweight communication protocols [5]. Promising opportunities exist for the development of IoT-based healthcare technology in terms of social effect, economic advantages, and technological improvements. The IoMT transforms [6, 7] healthcare by utilizing IoT technology to improve patient care and medical services. The interconnection of different medical devices/sensors forms an IOMT and is shown in Figure 7.1.

DOI: 10.1201/9781003640325-7

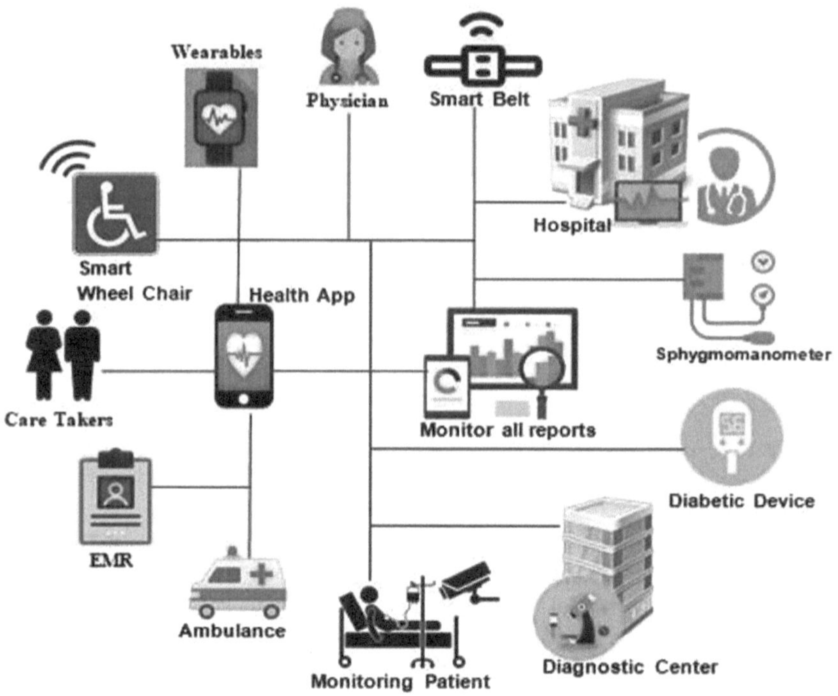


*Figure 7.1* Internet of medical things (IoMT).

## 7.2 DIGITAL FORENSICS

Digital forensics (DF) is a fascinating and crucial field that focuses on the recovery, investigation, and analysis of information found in digital devices and networks [8, 9] often in the context of cybercrimes or security breaches. It plays a pivotal role in modern law enforcement, cybersecurity, and legal investigations [10]. DF involves collecting, preserving, and analyzing electronic data to support investigations and legal proceedings. It includes several subdisciplines such as computer forensics, focusing on computers and storage devices, network forensics analyzing network traffic, mobile device forensics, and forensic data analysis [11]. Typically, it follows steps like identifying evidence, acquiring data, analyzing it systematically, and presenting findings in a clear, legally admissible manner. It is used in solving cybercrimes, corporate investigations, fraud detection, and incident response. The life cycle of DF is shown in Figure 7.2.

As shown in Figure 7.2, the DF life cycle [12] typically involves identification, preservation, analysis, documentation, and presentation of digital evidence to support investigations.

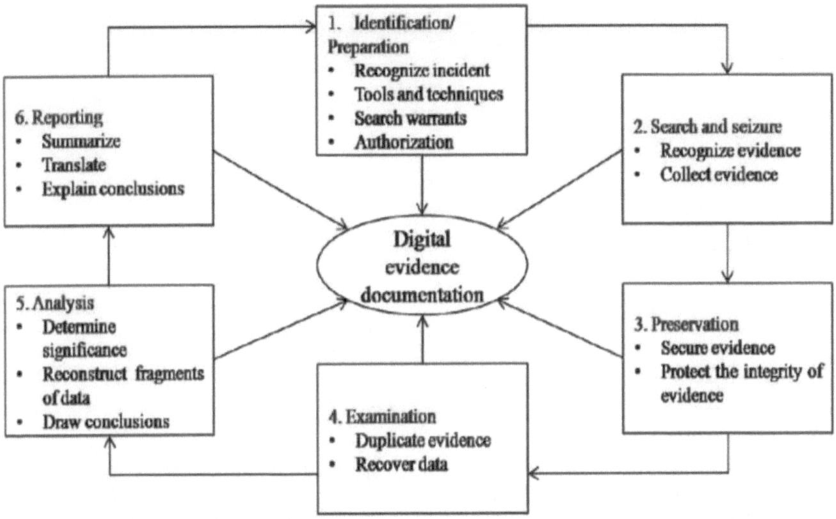


*Figure 7.2* Lifecycle of digital forensics.

i. **Identification:** This stage involves identifying the relevant devices, data sources, and potential evidence related to the incident or investigation.
ii. **Preservation:** Once identified, the next step is to preserve the integrity and authenticity of the evidence by creating copies or images of the data in a secure manner, ensuring no tampering or alteration occurs.
iii. **Analysis:** This involves examining the collected data to identify relevant information, patterns, and anomalies that can help determine the cause and scope of the incident or crime.
iv. **Documentation:** Thoroughly documenting all steps taken during the investigation, including evidence collection, analysis methods, and findings, is crucial for legal admissibility and future reference.
v. **Presentation:** Finally, the findings and evidence are presented in a clear and concise manner, often in the form of reports or presentations, to relevant stakeholders, such as law enforcement or legal teams.

### 7.2.1 Classifications of digital forensics

DF is a vast field with several specialized branches, each focusing on different types of digital evidence. The different types of DF [13] are shown in Figure 7.3. The following list shows the different types of DF.

i. **Computer forensics:** Focuses on recovering and analyzing data from computers, laptops, and storage devices such as hard drives, USBs, etc. It is commonly used in criminal investigations and data breaches.

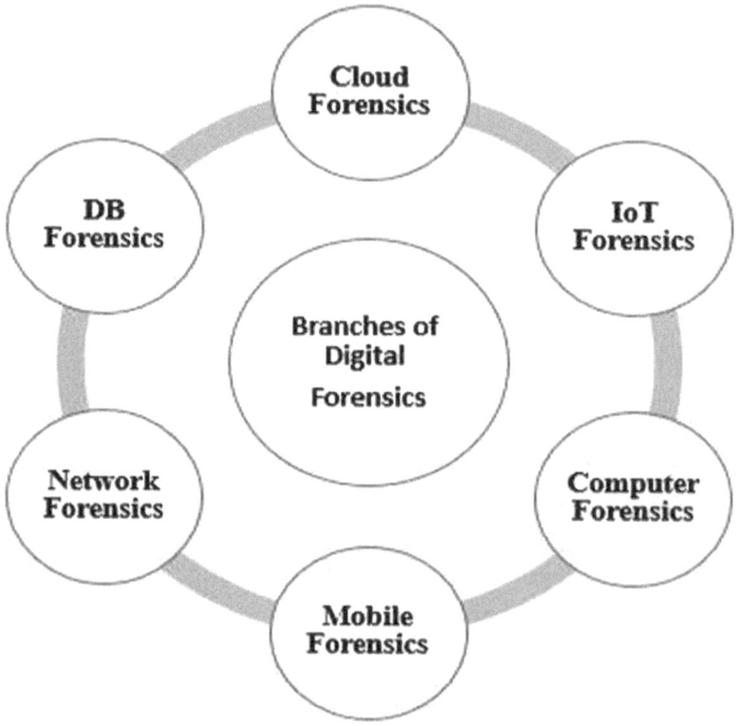


*Figure 7.3* Types of digital forensics.

ii. **Network forensics:** Involves monitoring and analyzing network traffic to identify intrusions, attacks, or unauthorized activities. It is crucial for cybersecurity and tracking cybercriminals.
iii. **Mobile device forensics:** Deals with extracting and examining data from mobile devices, such as smartphones /tablets, including messages, call logs, and app data.
iv. **Database forensics:** Examines databases and the related metadata to uncover unauthorized activities, such as data tampering or breaches.
v. **Forensic Data Analysis (FDA):** Focuses on identifying patterns, anomalies, and trends within large data sets, often used to detect financial fraud or insider threats.
vi. **Memory forensics:** Analyzes a computer's volatile memory (RAM) to uncover details about running processes, malware, or other in-memory artifacts.
vii. **Cloud forensics:** Investigates data stored on cloud platforms to trace cyber incidents and identify evidence.

### 7.2.2 Applications of digital forensics

DF is indispensable in the modern digital age, ensuring accountability, security, and justice across diverse fields [14]. It has a wide range of applications across various sectors. The various applications of DF are listed below.

i. **Law enforcement:** Investigating cybercrimes, such as hacking, identity theft, online fraud, recovering deleted or hidden evidence from digital devices to solve crimes, tracing illegal activities on the dark web.
ii. **Corporate investigations:** Detecting employee misconduct, such as intellectual property theft or policy violations, investigating financial fraud, embezzlement, analyzing insider threats or data breaches in organizations.
iii. **Cybersecurity:** Identifying vulnerabilities and sources of attacks on IT systems, analyzing malware to understand its origin and impact, and conducting incident response to mitigate and prevent security breaches.
iv. **Legal proceedings:** Collecting and analyzing digital evidence for court cases, ensuring that digital evidence complies with legal and regulatory standards, reconstructing timelines and events for use in litigation.
v. **Tele healthcare:** In telehealth, specific forensic techniques are employed to ensure the security, integrity, and reliability of digital evidence, investigating breaches or unauthorized access to telehealth systems and protecting medical records and sensitive information from tampering.
vi. **Insurance and financial fraud:** Applications include uncovering fraudulent claims in insurance processes, detecting unauthorized transactions or money laundering activities, providing digital evidence for auditing purposes.
vii. **Military and national security:** Investigating cyber warfare and espionage activities, securing classified information and communication networks, monitoring and analyzing cyber threats to national infrastructure.
viii. **Education and research:** Supporting academic research on DF methodologies, educating future forensic analysts and law enforcement professionals, developing innovative tools and techniques for forensic investigations.

### 7.2.3 Digital forensics tools

DF tools are hardware and software tools [15] that can be used to aid in the recovery and preservation of digital evidence. Law enforcement can use DF

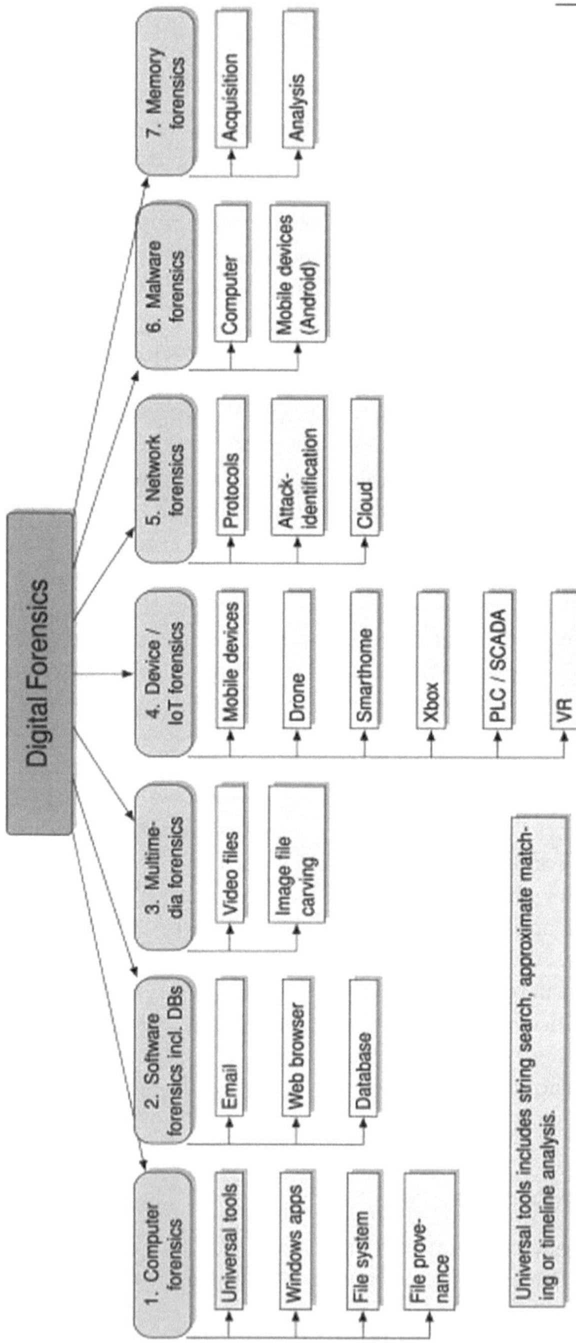


*Figure 7.4* Digital forensics tools.

tools to collect and preserve digital evidence and support or refute hypotheses before courts. The various types of DF tools are depicted in Figure 7.4, which includes the Sleuth Kit, Wireshark, Autopsy, SIFT, Paladin, Xplico, ExifTool, and Magnet RAM Capture, etc. Forensic imaging of the systems being investigated, image processing, and producing a report with the information gathered are all steps in the forensic analysis process. Security analysts and investigators can gather forensic data from computer devices, transform it into common formats for study, and filter it to find pertinent information with the aid of DF technologies.

DF tools are essential for investigating and analyzing electronic devices and digital data. They help forensic experts extract, preserve, and analyze evidence in legal cases, cybersecurity incidents, and more. Table 7.1 shows DF tools, known for their capabilities in data analysis, incident response, and evidence collection. Each tool has its unique features and areas of expertise. Choosing the right DF tool depends on several factors such as type of investigation, the devices involved, specific goals, etc.

## 7.3 DIGITAL FORENSICS IN IOMT

The IoMT has revolutionized healthcare by connecting medical devices, sensors, and systems, enabling real-time monitoring, efficient diagnostics, and personalized treatments [16]. However, this interconnected ecosystem also introduces significant challenges in security, privacy, and DF. DF in the IoMT is a critical aspect of ensuring the security and integrity of connected medical devices and the sensitive data they handle. The need for security/ privacy/DF n IoMT is shown in Figure 7.5. Since patient EHRs are currently one of the primary targets for malevolent attackers, investigators must also ensure data owners' privacy throughout the investigative process [17]. Three steps are suggested for DF because IoT is primarily cloud-based. Users' devices come first, followed by the network over which the data are transferred, and lastly, cloud servers. The chain of custody must be followed in order for any digital evidence that is retrieved to be trustworthy, genuine, comprehensive, credible, and admissible before it can be used as evidence in court.

i. **Incident response:** When data breaches or system compromises occur, DF helps identify the source of the attack, the methods used, and the extent of the damage.
ii. **Data protection and compliance:** Ensuring that sensitive patient information is handled in compliance with regulations like HIPAA or GDPR. Forensics can verify that no unauthorized access or tampering has occurred.
iii. **Malware detection:** Identifying and analyzing malware that may target telehealth platforms, such as ransomware or spyware, to prevent future incidents.

*Table 7.1* Digital forensic tools

| *Tool Category* | *Tool Name* | *Description* |
|---|---|---|
| Disk imaging and data acquisition | FTK Imager | Creates forensic images of storage devices, preserving data integrity |
| — | EnCase | A commercial platform for data acquisition, analysis, and reporting |
| — | Cellebrite UFED | A software application for collecting, preserving, and analyzing digital evidence from various devices |
| Forensic analysis and investigation | Autopsy | An open-source platform for analyzing disk images and conducting forensic investigations |
| — | Forensic Toolkit (FTK) | A commercial digital forensics platform for analyzing and investigating digital evidence |
| — | Magnet AXIOM | A digital investigation platform for obtaining and analyzing forensic data |
| — | X-Ways Forensics | A tool for analyzing digital evidence and recovering data |
| Network forensics | Wireshark | A network protocol analyzer for capturing and examining network traffic |
| — | Xplico | A network forensic analysis tool designed to extract data from network traffic |
| — | NetworkMiner | A network forensic tool for analyzing network traffic and identifying devices |
| Other tools | Volatility | A tool for analyzing memory images |
| — | Registry Recon | A tool for extracting and analyzing Windows registry hives |
| — | SIFT Workstation | A virtual appliance containing a suite of forensic tools |

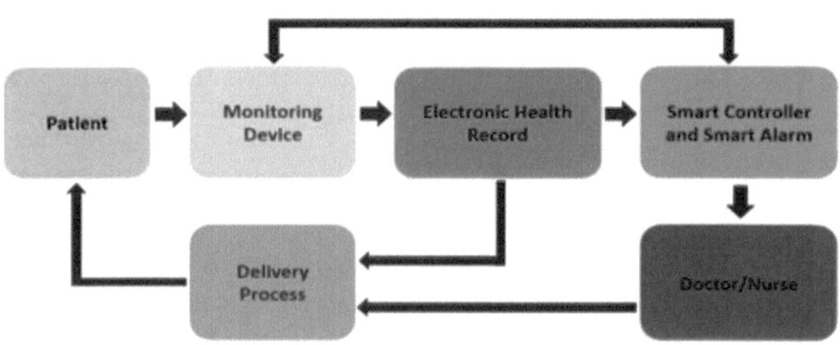


*Figure 7.5* Need for security/privacy/digital forensics in IoMT.

iv. **Auditing and monitoring:** Analyzing system logs and network activity to detect anomalies, unauthorized access, or suspicious activities in real time.
v. **Cloud and remote access forensics:** Investigating breaches in cloud systems that store medical records or telehealth data. It ensures that remote consultations are secure and free from interference.
vi. **Device and wearable forensics:** Examining telehealth devices, such as health monitors and wearables, for signs of tampering or misuse, ensuring the accuracy and authenticity of health data.
vii. **Fraud detection:** Identifying fraudulent activities, such as false insurance claims or unauthorized use of telehealth services, using forensic techniques.

The three-tiered architecture of DF using device/things forensics, network forensics and cloud forensics is shown in Figure 7.6.

Apart from DF, AI/ML techniques [18] are transforming the healthcare industry by enhancing clinical diagnostics, healthcare management, and public health infrastructures. Drug development, disease diagnosis, and effective hospital resource utilization are just a few of the healthcare uses of AI and ML. By strengthening their abilities and promoting patient outcomes, service quality, and the overall effectiveness of the healthcare system, AI and ML has the potential to support healthcare providers, and thereby, it can save costs and improve everyone's health. Large volumes of healthcare data

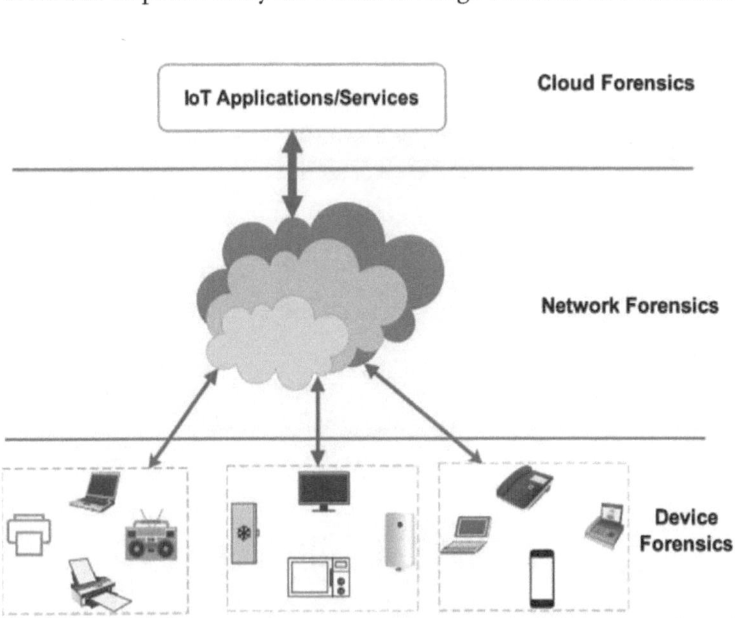


*Figure 7.6* Three tier digital forensics in internet of medical things.

can be analyzed by AI and ML, which can also spot trends and help with activities like image processing and repetitive task automation. Moreover, AI/ML techniques can facilitate natural language processing, which makes it easier for medical professionals to access and analyze patient data through natural language interface. Though AI and ML are at their early stage, they have potential applications in IoMT for medical therapeutics in near future. Wireless body sensors use ML techniques like support vector machines and decision trees to gather healthcare data using smart technologies [19]. These ML methods help in the diagnosis and prognosis of diseases in order to provide highly accurate predictions and classifications. For later usage, the processed data will be kept on cloud storage.

The layered architecture of IoMT is shown in Figure 7.7. The biomedical sensors, wireless sensors, and recorded data are represented by the perception layer. The gateway layer is in charge of moving the gathered data to a long-range or short-range communication network, where it is stored in a network server or IoTs server at the data storage layer. Finally, the application layer, which is an application server that runs user applications, monitors, controls, etc. with the aid of cloud, edge, or fog computing, allows access to or visualization of the stored data. The healthcare technology has greatly evolved with the integration of AI/ML techniques into IoMT for data management [20]. Massive volumes of patient data are produced by IoMT devices and saved in electronic health records (EHRs), including vital signs and medication adherence records.

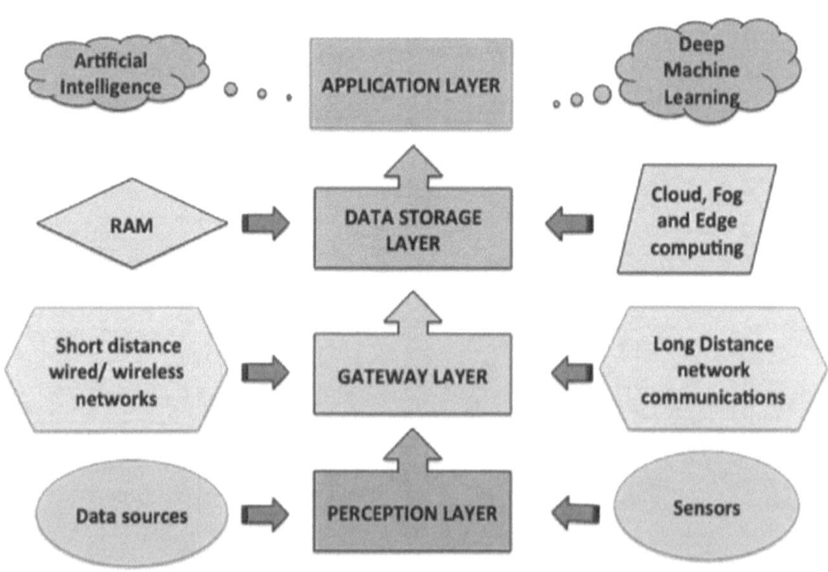


*Figure 7.7* Architecture of IoMT.

AI/ML techniques can help medical practitioners and healthcare providers with early disease detection, appropriate treatment regimens, and predictive healthcare by analyzing, interpreting, and extracting useful features from IoMT data and thereby meeting the demands of each patient. Furthermore, protocols that include ML into IoMT increase decision support systems, expedite diagnosis, and constantly improve health. However, as sensitive medical data serves as the foundation for well-informed medical decisions and customized treatment plans, this integration also places a high priority. The healthcare system may be completely transformed by including data processing and machine learning (ML) into the IoMT by enabling remote healthcare system.

## 7.4 RELATED WORK

The IoMT and IOT-based health care systems incorporate the following AI approaches. The study provided a comprehensive analysis of the advancements made in wearable IoMT for healthcare systems, with an emphasis on how well they work for illness detection, prevention, and surveillance. It explores the approaches used by researchers to improve the general accuracy, effectiveness, and safety of the healthcare system. The essay also discusses the opportunities and challenges of creating AI-powered IoT-based healthcare systems [21]. It recognizes that wearable medical sensors and IoTs-based health monitoring systems make it possible to provide remote healthcare services, which maximizes the use of vital hospital beds and lowers costs. The concept of IoMT and its impact on healthcare operations, including increased efficacy, cost savings, and better patient outcomes, were explored in the article. It explores IoMT's design, technologies, real-world applications, security frameworks, and challenges.

AI-based Internet of Things (AIoT) can be used to create smart environments for the elderly and infirm. These environments can help with geriatric support, vulnerability analysis, disease diagnosis, appointment scheduling, after-care assistance, and regular vital sign monitoring. The study emphasized the need for additional research to completely comprehend the impact and effect on different IoT applications while highlighting the possible problems and inconsistencies with the IoMT strategy [22]. Hence, AI can be applied to IoMT and point-of-care devices in cutting-edge healthcare fields like diabetes treatment, cancer detection, and heart monitoring. The application of AI/ML techniques in IoMT is shown in Figure 7.8.

Although quality issues still exist, the medical sector's data interpretation is being improved by the IoTs and medical data analytics. For reliable quality in accuracy, latency, and reaction time, deep learning is essential. DF in the context of the IoMT involves specialized tools [23] and techniques to investigate and secure medical devices and their data. Some of the existing research works carried out on the application of DF tools and techniques in healthcare/ IOMT are summarized in Table 7.2.

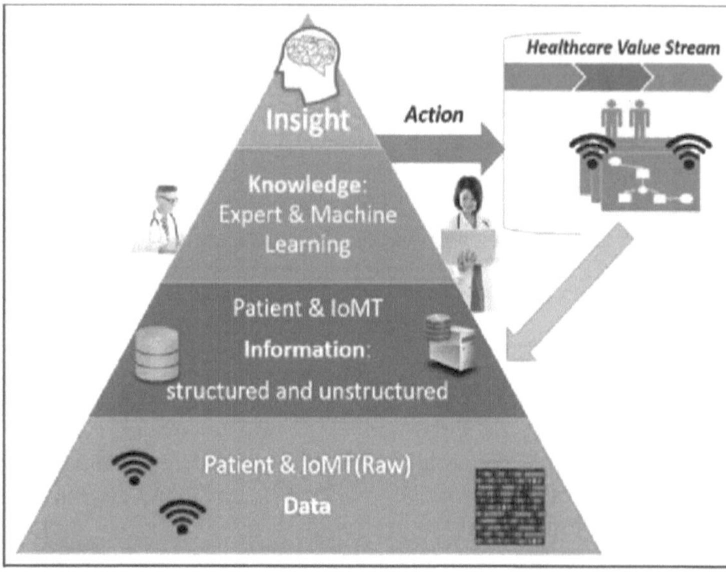


*Figure 7.8* Applying AI/ML techniques in IoMT.

## 7.5 MACHINE LEARNING IN TELEHEALTHCARE

Machine learning (ML) is significantly enhancing the IoMT for telemedicine, leading to improved healthcare delivery and patient outcomes. The integration of ML within the IoMT has significantly enhanced telemedicine applications, enabling improved patient monitoring and disease prediction [24]. These advancements are transforming telemedicine by providing real-time patient data, improving diagnostics, and enabling personalized treatments. The integration of ML in IoMT for telehealthcare is shown in Figure 7.9.

The three tiers of traditional telemedicine are:

**Tier 1:** Thing layer (wireless (body) sensors)
**Tier 2:** Network layer (fog) gateway, and
**Tier 3:** Data management layer/ML layer

The hospital/healthcare is fundamentally a component of the cloud computing infrastructure and telemedicine system. Given that the client is represented by Tiers 1 and 2 of remote healthcare monitoring, the server is represented by Tier 3.

*Table 7.2* Types of digital forensics tools

| *Category* | *Name of the Tool* | *Capability of the Tool* |
|---|---|---|
| Device (incl. IoT forensics) | FSNView | To document the metadata of a single disk image, which is done by using many different storage system parsers on the same disk image |
| Computer forensics | Mrsh_net | An extension to the mrsh_v2 tool to aid in the speed of approximate matching. This is done by implementing a single large Bloom Filter |
| Memory forensics | Sdkernel | A tool designed to identify the kernel version from the kernel image on the disk |
| Memory forensics | Robust Linux memory acquisition | The kernel module LKM injects the acquisition module into the existing system kernel in order to acquire the memory |
| Software forensics incl. DBs | Sifter | To rank the forensic importance of string searches and have implemented as a Sifter. The ranking is done by 18 factors such as Recency-Created and Recency-Modified |
| Multimedia | Forensic analysis of video file formats | To extract file format structures and metadata for various cameras and phones. The parsers were shown to extract enough information |
| Software forensics (DBs) | Forensic2020 | To serve as a bootable environment, which is a controlled environment where the triage software runs in a known-safe operating system |
| Memory | linux_compressed swap linux_ duno_maps | outputs statistical information on the state of frontswap and zswap and also extracts all compressed pages to disk in their uncompressed form |
| Software forensics (DBs) | OpenLV | To quickly and safely interact with collected evidence, as if they had sat down at the Computer Forensics when evidence was collected |
| Computer forensics | AFEIC: Advanced forensic Ext4 inode carving | File carving module that was built to work with The Sleuth Kit in order to perform a search for inode entries of files on the system without requiring the information from the superblock |
| Malware forensics | BinComp | BinComp uses an idea of layers of which the first is a supervised compilation process, second extracts the given features, the third identifies compiler version and optimization level form the sematic features of the compiler function |
| Memory forensics | Winpmem and Pmem | To capture the entire system memory and allow the extraction of ACPI tables from a memory image, and scanning the respective tables for potential rootkit |
| Software forensics (DBs) | Privacy Preserving Email Forensics (PPEF) | Autopsy plug-in that allows for the searching of sensitive email while maintaining the privacy of the owner |

(*continued*)

*Table 7.2 (Cont.)*

| *Category* | *Name of the Tool* | *Capability of the Tool* |
|---|---|---|
| Device (incl. IoT forensics) | ConvertPDML | To parse relevant WhatsApp information from a PDML file and display it in HTML |
| Network forensics | Synchronisation Service Evidence Retrieval Tool | SSERT-remotely recover of digital evidence from folders shared between Sync thing |
| Malware forensics | Simple Set Comparison Tool | Phishing investigators can quickly identify and focus on phish targeting a particular brand |
| Software/DB forensics | Browser Storage Extractor (BrowStEx) | A web storage for data artifacts from data from web browser tools such as Web Historian, NetAnalysis and WEFA |
| Computer forensics | Mrsh-cf | Similarity hashing/approximate matching tool equal to mrsh-net but uses Cuckoo filter instead of Bloom filter with less memory |
| Computer forensics | MetroExtractor | Gathers static and volatile forensic artefacts in Windows 9 apps. Vlatile artifacts extract from hibernation and swap on storage media |
| Computer forensics | Litigation Hold Verification Tool | To deter mine spoliation and fake evidence provided by a litigant party |
| Network forensics | Hviz | An interactive visualization approach to represent the event timeline of HTTP/HTTPS activities of a workstation in a comprehensible manner |
| Device/IoT forensics | Control Program Logic Change Detector | CPLCD works with a set of detection rules (DRs) to detect and record undesired incidents on interfering normal operations of PLC |
| Software/DB forensics | EDBForensic | A tool to facilitate the recovery of deleted records and tables from an extensible storage engine (ESE) database |
| Software/DB forensics | InVEST: Intelligent visual email search and triage | A tool which allows for multiple emails to be analyzed and indexed with the goal to reduce the number of emails that need to be viewed in detail |
| Network forensics | TLS Key Extractor (TLSkex) | A tool to extract the master key of a TLS connection at from a virtual machine's main memory independent of the encryption algorithm |
| Memory forensics | Psquickscan Psscan | A plugin for an experimental framework that scans the memory of pool tags as opposed to scanning the entirety of virtual memory |
| Software/DB forensics | Database Image Content Explorer (DICE) | Restore deleted and de-allocated data across a variety of different Database Management Systems (DBMSes) |
| Network forensics | Covert6 | Create covert channels in IPv6 thereby providing corroboration of its existence, in a simulated enterprise infrastructure with routers, firewalls |

*Table 7.2 (Cont.)*

| *Category* | *Name of the Tool* | *Capability of the Tool* |
|---|---|---|
| Network forensics | Kumodd | Cloud drive acquisition |
| Computer forensics | Advanced Automated Disk Investigation Toolkit (AUDIT) | Integrate and configure the tools automatically for the purpose of both general and specific investigations, searching the disk for evidence in graphics files, emails, documents, and "hidden" locations |
| Malware forensics | AMExtractor | AMExtractor, a tool for acquiring volatile physical memory from a wide range of Android devices and supports rootkit detection |
| Memory forensics | Layout Expert | Calculate memory layout of critical kernel structures at runtime on the target system without extra tools, such as compiler tool chain |
| Memory forensics | BinGold | The tool accurately and automatically recovering the semantics of a binary code |
| Software/DB forensics | Forensic Email Analysis Tool | A tool which allows for multiple emails to be analyzed and indexed in order to reduce the number of emails that need to be viewed in detail |
| Device/IoT forensics | DRone Open-source Parser (DROP) | Parses proprietary DAT files extracted from the drone's nonvolatile internal storage |
| Malware forensics | Lua dissector | Protocol dissector in Wireshark using Lua coding language |
| Software/DB forensics | Digital Forensics Framework (DFF) plugin | Investigate whether a technically secure selective deletion is possible |
| Device/IoT forensics | Cutter | Extracts SMTP configuration from the network log and parses its to obtain email addresses, username and password |
| Device/IoT forensics | N/A | Allows direct network-based communication with the PLC (no intermediate server is needed) |
| Device/IoT forensics | Cloud-based IoT Forensic Toolkit (CIFT) | Identification, acquisition and analysis of both native artifacts from the cloud and client-centric artifacts from local devices |
| Computer forensics | Automated Provenance (AutoProv) | Recreate the provenance of a file of interest on a forensic image |
| Multimedia forensics | Decision Theoretic carving program (DECA) | Designed for fast carving of large non- fragmented JPEGs like high resolution pictures produced by DSLR cameras |

*(continued)*

*Table 7.2 (Cont.)*

| *Category* | *Name of the Tool* | *Capability of the Tool* |
|---|---|---|
| Memory forensics | Heapinfo Heapdump Heapsearch Heaprefs | heapinfo: provides an abstract overview over the number of arenas, chunks and their sizes. heapdump: dumps all allocated and freed chunks to disk in separate files for further analysis. heapsearch: searches all chunks for the given string, regex or pointer(s). heaprefs: examines the data part of the given chunk(s) for any references to other chunks. |
| Malware forensics | AndroParse | Analysis of Android app using the parser to extract 4 most common features of an Android app: permissions, APIs, strings and intents |
| Software/DB forensics | MongoDB Deleted Data Recovery Tool | Recovery of deleted data from a MongoDB |
| Device/IoT forensics | Forensic Evidence Acquisition and Analysis System (FEAAS) | FEAAS consolidates evidentiary data into a readable report that can infer user events (like entering or leaving a home) and what triggered an event |
| Malware forensics | Fordroid | An inter-component static forensic tool for Android applications which automatically identifies sensitive information is stored in local storage |
| Network forensics | Wifimit | The package combines several existing tools and attack strategies to bypass the wireless security mechanisms like WEP, WPA, and WPS |
| Computer forensics | Timeline2GUI | Used to analyse CSV log file by Log2Timeline |
| Device/IoT forensics | Plugins/Autospy plugins | Analysis parsing plugins – 3 plugins and 1 standalone Plugin extract from Qbee camera – extract cloud credentials |
| Computer forensics | Sync Triage | The plugins create a list of synced devices which includes details about the inferred device but also the provenance |
| Computer forensics | NTFSObjIDParser | The prototype correlates Object ID entries with the MFT record found in the entry reference by parsing the MFT record's SIA, FNA and OIA |
| Memory forensics | Winesap (Volatility plugin) | Analyzes the registry-based Windows Auto Start Extendibility Points (ASEPs) in a memory dump |
| Software/DB forensics | Bring2lite | To connect recovered data to its according database schema and table. Hence the context and the data types of each record field are known |

Table 7.2 (Cont.)

| Category | Name of the Tool | Capability of the Tool |
|---|---|---|
| Memory forensics | Hooktracer | Performs post-processing of api hooks-generated output in conjunction with our own memory analysis algorithms |
| Device/IoT forensics | NAVER Clova | Designed to collect command history artifacts directly through the communication with the cloud |
| Software/DB forensics | Database Forensic File Format (DB3F) Database Forensic Toolkit (DF-Toolkit), | Database Forensic Toolkit (DF- Toolkit): used to view and search data stored in DB3F. DF-Toolkit: to view and filter DBMS forensic artifacts stored in DB3F |
| Software/B forensics | AFF4 evidence container | It provides the same logical imaging primitives as existing approaches, with the advantages of deduplicated content storage, etc |
| Memory forensics | Ptenum | Able to detect executable pages despite any intentional (or unintentional) hiding technique |
| Memory forensics | Vivedump | Used in the analysis of memory dumps of HTC Vive VR systems and share related datasets. It will output a textual of all evidence data |
| Device/IoT forensics | Digital Drone Forensic application | Primary focus on analyzing the essential log parameters of drones |
| Malware forensics | BotDAD | The module starts with parsing the PCAP file and generates the CSV file for both request and response features |

### *Tier 1: Thing layer (edge) for data collection*

Vital signs for personal healthcare are gathered from patients' gadgets in this tier. These medical devices have a variety of sensors that track physiological parameters like blood pressure and ECGs. Every sensor transmits a signal, which is then processed to yield the outcomes and the following data collected from various sensors into the pool.

- *i. Blood pressure sensor*
- *ii. SPO2 sensor*
- *iii. ECG/EEG/EMG sensors*
- *iv. Temperature sensor*

### *Tier 2: Network layer (fog) for data communication*

After receiving the data from the previous layer, this layer alerts the user's designated personal devices. Additionally, using an external gateway that enables long-distance connection, this layer is in charge of routinely

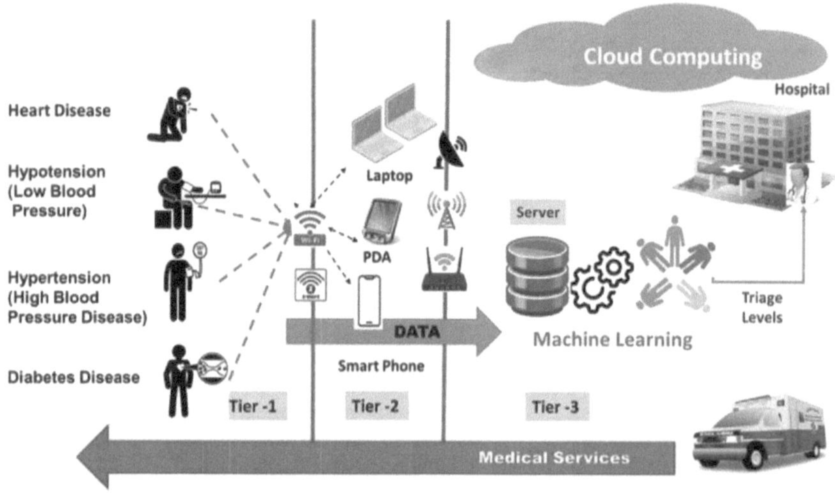


*Figure 7.9* Integrating ML in IoMT for telehealthcare.

transmitting data to the distant server. Since the gateway connects the public access network to the home networks, data are sent to a central server or hospital by the gateway's components.

### *Tier 3: Data management/ML layer/processing/storage layer*

The last layer is where the ML/data processing and storage process is carried out. Sensors and server-based devices are among the medical sources in the system. Real-time data delivery is provided. Doctors can, however, examine data in real time by utilizing the remote control. This layer may have cloud for data storage and infrastructure for processing.

#### ML layer:

This ML layer is used to analyze large volumes of real-time medical data collected from connected devices, identify patterns, predict potential health risks, and provide insights to healthcare providers for better decision-making and personalized patient care; essentially, it leverages ML algorithms to extract meaningful information from the raw data, enabling proactive healthcare management and improved patient outcomes.

#### Application layer:

The application layer in IoMT is primarily used for data transmission and processing of medical information collected from connected medical devices, enabling features like real-time patient monitoring, remote patient care, early disease detection, and facilitating communication between medical devices and healthcare systems; essentially, it allows for the practical application [25] of the data gathered by IoMT devices through functionalities like data analysis, alerts, and integration with healthcare platforms.

**Applications:**

1. **Remote monitoring/diagnosis:** ML algorithms analyze data from IoMT devices to diagnose diseases remotely. This allows healthcare providers to offer timely and accurate diagnoses without the need for in-person visits.
2. **Patient monitoring:** IoMT devices equipped with ML continuously monitor patients' vital signs and health metrics. These data are analyzed in real time to detect anomalies and alert healthcare providers, ensuring prompt intervention.
3. **Personalized treatment:** ML tailors treatment plans based on individual patient data collected from IoMT devices. This personalized approach improves the effectiveness of treatments and enhances patient care.
4. **Emergency response:** ML-based telemedicine frameworks prioritize remote patients with chronic diseases for emergency healthcare services. This ensures that patients with urgent needs receive timely medical attention.
5. **Data security:** ML enhances the security of IoMT systems by detecting and mitigating cyber threats, ensuring that patient data is handled securely and in compliance with privacy regulations.

These advancements facilitate timely medical interventions and personalized healthcare solutions. However, several limitations [26] persist that hinder the full realization of these technologies.

**Limitations and challenges of machine learning in IoMT**

While the potential of ML in IoMT for telemedicine is substantial, addressing these limitations is crucial for enhancing the effectiveness and accessibility of healthcare solutions. Future research should focus on developing cost-effective strategies and improving data security measures to overcome these challenges [27].

i. **Data privacy concerns:** The integration of IoMT raises significant issues regarding patient data security and privacy, necessitating robust encryption and regulatory compliance.
ii. **Implementation barriers:** Socioeconomic factors, such as high costs and technological access in less-developed regions, limit the widespread adoption of these systems.

iii. **Device reliability:** Challenges related to sensor accuracy and data transmission speed can affect the reliability of health monitoring systems.
iv. **Interoperability:** Diverse healthcare devices and systems often lack compatibility, complicating data sharing and integration.
v. **Energy consumption:** Many IoMT devices are constrained by battery life, which can limit the deployment of complex ML algorithms.
vi. **Limited data availability:** Insufficient data can hinder the training of effective ML models, leading to biased or inaccurate predictions.
vii. **Cloud Integration:** The combination of IoMT with cloud computing enhances data storage and processing capabilities, facilitating better patient interactions and diagnostic accuracy.

While the potential of ML in IoMT for telemedicine is substantial, addressing these challenges is crucial for enhancing the effectiveness and accessibility of healthcare solutions. Future research should focus on developing cost-effective strategies and improving data security measures to overcome these challenges [28]. Implementing ML in the IoMT for telemedicine presents several challenges and limitations that must be addressed to enhance healthcare delivery. These challenges include data security, privacy concerns, interoperability, and the need for efficient algorithms capable of handling large volumes of data [29].

**Addressing the challenges**

- **Enhanced security protocols:** Implementing advanced cybersecurity measures, such as data encryption and two-factor authentication, can mitigate risks.
- **Development of novel architectures:** Exploring new ML architectures and optimization techniques can improve model efficiency and adaptability in low-resource environments.
- **Standardization efforts:** Promoting interoperability standards among IoMT devices can facilitate seamless data exchange and integration.

## 7.6 DIGITAL FORENSICS IN TELEHEALTHCARE

DF in tele-healthcare [30] serves as a critical safeguard to ensure the security and integrity of patient data, systems, and networks. DF supports the trustworthiness of tele-healthcare, making it a safer and more reliable option for remote healthcare delivery. IoMT forensics [31, 32] is essential for protecting patient safety, maintaining trust in medical technologies, and ensuring compliance with healthcare standards. The various DF tools used in tele-healthcare are shown in Figure 7.10. The performance metrics of NB, RF, and LR algorithms in IoMT and DF/IoMT environments are tabulated in Table 7.3 and plotted in graph shown in Figure 7.11.

### 7.6.1 Digital forensics in telehealthcare

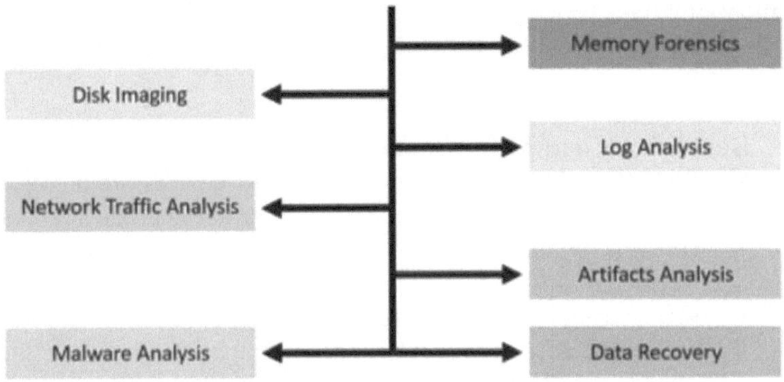


*Figure 7.10* Digital forensics tools in telehealthcare.

*Table 7.3* Performance metrics for conventional and DF/IoMT methods

| | *With conventional IoMT method* | | | | *With DF/IoMT method* | | | |
|---|---|---|---|---|---|---|---|---|
| *Algorithm* | *Accuracy* | *Precision* | *Recall* | *F–Score* | *Accuracy* | *Precision* | *Recall* | *F–Score* |
| Naive Bayes | 0.70 | 0.77 | 0.73 | 0.72 | 0.61667 | 0.67238 | 0.61212 | 0.68009 |
| Random Forest | 0.7222 | 0.73 | 0.72 | 0.72 | 0.71666 | 0.77658 | 0.66667 | 0.70705 |
| Logistic Regression | 0.75 | 0.76 | 0.75 | 0.75 | 0.65 | 0.67426 | 0.67 | 0.66175 |

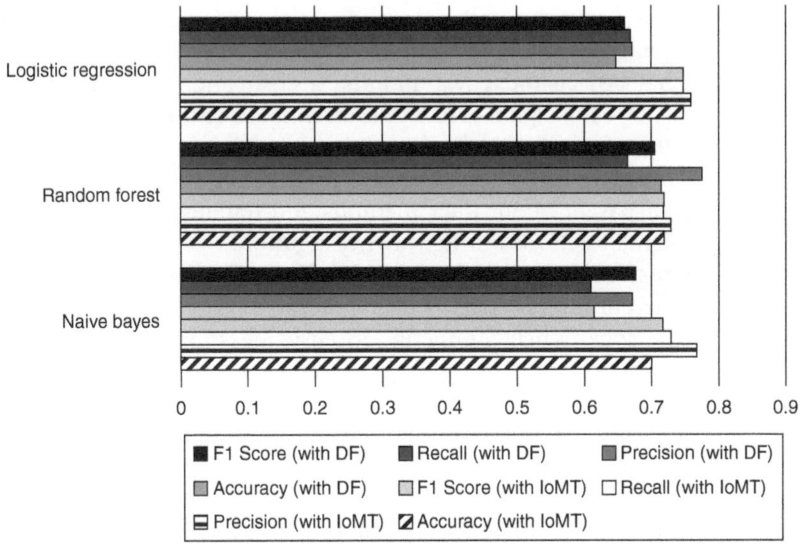


*Figure 7.11* Performance comparison of IoMT vs DF/IoMT.

## 7.7 AI ETHICS

In the context of IoMT and DF, ethical considerations are paramount, encompassing data privacy, patient confidentiality, and the responsible use of collected evidence. The following is the ethical considerations [33] for DF in IoMT.

i. Data privacy and patient confidentiality
   - **Protecting sensitive information:** IoMT devices often collect and transmit highly sensitive medical data, making privacy a critical concern. Digital forensic investigations must prioritize the protection of this data, ensuring it's handled ethically and legally.
   - **Minimizing data collection:** Forensic specialists should only collect the data necessary for the investigation, avoiding unnecessary data collection and storage.
   - **Anonymization and pseudonymization:** Techniques like anonymization or pseudonymization should be employed to protect patient identities when sharing or analyzing data.
   - **Data security:** Robust security measures are essential to prevent unauthorized access, modification, or disclosure of sensitive medical data during storage, transmission, and analysis.

ii. Legal and ethical challenges
   - **Compliance with laws and regulations:** Digital forensic investigations must adhere to all applicable laws/regulations, including data protection laws like HIPAA (US) and GDPR (Europe).
   - **Obtaining consent:** When possible, obtaining informed consent from patients or their legal representatives before conducting digital forensic investigations is crucial.
   - **Chain of custody:** Maintaining a clear and verifiable chain of custody for digital evidence is essential to ensure its integrity and admissibility in legal proceedings.
   - **Transparency and accountability:** Forensic specialists should be transparent about their methods and findings, and accountable for their actions during the investigation.
   - **Cross-border investigations:** IoMT devices can be used across different jurisdictions, which can lead to legal and jurisdictional challenges when conducting forensic investigations.

iii. Ethical principles for DF
   - **Integrity:** Maintaining the integrity of digital evidence is paramount, ensuring that it remains unaltered and reliable.
   - **Objectivity:** Forensic specialists should approach investigations objectively, without bias or preconceived notions.

- **Confidentiality:** Protecting the confidentiality of sensitive information is a fundamental ethical principle.
- **Competence:** Forensic specialists should possess the necessary skills and knowledge to conduct investigations effectively and ethically.
- **Honesty:** Forensic specialists should be honest and transparent in their findings and reporting.

## 7.8 CURRENT TRENDS AND FUTURE CHALLENGES

DF in the IoMT faces challenges including data security, privacy concerns, device heterogeneity, limited processing power, and the need for specialized tools and procedures to collect and analyze data from diverse medical devices and cloud environments. It faces challenges including data collection from diverse and resource-constrained devices, data integrity and privacy concerns, and the need for specialized expertise and tools. The current trends in DF, shaping the field in 2025 are listed below. The future trends in DF in IoMT are depicted in Figure 7.12.

i. **AI and machine learning integration:** Artificial intelligence is being used to automate forensic processes, analyze large datasets, and identify patterns or anomalies more efficiently. This reduces manual workload and enhances accuracy.

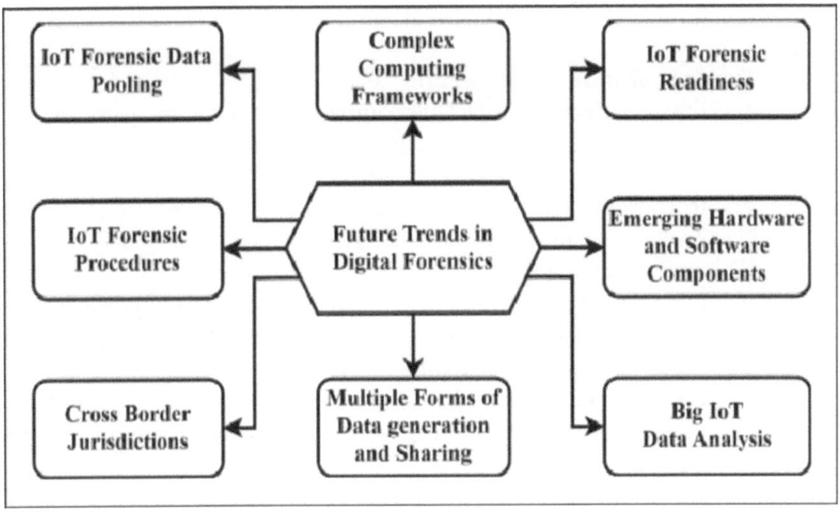


*Figure 7.12* Future trends in digital forensics.

ii. **Cloud forensics:** With the growing reliance on cloud storage, forensic experts are developing specialized tools to investigate data breaches and recover evidence from distributed cloud environments.
iii. **Mobile and IoT forensics:** As mobile devices and IoT devices become more prevalent, forensic techniques are adapting to extract and analyze data from these sources, including wearables and smart home devices.
iv. **Deepfake detection:** The rise of deepfake technology has led to the development of tools to identify and analyze manipulated media, ensuring the authenticity of digital evidence.
v. **Blockchain forensics:** With the increasing use of cryptocurrencies, blockchain forensics is gaining importance in tracking transactions and uncovering financial crimes.
vi. **Quantum-resistant forensics:** As quantum computing advances, forensic methods are being updated to address potential threats to encryption and data security.
vii. **Remote forensics:** The shift to remote work has increased the need for forensic tools that can investigate incidents without physical access to devices or networks.
viii. **Ethical AI and data privacy:** Forensic practices are focusing on maintaining ethical standards and ensuring compliance with data privacy regulations during investigations.

These trends highlight the dynamic nature of DF and its critical role in addressing modern cybersecurity challenges. While these challenges are significant, they also present opportunities for innovation in telemedicine. Addressing these limitations can lead to more effective and secure healthcare solutions, ultimately improving patient outcomes.

i. Data acquisition and collection
   - **Diverse devices:** IoMT encompasses a wide range of devices with varying capabilities and data formats, making it difficult to develop a universal forensic approach.
   - **Resource constraints:** Many IoMT devices have limited storage, processing power, and connectivity, making data collection and analysis challenging.
   - **Data volatility:** IoMT devices often store data temporarily or in volatile memory, which can be lost or modified easily, requiring rapid data acquisition and preservation.
   - **Data format diversity:** IoMT devices use various data formats, including sensor data, images, and logs, which can be difficult to extract and analyze.
   - **Data volume:** The sheer volume of data generated by IoMT devices can be overwhelming, requiring efficient data collection and storage techniques.

ii. Specific challenges in IoMT forensics
   - **Device diversity:** IoMT encompasses a wide range of devices, each with its own unique characteristics and data storage mechanisms, posing challenges for forensic analysis.
   - **Real-time data:** IoMT devices often generate real-time data, requiring forensic specialists to develop techniques for capturing and analyzing this data in a timely and accurate manner.
   - **Interoperability:** IoMT devices may communicate with various systems and devices, requiring forensic specialists to understand the interoperability aspects of these systems.
   - **Lack of standards:** The IoMT field is relatively new, and there are still gaps in standards and best practices for DF.

iii. Data integrity and chain of custody
   - **Data alteration:** IoMT devices are susceptible to data tampering and modification, making it crucial to ensure the integrity of collected evidence.
   - **Chain of custody:** Establishing a clear chain of custody for evidence collected from IoMT devices is essential for legal admissibility.
   - **Data synchronization:** IoMT devices often synchronize data with cloud services, making it difficult to determine the origin and authenticity of data.

iv. Specialized expertise and tools
   - **Lack of skilled professionals:** There is a shortage of forensic professionals with the expertise to conduct IoMT investigations.
   - **Need for specialized tools:** IoMT forensic investigations require specialized tools and techniques that are not readily available.
   - **Training and education:** Forensic professionals need to be trained on the latest IoMT technologies, forensic techniques and tools.

v. Ethics, privacy and compliance:
   IoMT devices often collect sensitive patient data, requiring strict adherence to privacy regulations such as HIPAA/GDPR. Also, techniques for anonymizing patient data to protect privacy while allowing forensic analysis are needed. IoMT forensics must comply with relevant regulations and standards, such as those related to data security and privacy.

## 7.9 CONCLUSION

In this book chapter, the digital Forensic techniques are applied to enhance personalized healthcare systems within the framework of the IoMT towards smart Tele-healthcare. Since AI and ML fosters trust and guarantees decision-making authority, it is regarded as significant in healthcare applications. The use of DF in IoMT has facilitated the development of AI/ML methods for robotic surgery, personalized treatment, prediction methods, and the diagnosis of cardiac disease. In the context of IoMT, digital forensic techniques are used to improve customized healthcare systems. These DF techniques will help the healthcare providers/physicians to make the transparent and best decision in telehealthcare system. Hence, DF is much impactful in tele-healthcare applications because it ensures integrity, confidentiality, and availability of healthcare/personal records and builds confidence. Hence, DF techniques in IoMT are analyzed to telemedicine applications such as robotic surgery, personalized health care, prediction techniques, and cardiac disease detection.

## REFERENCES

[1] Sadeghi-Niaraki, A. (2023). Internet of Thing (IoT) review of review: Bibliometric overview since its foundation. *Future Generation Computer Systems*, *143*, 361–377.

[2] Hemalatha, R. J., Akila, D., Balaganesh, D., & Paul, A. (Eds.). (2022). The Internet of Medical Things (IoMT). Wiley. https://doi.org/10.1002/9781119769200

[3] Mariappan, R. (2024). Extensive review of literature on explainable AI (XAI) in healthcare applications. *Recent Advances in Computer Science and Communications*, *18*(1), E200324228159. https://doi.org/10.2174/0126662558296699240314055348

[4] Vishnu, S., Ramson, S. R. J., & Jegan, R. (2020). Internet of Medical Things (IoMT) – An overview, 5th International Conference on Devices, Circuits and Systems (ICDCS). In 2020 5th Intl Conference on Devices, Circuits and Systems (ICDCS). IEEE. https://doi.org/10.1109/icdcs48716.2020.243558.

[5] Khaled, A. E. (2022). Internet of Medical Things (IoMT): Overview, taxonomies, and classifications. *Journal of Computer and Communications*, *10* (8), 64–89. 10.4236/jcc.2022.108005

[6] Moutaib, M., Ahajjam, T., Fattah, M., Farhaoui, Y., & Aghoutane, B. (2022). Internet of medical things. In Networking Technologies in Smart Healthcare (pp. 79–96). CRC Press. https://doi.org/10.1201/9781003239888-4

[7] Gatouillat, A., Badr, Y., Massot, B., & Sejdic, E. (2018). Internet of Medical Things: A review of recent contributions dealing with cyber-physical systems in medicine. *IEEE Internet of Things Journal*, *5* (5), 3810–3822. https://doi.org/10.1109/jiot.2018.2849014.

[8] Årnes, A., Haas, P., Vigna, G., & Kemmerer, R. A. (2007). Using a virtual security testbed for digital forensic reconstruction. *Journal in Computer Virology*, 2, 275–289.

[9] Aitken, C., & Taroni, F. (2004). *Statistics and the Evaluation of Evidence for Forensic Scientists*, 2nd ed. Hoboken, NJ: Wiley.

[10] Alva, A., & Endicott-Popovsky, B. (2012). Digital evidence education in schools of law. *Journal of Digital Forensics*, 7 (2), 183–192.

[11] Altheide, C., & Harlan, C. (2011). *Digital Forensics with Open Source Tools*. Rockland, MA: Syngress, Elsevier.

[12] Pollitt, M. (2010). A history of digital forensics. In: Chow, KP., Shenoi, S. (eds) Advances in Digital Forensics VI. Digital Forensics. IFIP Advances in Information and Communication Technology, vol. 337. Springer, Berlin, Heidelberg. https://doi.org/10.1007/978-3-642-15506-2_1

[13] Alazab, M., Abu Khurma, R., Awajan, A., & Wedyan, M. (2022). Digital forensics classification based on a hybrid neural network and the salp swarm algorithm. *Electronics*, *11*(12), 1903. https://doi.org/10.3390/electronics11121903

[14] Beebe, N. (2009). Digital Forensic Research: The Good, the Bad and the Unaddressed. In: Peterson, G., Shenoi, S. (eds) Advances in Digital Forensics V. Digital Forensics 2009. IFIP Advances in Information and Communication Technology, vol 306. Springer, Berlin, Heidelberg.

[15] Wu, T., Breitinger, F., & O'Shaughnessy, S. (2020). Digital forensic tools: Recent advances and enhancing the status quo. *Forensic Science International Digital Investigation*, 34, 300999. https://doi.org/10.1016/j.fsidi.2020.300999

[16] Razdan, S., & Sharma, S. (2021). Internet of Medical Things (IoMT): Overview, emerging technologies, and case studies. *IETE Technical Review*, *39* (4), 775–788. https://doi.org/10.1080/02564602.2021.1927863

[17] Wal, P., Wal, A., Verma, N., Karunakakaran, R., & Kapoor, A. (2022). Internet of medical things – The future of healthcare. *The Open Public Health Journal*, *15* (1), 1–9. https://doi.org/10.2174/18749445-v15-e221215-2022-142

[18] Manickam, P., Mariappan, et.al.,(2022). Artificial intelligence (AI) and IoMT assisted biomedical systems for intelligent healthcare. *Biosensors*, *12*(8), 562. https://doi.org/10.3390/bios12080562

[19] Muheidat, F., & Tawalbeh, L. A. (2023). AIoMT artificial intelligence (AI) and internet of medical things (IoMT). In *Elsevier-Computational Intelligence for Medical IoT (MIoT) Applications* (pp. 33–54).

[20] Mehta, R., Prasad, V. K., Mishra, S., Tanwar, S., & Patel, Y. (2023). Evolving technologies: IoT and artificial intelligence for healthcare informatics. In Institution of Engineering and Technology eBooks (pp. 231–254). https://doi.org/10.1049/pbhe041e_ch8

[21] Muheidat, F.,&Tawalbeh, L. A. (2023). AIoMT artificial intelligence (AI) and internet of medical things (IoMT). In Elsevier eBooks (pp.33–54). https://doi.org/10.1016/b978-0-323-99421-7.00013-1

[22] Pandiaraj, M., Siva, A., Mariappan., S., Murugesan., S. , Hansda., A., Kaushik., R., Shinde., S. P. (2022). Artificial intelligence (AI) and internet of medical things (IoMT) assisted biomedical systems for intelligent healthcare. *Biosensors*, *12*(8) 562. doi:10.3390/bios12080562

[23] Dubettier, A., Gernot, T., Giguet, E., & Rosenberger, C. (2023). File type identification tools for digital investigations. *Forensic Science International Digital Investigation*, 46, 301574. https://doi.org/10.1016/j.fsidi.2023.301574

[24] Binbusayyis, A., Alaskar, H., Vaiyapuri, T. *et al.* (2022). An investigation and comparison of machine learning approaches for intrusion detection in IoMT network. *Journal of Supercomputing*, *78*, 17403–17422. https://doi.org/10.1007/s11227-022-04568-3

[25] Dwivedi, R., Mehrotra, D., & Chandra, S. (2021). Potential of internet of medical things (IoMT) applications in building a smart healthcare system: A systematic review. *Journal of Oral Biology and Craniofacial Research*, *12*(2), 302–318. https://doi.org/10.1016/j.jobcr.2021.11.010

[26] Bharathi, M., & Amsaveni, A. (2021). Machine learning with IoMT: Opportunities and research challenges. In *Internet of Things* (pp. 235–252). Springer. https://doi.org/10.1007/978-3-030-63937-2_13

[27] Baig, Z. A., Szewczyk, P., Valli, C., Rabadia, P., Hannay, P., Chernyshev, M., ... & Peacock, M. (2017). Future challenges for smart cities: Cyber-security and digital forensics. *Digital Investigation*, *22*, 3–13. www.sciencedirect.com/science/article/pii/S1742287617300579

[28] Casino, F., Dasaklis, T. K., Spathoulas, G. P., Anagnostopoulos, M., Ghosal, A., Borocz, I., Solanas, A., Conti, M., & Patsakis, C. (2022). Research trends, challenges, and emerging topics in digital forensics: A review of reviews. *IEEE Access*, *10*, 25464–25493. https://ieeexplore.ieee.org/document/9720948

[29] Kebande, V. R., & Awad, A. I. (2024). Industrial internet of things ecosystems security and digital forensics: Achievements, open challenges, and future directions. *ACM Computing Surveys*, *56*(5), 1–37. https://dl.acm.org/doi/10.1145/3635030

[30] Yaacoub, J.-P. A., Noura, H. N., Salman, O., & Chehab, A. (2022). Advanced digital forensics and anti-digital forensics for IoT systems: Techniques, limitations and recommendations. *Internet of Things*, *19*, 100544. www.sciencedirect.com/science/article/pii/S25426605

[31] Mulchay, C., & Knuth, S. (2023). Best practices in tele-forensic methods of gathering data. *Journal of Forensic Social Work*, 7(2), 3–17. https://doi.org/10.15763/issn.1936-9298.2023.7.2.3-17

[32] Ellouze, N., Rekhis, S., & Boudriga, N. (2016). Forensic investigation of digital crimes in healthcare applications. In Advances in data mining and database management book series (pp. 169–210). https://doi.org/10.4018/978-1-7998-3025-2.ch017.

[33] Rezaei, M., Jafari-Sadeghi, V., Cao, D., & Mahdiraji, H. A. (2021). Key indicators of ethical challenges in digital healthcare: A combined Delphi exploration and confirmative factor analysis approach with evidence from Khorasan province in Iran. *Technological Forecasting and Social Change*, *167*, 120724. https://doi.org/10.1016/j.techfore.2021.120724

Chapter 8

# AI-driven forensics in IoMT

## Strengthening security, legal compliance, and ethical governance

*Vijaishree Dubey Pandey, Vijeta Verma, Rituraj Sinha, and Shashank Solanki*

## 8.1 INTRODUCTION

Modern digital evidence problems have become complex, leading investigators to improve their investigative process by integrating artificial intelligence (AI) technology into forensic systems. Criminal investigators encounter digital evidence in their work more often, so they introduce modern systems for their investigations Investigation teams must sustain security measures for evidence through established digital evidence procedures, which enable appropriate findings before the court requests investigation materials because of progressing digital technology. According to Ref [1], forensic investigators must arrange the elements of a digital database chronologically when they need to show specific incidents. During the last decade, investigators used forensic-led principle-based digital investigation systems, which helped technology achieve unprecedented advances. The primary technology achievement in addressing major cybercrime operations belongs to software analysis development. The development of digital forensic technology advances because AI and machine learning speed up system data processing for evidence acquisition [2].

Data science analytics monitoring systems reach success points when social network systems integrate with author identification bodies, according to the findings of [3]. Organisations reach their investigative levels with the help of expert data analysis methods when such techniques help probable cause investigations find new patterns. AI delivers fast-resolution methods for handling size-related problems that appear during investigations of extensive electronic evidence in digital forensics cases. The computer software needs predefined development programs that address all operational data types. Big data analysis techniques like MapReduce allow modern developers to improve law enforcement cases using AI algorithms that examine evidence from databases, network information, and digital photo assets. The innovation delivered two key advantages for evidence verification operations and expedient digital evidence processing. The advanced system executes human relational studies through its well-defined operational functions and writes

DOI: 10.1201/9781003640325-8

pattern matching to detect authors during source validation operations. According to Ref [4], the police gained positive results from their forensic examinations with the support of dependable AI solutions.

Further, the IoMT led to a fundamental transformation of healthcare systems by enhancing the investigation of medical information and the methods of delivering healthcare treatment and control capabilities. Medical facilities built an extensive network comprising multiple security points of vulnerability. Healthcare digital innovation emerged by merging the Internet of Medical Things smartphones and smart devices with cloud services, enabling access to healthcare treatments that boost patient health outcomes [5]. The more extended deployment of IoMT devices leads to accelerated device interconnectivity and exposes possible security vulnerabilities to hackers [6].

IoMT technology delivers three fundamental advantages to healthcare: pandemic management, real-time supervision, and personalised medical services. IoT devices and their related data have become prevalent throughout networks to present total solutions for resolving the associated security challenges. Medical experts [7] explain how strong response protocols in IoT-generated monitoring systems are necessary due to emerging vaccine-resistant strains. Edge devices connect to healthcare data infrastructure, escalating security exposure to sensitive health information because of malicious programs, ransomware breaches, and data theft acts, as described by [8]. Security measurement elevation must advance to work toward monitoring all challenges facing the complete IoMT system environment.

Security challenges found in IoMT systems stem from three basic forms: faulty devices combined with insecure data transfer protocols and unacceptable data storage systems. A proper solution emerges from hardware remediation, improved software stability, authentication upgrades, encryption control, and software updates. Protecting the environment requires two essential components: safe communication protocols and intrusion detection systems. At its best, patient care requires every strategic plan component to be implemented effectively [9].

The Healthcare transformation occurs through IoMT, which connects devices to sensors that generate health process information before guiding this information in the proper direction. According to Ref [10], medical diagnosis performance increases in the digital healthcare ecosystem because its electronic delivery system improves operational efficiency and supports better remote care monitoring and superior healthcare diagnostics. Strong forensic methods must be implemented to enable widespread IoMT deployment because security threats and data tampering appear while adopting this technology [11]. Cyberattacks against IoMT equipment and their linked networks continue to increase, so healthcare providers must immediately establish security measures alongside incident response systems. Unique forensic technology requires immediate development because real-time data transmission interacts with privacy regulations that define the IoMT technological setting [12].

Through its integration with IoMT forensic operations, AI creates solutions that provide operational performance improvements and highly precise results at scale. Several AI systems unite to detect irregularities and speed up evidence acquisition while conducting data analysis [13]. To handle security incident reconstruction processes, the system performs fast data processing that acts crucially in breach investigation and cyber assault response management stages. AI implementation within IoMT performs two vital security operations: danger discovery and threat response guidance. Prediction-based vulnerability assessments through the system detect platform weaknesses in devices and network and data system vulnerabilities. AI develops robust security structures that use real-time control performance assessment to create established procedural systems. Security protocols applied by these systems provide primary defences that protect patient data and devices used in IoMT [14].

Synthetic intelligence methods now detect top-level cyber threats by combining machine learning, deep learning, and natural language processing systems. When dealing with advanced persistent threats, AI-based systems achieve optimal results [15]. Through designed algorithms, management security policies receive recommendations for needed security control adjustments to handle current threats. Security systems using AI technology automatically detect how to adapt their digital surveillance capabilities without changing staffing expenses. The Random Forest algorithm is a machine learning technology that develops self-protecting security alerts for defending assets from active cyberattacks while providing unknown threat identification capabilities [16].

AI-based forensic tools are essential to combat the security vulnerabilities affecting Internet of Medical Things devices and their network infrastructure. AI improves fundamental crime investigation functions because automated anomaly searches within the system lead investigators to discover evidence more rapidly. AI performs two duties: surveying medical devices throughout networks and examining device susceptibilities to preserve medical system security and protect patient privacy. AI development enables IoMT forensics by strengthening cyber threat protections to reach the maximum potential benefits of connected healthcare, according to [17].

This research aims to create an AI-run forensic system that will solve all complexities alongside security and ethical problems within the Internet of Medical Things infrastructure [18]. This research studies existing forensic solutions because medical device diversity and enormous fast data transfer demands create important obstacles for IoMT infrastructure. The assessment of various threats, such as breaches, intrusions and tampering, must be adequately conducted in security research for Internet of Medical

Things systems to develop preventive security measures and emergency response plans [19].

## 8.2 AI IN IOMT FORENSIC INVESTIGATIONS: AN OVERVIEW

AI technology allows forensic science to produce better results during crime scene assessments, evidence confirmation, and suspect investigation procedures. The system achieves peak performance by examining extensive datasets to generate patterns that provide exact results, which create faster investigations [20]. The new digital evidence technologies require complex management capabilities that AI demonstrates a strong potential to handle correctly. Established AI principles connected to digital forensics procedures enable organisations to process information quickly and detect evidence better. US federal entities, state departments, and departmental bodies have authorised AI digital forensics enhancements [21].

AI and automation deployment in forensic applications yield three principal advantages: higher operational excellence, economic resource savings, and decreased error rates. Organisations create higher profits through investments in automation since operational costs remain below the prices of manual human workers [22]. Limited operational budgets show that AI works perfectly for forensic laboratories because it combines economic advantages with enhanced analytical capabilities. When human operational knowledge is combined with AI, it results in exceptional success during crime investigation processes because the system aligns expert skills with established techniques and functional disciplinary understanding. Teamwork between personnel helps increase the detection ability of digital evidence and strengthens cyber network security The research-based analysis of AI operational boundaries needs extensive investigation to establish a complete understanding [23].

AI automation facilitates forensic scientists in tackling complex issues in their available time while automation responsibilities run independently. AI systems gain anomaly recognition capabilities during training, eventually producing reports while labelling evidence and executing work tasks with higher speed [24]. Implementing new efficiency technology diminishes investigative operation time and human error to produce accurate, dependable outcomes. Digital forensic staff leverage automated instruments to perform three basic tasks: collecting evidence, building documentation, and processing evidence during the development of automated analytics solutions. The operational benefits of AI forensic software include two main advantages: enhanced accuracy of trustworthy results and improved specific field performance. Experts use AI techniques in digital evidence assessments to process enormous amounts of digital data quickly and precisely, as described [25].

Automated systems require additional development to convert observed data into textual outputs. ART at maximal capability uses contextual evaluation procedures to extract the exact meanings of digital evidence from details to produce precise outcome analysis. The continuous research in digital forensics develops because digital evidence remains the essential foundation for criminal investigation evidence [26]. Forensic investigation deployments using AI technology reduce case duration while producing superior operational outcomes. Discoveries emerge for forensic technologies through AI technical advances.

Also, AI produces innovations that help users establish quick threat detection methods and produce predictive capabilities above standard security operations. Information technology assessment threats serve as investigator systems that increase modern digital cyber security response times when combined with threat detection procedures [27]. The optimal AI performance entails recognising abnormal pattern sequences followed by quick precision solutions that address prolonged sophisticated security threats via automated system vulnerability identification. The defence systems built with natural language processing algorithms unite deep learning models and machine learning capabilities to develop time-critical protective measures for essential data and network systems. AI maintains operational security capabilities that let it manage and find security alerts in constantly evolving environments [28].

Institutions can detect system abnormalities and malware categories through AI network defence tools to prevent cyber threats. Today, AI systems identify exact patterns through extensive database checks. Today's investigation systems use AI to execute faster assessments of critical infrastructure through network evaluations. AI develops efficient and affordable crisis solutions that defend various sectors, including engineering and cyberspace medicine [29].

Networks running machine-learning-based integrated systems face security issues because AI has spread widely across multiple life domains. Security systems must develop new safety protocols persistently to decrease the frequency of cyberattacks. The implementation of proactive AI solutions needs precise execution for cybercrime conflict because AI technologies develop both discovery tools and protective tools [30]. Experts recognise AI fundamental principles as essential for cyberspace information security solution development since they assume the next breakthroughs will emerge from AI research. Systems employing AI -based autonomic computing operate independently through self-managing features that enable automatic adjustment and perform self-detection and self-repair functions to enhance fault tolerance and decrease adaptability requirements—the constant need for AI system advancement results from the escalating cyber dangers in the environment [31]. Programmable security requirements need to exist for AI systems because their built-in adaptive skills activate automatically.

Technology security systems operate fast detection programs and automatic response capabilities to ensure AI systems comply with digital security requirements. Active surveillance is required for AI tools, and systems need to run automatically when emergencies occur, as ethical rules and privacy legislation must remain balanced during system upkeep.

AI systems that merge with automated forensic evaluations mark a revolutionary change because they improve investigation precision while speeding up procedures and generating universality across all sectors. The combination of AI algorithms both automates evidence processing and reduces worker errors while improving laboratory work efficiency. Digital forensics investigation speeds up and produces target-focused results because AI systems generate precise answers from extensive data source inputs[32]. The AI adaptive learning method accumulates continuous patterns to deliver expert-level scholarly knowledge which helps forensic experts handle changing threats and requirements.

AI reaches successful outcomes in forensic evaluations only when it collaborates with skilled human specialists. Specialists use their contextual information to interpret data-based observations following machine intelligence and human expertise collaboration. AI systems collaborate with human operators to facilitate collaborative tasks that blend their respective skills into developing dependable forensic methods. Field experts have the capability to improve AI-generated output using their professional expertise to produce accurate and meaningful results [33]. The team collaboration strengthens the investigations and displays complete control over all important forensic decision-making processes. Verifiable statistical patterns that stem from impression and pattern evidence enable forensic investigators to produce unbiased results [34].

They explain that AI and automation implementation deliver two primary advantages for forensic assessment: enhanced productivity with higher quality outputs and decreased operational expenses. Organizations tend to select automated systems because of their reduced costs [35]. The automated solutions process diverse information categories above basic text translation capabilities. Law enforcement digital forensics enhanced by AI applications leads to higher investigation accuracy. It generates more resolved cases based on the research of AI operating in forensic assessments to bring substantial shifts that challenge cybersecurity operations and influence investigations conducted by law enforcement and legal processes. AI processes allow for improving human performance combined with better threat management procedures to create impartial forensic systems that develop strong public security frameworks [36].

The full readiness of AI-driven automated forensic evaluations depends on ongoing research-based development attempts. AI-based digital forensics research requires a remedy to existing deployment problems, and advanced implementation methods and optimised existing technical solutions must be established [37]. Scientists must evaluate all aspects of the technology to reach maximum operational capability because AI produces objective data that removes forensic subjectivity. Security measures deployed to forensic investigation capabilities and cybersecurity protection will experience substantial improvement. Introducing AI-powered automated forensic systems will produce significant modifications that will transform all areas of forensic work [38].

## 8.3 SECURITY CHALLENGES IN IOMT FORENSICS

Medical devices and health systems connect through Internet of Medical Things technology to transmit data for modern healthcare, including remote patient supervision and enhanced care delivery. The extensive interconnected nature of medical devices brings significant security risks that need thorough attention to protect medical data confidentiality, availability, and integrity. IoMT security and privacy challenges are hindered by institutions' limited ability to monitor components and enforce security policies. At the same time, its network-based device connection systems present data collection and decision-making enhancement capabilities [39]. Understanding these issues will enable the complete realisation of IoMT technology capabilities. The IoMT data contains multiple elements, including patient information and medical records, vital parameters, diagnosis outputs, and sensor measurement results. Multiple healthcare sources, including wearable devices, remote monitoring systems, and electronic health records, send data to cloud storage, which healthcare providers access data security has become more vulnerable because the IoMT advances healthcare data toward complete digitisation and extends its distribution across various locations and its frequent movement. Protecting sensitive data requires priority because privacy concerns are extreme The healthcare system uses patient information from this data to maintain transparency throughout all phases of patient tracking. Smartphones and other smart devices now represent a significant problem for healthcare privacy breaches. IoMT data, with its extensive distribution and complexity, establishes conditions that make security threats highly likely to occur [40].

Security threats within the IoMT data landscape include malware, ransomware data breaches and denial-of-service attacks, which break patient privacy and affect healthcare services while putting lives in danger from network issues and hacking. The practice of third-party control over patient data has revealed security vulnerabilities, according to [41]. Patient data protection becomes more difficult because information volumes rise steadily. A proper solution to combat dangers should use technical solutions, administrative practices, and physical defence methods. A complete security strategy must evaluate vulnerabilities across the entire data management period, from device collection to processing. Properly defending IoMT systems requires multiple protective methods, including robust authentication systems, encryption protocols, and continuous software developments to counter hacking attempts. Healthcare data breaches continue to increase, so healthcare organisations require better approaches to protect their information. Patient security is crucial because healthcare organisations gather sensitive data for network server storage to deliver healthcare services [42]. High trust levels in the sensitive information processing healthcare smartphone network represent the most essential priority. Organisations in healthcare need to meet the standards of HIPAA and GDPR to protect sensitive information and must face penalties when data breaches occur. Healthcare organisations must implement security protocols to give patients the right to access their information while acquiring their permissions for data utilisation.

Medical technology now benefits from the Internet of Things convergence to create the Internet of Medical Things that integrates multiple medical systems for better patient outcomes, operational efficiency, and remote healthcare control. The surge of Internet of Medical Things devices, between wearable fitness trackers and implantable medical devices, has led to massive flows of sensitive patient information that require strong defensive techniques to block improper data access and protect against data breaches and cyberattacks. Advanced digitisation and growing smartphone and smart device diffusion continue to increase the vulnerability landscape [43]. The safety of IoMT devices requires exceptional attention since security breaches can lead to multiple severe consequences, which range from privacy breaches to monetary losses and jeopardised patient safety and may even result in fatalities.

Malware injection attacks target IoMT devices because of their built-in design and configuration weaknesses. Unlawful perpetrators gain control through these attacks to steal sensitive data, disrupting regular device operations. IoMT devices suffer from multiple cyber threats because insufficient security controls allow attackers to launch attacks through weak authentication and encryption. The risk level remains high because IoMT devices connect numerous devices, which allows a single breached device to expose the entire network. The accelerating growth of IoT equipment has generated numerous security weaknesses that create issues for data handling and storage functions. Security precautions need immediate implementation because malware injection attacks against IoMT devices create severe consequences, such as security breaches, device malfunctions, and patient safety risks [44].

IoT device proliferation generates various security vulnerabilities that attract cybercriminals with opportunistic intentions. The inadequate security parameters and different designs, coupled with the restricted functionalities of these devices, make them vulnerable to various threats. IoMT devices attract hackers due to their large quantities of persistent internet connectivity, multiple vulnerabilities, and basic and unsecured setups. The specific development of malicious software targeting such devices resulted in complicated obstacles for existing intrusion detection methods [45]. The protection of IoMT devices has become essential because their adoption rate continues to rise quickly.

The forensic analysis of IoMT requires immediate attention because malware attacks and data breaches affect the limited capabilities of these devices, which operate on various platforms. The extensive data range and undefined network structure make traditional forensics techniques inadequate. Digital investigations become more complicated due to the absence of standard procedures and tools, which forces forensic investigators to produce new methods to handle digital evidence acquisition analysis and interpretation steps [46]. All IoT devices generate essential evidence artefacts that help investigators conduct their work. Investigators must understand undisclosed resources and their strategies to recover artefacts from these devices.

IoMT forensics uses incident response strategies and data collection activities before performing evidence analysis to address data breaches and malware attacks. During incident response, teams must detect security threats; afterwards, they separate them from the systems and eliminate dangers before maintaining evidence integrity. A comprehensive data collection process requires investigators to collaborate to acquire data from IoMT systems and IT infrastructures through multiple methods. Foreign examiners encounter difficulties dealing with the diverse range of IoT devices because of their heterogeneous nature. Evidence analysis involves examining acquired data to detect intrusive codes while following attacker actions until investigators establish the size of the incident impact. The sought objective entails obtaining complete insight into incidents, allowing organisations to implement remediation measures that strengthen their protective measures [47].

Further, the healthcare industry transformed significantly by adopting medical things-connected technology because doctors now monitor patients remotely while creating individual care plans and providing better diagnosis capabilities. The interconnection of various devices has created substantial security risks through which cyber attackers view IoMT devices as desirable targets. Security breaches need comprehensive forensic investigations to help investigators find essential causes, identify damages, and gather legal evidence, as detailed in [48]. The variety of IoMT platforms, data locations, and multiple communication protocols create substantial problems for collecting evidence. To efficiently retrieve and analyse essential information, investigators require extensive knowledge of different device constructs alongside data formats. IoMT systems spread data storage points between device-based storage cloud storage and local server storage, making it hard to locate and obtain full data access [49].

The reduced capabilities of several IoMT devices, such as their limited processing potential and restricted data storage capacities, negatively affect traditional forensic examination methods. The insufficient capabilities of these devices prevent them from running advanced forensic tools and maintaining abundant data storage, which complicates obtaining the entire unmodified device memory snapshot. Network segmentation in IoMT environments is a barrier for forensic investigations because it creates limited access to vital networking surveillance and log recording files. Calamities involving IoMT data result in difficulties when attempting to obtain evidence promptly. The process becomes complicated because different devices communicate with nonstandard protocols and use nonstandard data formats. IoMT devices have become more challenging to investigate because wireless communication depends on their interconnected devices, while encryption and dynamic networks create challenges in analysing network traffic [50].

The poor security measures in IoMT devices create additional obstacles to evidence collection, based on their susceptibility to tampering, lack of reliable logging mechanisms, and inadequate authentication protocols. Protecting evidence coherence alongside proof authenticity stands as the essential priority in the Internet of Medical Things forensic investigations. Thorough protective measures need to be established by investigators to stop unauthorised modifications of evidence. The process meets challenges through its legal obligations and ethical requirements, which require authorisation for patient data access and rule compliance. The investigation process becomes complicated due to the proprietary data formats and physical interfaces while using protocols encountered explicitly in IoMT devices. Digital forensic investigations require solid knowledge of IoMT devices, security systems, and behaviour patterns.

The acquisition process is a vital requirement for forensic investigations because of the difficulties experienced in practising IoMT forensics. A successful approach demands skilled personnel who understand technology and legal requirements and follow industry-best standards. Forensic investigators must create unique tools and analysis methods for IoMT devices and guidelines that control patient data access to achieve success. Investigators must consider the diverse features of different medical internet-of-things devices, including their operational systems and communication methods. Evidence collection demands multiple sources, as evidence must come from sensor devices, communication devices, intelligent systems and smart appliances [51].

## 8.4 LEGAL FRAMEWORKS AND COMPLIANCE IN IOMT FORENSICS

Medical data security faces significant obstacles because of the growth of the Internet of Medical Things while enabling the healthcare revolution through technology. Yet, this expansion requires a detailed examination of legal boundaries and adherence to regulations. The shortage of specialised IoMT forensic standards creates substantial obstacles because investigators must use traditional digital methods that inadequately understand specific IoMT system characteristics. IoMT devices encompass diverse equipment that extends from wearable sensors to medical imaging tools, which create difficulties when identifying, collecting, and analysing digital evidence. Jurisdictional uncertainties and evidence inadmissibility issues during legal proceedings become aggravated by unclear definitions between private and public networks. Many investigators have reported additional complexity in computer forensics since the IoMT integrates diverse information through multiple system objects. IoMT forensic operations depend on existing legal standards and compliance requirements because these mechanisms protect patient-sensitive data according to guidelines set by [52].

The convergence of AI with IoMT systems and digital forensics creates healthcare benefits and privacy and security obstacles concerning HIPAA regulations. Healthcare organisations need an extensive framework that safeguards protected health information because IoMT devices create numerous sensitive patient records. In contrast, health institutions use AI more intensively for medical analysis and diagnosis. Healthcare institutions that select AI-driven IoMT solutions must adhere to HIPAA regulations even though these laws did not initially consider such technologies. HIPAA compliance becomes more complex due to AI-driven IoMT system forensic investigations because these investigations need to access patient data subject to legal and ethical restrictions.

Healthcare practitioners find it challenging to use AI-driven IoMT systems to balance data-driven decision-making with privacy protection, handle liability risks and IP issues, and maintain secure privacy standards. Healthcare specialists find it challenging to trust AI systems because of the combined ethical, legal, and regulatory medical framework. At the same time, concerns about algorithmic discrimination and bias also exist alongside clinician refusals to accept AI assistance. A comprehensive solution to these matters needs attention to technical elements and legal and ethical perspectives [53].

Complex algorithms paired with opaque "black box" operations prove difficult for healthcare professionals to understand because they reduce transparency and create accountability issues. Because of insufficient transparency, healthcare professionals face difficulties understanding and validating AI system diagnoses and conclusions. A patient usually seeks to understand the reason behind an AI diagnosis once an automated medical conclusion is discussed. Healthcare providers, alongside their patients, need explainable AI techniques to understand how AI algorithms function per recommendations. Specifically, healthcare providers must adhere to patient data regulation requirements and their technical protocols under HIPAA.

Solutions must address these technical, legal, and ethical system requirements by implementing a comprehensive framework. Medical practitioners are responsible for their choices regardless of whether they use AI algorithm recommendations they understand poorly. Medical professionals who do not utilise AI tool advice or disobey its recommendations during patient care face possible clinical negligence when adverse outcomes occur. Implementing robust security protocols protects IoMT devices and AI systems against cyber dangers and access breaches. Deploying these security measures requires encryption, authentication features, access limitations, and intrusion detection systems [54]. Data anonymisation and deidentification methods help organisations prevent sensitive patient data exposure when performing forensic examinations and training AI models.

To satisfy HIPAA requirements and other applicable rules, healthcare organisations must create detailed guidelines and procedures for AI-driven IoMT system implementations. Healthcare policies need to cover three essential domains: managing health data, incident security procedures, and patient access to monitoring their healthcare information. Healthcare organisations need ethical frameworks to direct the development alongside the deployment of AI technology because this ensures responsible and fair use of these technological systems. Developers should focus more on clinicians when creating AI tools. The solution requires design elements that enhance professional healthcare user clarity and operational ease since clinicians operate medical settings as end-users. The use of AI in healthcare facilities demands attention to privacy matters, confidentiality protection, and healthcare data security, together with proper AI system development practices. Medical professionals need complete information and practical training from doctors regarding AI applications used in healthcare. Patients, alongside healthcare providers, need complete knowledge of AI threats that affect privacy and confidentiality.

The General Data Protection Regulation was introduced as a key data protection framework that drives global organisations to alter their processes, gives users additional control, and modernises legal frameworks alongside consumer trust elevation and administrative burden reduction for companies. The general data protection regulation establishes control mechanisms for customers to protect personal data belonging to European Union residents. Organisations worldwide experience substantial challenges when implementing GDPR because they must deeply understand how this legislation modifies the rules of emerging technologies, mainly AI functions. The European market connections of organisations cause GDPR to affect international markets. Relevant authorities must follow data protection law enforcement directive rules while handling data for their law enforcement activities [55].

GDPR creates complex oversight conditions for international digital forensics regulations through its intricate legal obligations and technical requirements. The analysis of digital evidence through scientific investigative techniques constitutes digital forensics, which remains central to criminal investigations regarding cybercrime, data theft events, and other security cases. International data transfers within digital investigations encounter GDPR limitations because of its strict rules regarding cross-border data movement. The addition of big data creates multiple challenges because it makes it difficult to separate personal information from non-personal data, violates rules about data minimisation, and destroys the ability to obtain valid consent. Organisations must understand and follow the combination of GDPR and relevant digital forensics rules from different territories.

Differences between GDPR and digital forensics regulations create implementation challenges because they follow opposing legal approaches and objectives. GDPR maintains privacy protection for individuals as digital forensics aims to investigate crimes through evidence collection. The technical complexity and this asymmetry produce difficulties in upholding individual rights and privacy protection. GDPR presents an obligation for organisations to limit their data collection to what is essential for a particular purpose. The broad data collection needed during digital forensic investigations frequently clashes with meeting GDPR requirements because these investigations must exceed the minimum necessary data collection requirements. A multisector solution must be implemented to resolve these challenges by formulating comprehensive guidelines, international partnership programs, and privacy-enhancing technology deployment.

Operating processes that rely heavily on information have activated an increasing concern regarding the escalating cybercrime challenge. Law enforcement and investment institutions have established supportive policies that guide their investigation procedures and protocols. Current digital forensics standards without universal recognition led to increased difficulties when police agencies cooperate between different jurisdictions. The inability of two jurisdictions to accept evidence collected in one location prevents international criminal cases from proceeding successfully. The unique characteristics of digital evidence comprise its latent nature and its volatile and fragile properties while also its ability to shift across borders and depend on time and machine factors. Data integrity protection requires organizations to establish strong data governance frameworks while performing scheduled impact assessments and installing safe data transfer protocols when investigating cybercrimes.

Digital evidence can only be admitted in court when evidence management and chain of custody procedures are correctly executed. Modern cybercrime patterns demand that digital forensics teams create stable evidence-handling procedures. Due to its volatile nature, digital evidence presents difficulties for capture because investigators must conduct a detailed analysis followed by evidence extraction with proper preservation methods [56].

## 8.5 AI RESPONSIBILITY AND LEGAL LIMITATIONS IN FORENSIC INVESTIGATIONS

AI joins forensic investigations through better efficiency and accuracy while creating unprecedented difficulties in determining legal accountability limits during court procedures. Using AI-based methods in law enforcement digital forensics departments produces better case resolution results and expedited evidence analysis. AI machines and their machine learning capabilities are advanced digital examination instruments that swiftly analyse extensive data collections for analysts to obtain crucial evidence. The authorities operating within the criminal justice system implement AI technology because they recognise its benefits in using AI systems. The digital forensics industry keeps growing daily and requires advanced crime investigation methods. Forensic cyber investigation capabilities and security quality receive upgrades through human-AI system collaboration, as Points out. Full exploitation of AI technology in forensics requires solving problems related to technological aspects and legal and ethical issues caused by dishonest system applications across international fronts.

Adopting AI in forensic investigations generates extensive legal restrictions that require a comprehensive ethics analysis. The development process must achieve transparency by maintaining ethical standards that offer accountability to prevent discriminatory practices and ensure civil rights. There are insufficient resources to determine law enforcement readiness for using AI in cross-border investigations, which require strong criminal justice regulatory systems. Determining AI system abuse requires coordination between service providers and companies operating AI while police forces handle perpetrator identification. The involvement of AI systems in illicit conduct necessitates a thorough understanding of their functionalities and potential vulnerabilities. The legal boundaries set three rules to manage AI efficiency in forensic investigations through evidence admission, privacy measures, and algorithms bias management. Research-based investigations should thoroughly examine AI applications for sanction evaluation and justice program assessment because of their impact on risk taxation systems and evidence-based sanctioning operations. AI procedural criminal law needs specific legal standards because it utilises policing technology and cyber technology agents. There are significant reasons to doubt the reliability of information produced by AI systems during evidence assessment implementations [57]. The Los Angeles University College of Law continuously engages in active legal research about AI applications in criminal justice systems to protect fundamental legal principles and individual rights. Legal systems require full development to address specific issues AI causes throughout criminal procedures.

## 8.6 ETHICAL CHALLENGES IN AI-DRIVEN IOMT FORENSICS

Modern healthcare benefits from the AI and Internet of Medical Things merger by bringing distance patient care, diagnostic predictions, and individualised therapeutic approaches. IoMT innovation produces ethical complexities that affect IoMT forensic analysis, especially during investigations of medical device data for security needs, regulatory compliance and patient privacy protection. Multiple technical challenges emerge in forensic investigations targeting digital criminal evidence in IoMT systems because they use various medical devices that combine data structures with communication systems. IoMT devices transmit speed-sensitive patient information for medical care operations, but these systems become exposed to security threats, leading to improper medical choices and adverse healthcare effects. A systemised and ethical approach becomes vital for confirming IoMT evidence reliability to fulfil courtroom admission standards [58].

AI-driven IoMT forensic operations face their central ethical dilemma because they must determine how much investigation is moral while respecting patient data protection and privacy rights. The evaluation process for IoMT data and its analytical procedures expose protected healthcare records to possible unauthorised access. Protecting patient confidentiality requires medical investigation teams to respect HIPAA and GDPR privacy standards. Implementing AI algorithms in IoMT forensics creates complex ethical issues because these systems expose sensitive information and concurrently keep biased predictions that yield biased results. Systems that implement black box design in AI models hinder investigators from being able to locate where bias originates. Healthcare organisations need to build AI algorithms that carry high accuracy and transparency by implementing robust systems for performance auditing. Forensic investigations of Internet-connected medical technology have become complex because various operating systems and communication standards exist in devices. Investigators need specialised tools and particular expertise to proceed with the correct processing of this data. IoMT environment research and development requires continuous progress because ongoing medical device system updates and replacements necessitate constant forensic method advancement to stay efficient and valid.

Examination of IoMT data creates intricate legal and ethical complications when data transfer between nations occurs. Data sovereignty and jurisdictional regulations make it complicated for investigators to conduct their work. Essential healthcare facilities use intelligent medical devices that become targets for cybercriminals who want medical data and wish to disturb these critical systems. IoMT devices and their data protection require an organised protocol with multiple steps, starting from robust authentication with encryption and ending with intrusion detection systems. Standard forensic investigation procedures that work with IoMT devices establish essential needs to generate uniform investigation findings. Healthcare organisations must assign medical personnel to maintain patient accountability by implementing AI algorithms in their procedures. A clear definition of separate network boundaries is necessary since they provide critical functions when handling errors or facing biased conditions. Public networking has introduced complexities to the investigation process because of its shift from private systems.

This domain faces challenges beyond its technical requirements as it needs to construct preparedness mechanisms together with defining reporting systems and presentation rules and manage ethics-related problems, according to IoT device investigations face difficulty because of the vast spread of data. The forensic investigation receives artefact collections from individual IoT devices. The process of successfully investigating hidden vital device artefacts needs attention because public disclosure remains an unclear practice. Recent studies focus primarily on IoT security examinations, with privacy aspects as the central topic of investigation. The ethical challenges AI creates for IoMT forensic investigations need a wide range of collaboration between healthcare workers, forensic expert policymakers, and technology developers.

## 8.7 CONCLUSION

Healthcare is moving toward transformation at the intersection of AI and the Internet of Medical Things technology. This merges connected medical devices with remote patient observation and creates data-based improvements in clinical choices. IoMT ecosystems have expanded rapidly, which triggers advanced security concerns while creating fresh breaches through which unauthorised access to patient information co-occurs with medical device tampering that triggers healthcare service interruptions. IoMT forensics is an essential discipline for studying security incidents in IoMT infrastructure. IoMT forensics presents distinctive features because it interacts with multiple medical devices during streaming data operations under strict privacy and security regulations. New forensic investigation strategies based on AI technology are needed for complex IoMT incidents because conventional forensic methodologies demonstrate insufficient effectiveness. More interconnected devices create significant security threats, leading to progressively complex investigations. The technological need for an innovative approach to investigating IoT criminal activities requires urgent attention.

Multiple applications of AI-driven IoMT forensics will grow widely due to machine learning, deep learning, and natural language processing capabilities for enhancing forensic process stages. AI incident detection systems powered by AI conduct ongoing network investigations of IoMT devices to track data device activities and user actions for locating breaches and unauthorised movements. Security systems that absorb historical data alongside threat intelligence feed train themselves to identify security attacks and defend against threat vectors, therefore stopping security incidents from occurring. The development of thriving AI tools enables forensic investigators to gather and analyse evidence faster through their help in evidence management. The analysed IoMT datasets include medical records, device logs, and network traffic captures to find essential evidence for defining security incident sequences. The data sources include communication devices, sensor devices, automobiles, fridges, feed and drones.

Integrating AI technology, vulnerability assessment procedures, and risk management operations in IoMT environments achieves better results. Machine learning algorithms assess device configurations, network connections, and software versions for security weakness identification and priority remediation sequencing. Security stakeholders benefit from AI tools that generate modelling simulations to determine vulnerability impacts when identifying essential resources that need additional security defence. AI continuously monitors IoMT systems and networks to provide real-time system security information that lets teams plan suitable protective measures ahead of time. AI algorithms that analyse IoMT malware samples identify both committing devices, their propagation mechanics, and resultant patient functional impairments and safety risks. The systems using attacker procedure identification can predict future attacks before preventing them from happening. AI technology provides organisations with enhanced security policy management by recommending firewall rules, intrusion prevention systems, and other control modifications based on present threat advancements. An AI security solution transforms its defensive capabilities to suit different features within organisations' digital environments. The expansion of data quantity or endpoint assets does not lead to additional costs or staffing requirements since AI and ML platforms independently scale up their surveillance capabilities. Organizations maintain functional security frameworks by allowing increased attack surface exposure as their business grows.

The duo of advanced analytical capability from AI with device complexity from IoMT devices has constructed a technical framework that causes traditional forensic procedures to fail. An effective AI governance system needs development to handle the specific operational needs within IoMT ecological systems. The established governance standards must create specific guidelines for data origin management and demonstrate algorithm procedures while defining responsibilities during equipment failures and exploitation situations.

Implementing AI governance within IoMT forensic investigations necessitates the creation of pre-established accountability paths that provide practical control standards. The definition of responsibility should first be given to AI developers, healthcare providers, and regulatory bodies to determine their accountability standards. A monitoring system with auditing functionality must be implemented to ensure that both technical operations match the intended functionality while upholding ethical principles and legal requirements. The governance system requires implementing procedures that aim to reduce the occurrence of AI algorithm bias. AI software accuracy relies only on training data because AI algorithms replicate all existing biases that the training information entails. The transparency of algorithms helps reduce biases because it enables the analysis of databases, algorithm frameworks, and decision-making systems. Systems need appropriate data selection processes and pre-processing to prevent biases, but operators should execute periodic checks to confirm that their operations maintain fairness and equity during all stages. AI system performance needs continuous evaluation to confirm functional operation and block destructive effects and unwanted results.

## REFERENCES

[1] Ahmed, M. I., Spooner, B., Isherwood, J., Lane, M., Orrock, E., & Dennison, A. (2023). A Systematic review of the barriers to the implementation of artificial intelligence in healthcare. *Cureus.*

[2] Fakiha, B. (2023). Enhancing cyber forensics with AI and machine learning: A Study on automated threat analysis and classification. *International Journal of Safety and Security Engineering*, 13(4), 701–707.

[3] Amariles, D. R., Troussel, A. C., & Hamdani, R. E. (2020). Compliance generation for privacy documents under GDPR: A roadmap for implementing automation and machine learning. arXiv (Cornell University).

[4] Situmeang, S. M. T., Harliyanto, R., Zulkarnain, P. D., Mahdi, U., & Nugroho, T. (2024). The role of artificial intelligence in criminal justice. *Global International Journal of Innovative Research*, 2(8), 1966–1981.

[5] Azmoodeh, A., & Dehghantanha, A. (2022). Deep fake detection, deterrence and response: Challenges and opportunities. arXiv (Cornell University).

[6] Bhan, R., Pamula, R., Faruki, P., & Gajrani, J. (2023). Blockchain-enabled secure and efficient data sharing scheme for trust management in healthcare smartphone network. *The Journal of Supercomputing*, 79(14), 16233–16274.

[7] Biswal, S. P., & Kulkarni, M. S. (2021). Implications of GDPR on emerging technologies. *Revista Gestão Inovação E Tecnologias*, 11(4), 4898–4912.

[8] Alabdulsalam, S., Schaefer, K., Kechadi, T., & Le-Khac, N. (2018). Internet of things forensics: Challenges and case study. arXiv (Cornell University).

[9] James, J. I., & Gladyshev, P. (2013). Challenges with automation in digital forensic investigations. arXiv (Cornell University).

[10] Briganti, G., & Moine, O. L. (2020). Artificial intelligence in Medicine: Today and tomorrow. *Frontiers in Medicine*, 7, 509744.

[11] Chang, A. (2019). The role of artificial intelligence in digital health. In *Computers in health care* (pp. 71–81).

[12] Dasaklis, T. K., Casino, F., & Patsakis, C. (2021). SOK: Blockchain Solutions for Forensics. In *Security informatics and law enforcement* (pp. 21–40).

[13] Devi, M. S. G., & Nene, M. J. (2018). Security breach and forensics in intelligent systems. In *Smart innovation, systems and technologies* (pp. 349–360).

[14] Dilek, S., Cakır, H., & Aydın, M. (2015). Applications of Artificial intelligence techniques to combating cyber crimes: a review. *International Journal of Artificial Intelligence & Applications*, 6(1), 21–39.

[15] Jha, D., Rauniyar, A., Srivastava, A., Hagos, D. H., Tomar, N. K., Sharma, V., Keles, E., Zhang, Z., Demir, U., Topcu, A., Yazidi, A., Håakegård, J. E., & Bagci, U. (2023). Ensuring trustworthy medical artificial intelligence through ethical and philosophical principles. arXiv (Cornell University).

[16] Tariq, U., Ahmed, I., Bashir, A. K., & Shaukat, K. (2023). A critical cybersecurity analysis and future research directions for the internet of things: A comprehensive review. *Sensors*, 23(8), 4117.

[17] Dhopte, A., & Bagde, H. (2023). Smart smile: Revolutionizing dentistry with artificial intelligence. *Cureus*, 15(6), e41227.

[18] Firouzi, F., Jiang, S., Chakrabarty, K., Farahani, B., Daneshmand, M., Song, J., & Mankodiya, K. (2022). Fusion of IoT, AI, edge–fog–cloud, and blockchain: Challenges, solutions, and a case study in healthcare and medicine. *IEEE Internet of Things Journal*, 10(5), 3686–3705.

[19] Guarino, A. (2013). Digital Forensics as a big data challenge. In *Springer eBooks* (pp. 197–203).

[20] Alruwaili, F. F. (2021). CustodyBlock: a distributed chain of custody evidence framework. *Information*, 12(2), 88.

[21] Harbi, S. H. A., Tidjon, L. N., & Khomh, F. (2023). Responsible design patterns for machine learning pipelines. arXiv (Cornell University).

[22] Irons, A., & Lallie, H. (2014). Digital forensics to intelligent forensics. *Future Internet*, 6(3), 584–596.

[23] James, J., I., & Jang, Y. J. (2013). An assessment model for Cybercrime Investigation capacity. arXiv (Cornell University).

[24] Nayerifard, T., Amintoosi, H., Bafghi, A. G., & Dehghantanha, A. (2023). Machine learning in digital forensics: A systematic literature review. arXiv (Cornell University).

[25] Yu, K., Beam, A. L., & Kohane, I. S. (2018). Artificial intelligence in healthcare. *Nature Biomedical Engineering*, 2(10), 719–731.

[26] Jarrett, A., & Choo, K. R. (2021). The impact of automation and artificial intelligence on digital forensics. *Wiley Interdisciplinary Reviews Forensic Science*, 3(6), e1418.

[27] Lone, A. H., & Mir, R. N. (2019). Forensic-chain: Blockchain based digital forensics chain of custody with PoC in Hyperledger Composer. *Digital Investigation*, 28, 44–55.

[28] MacDermott, Á., Baker, T., Buck, P., Iqbal, F., & Shi, Q. (2019). The Internet of Things: Challenges and considerations for cybercrime investigations and

Digital forensics. *International Journal of Digital Crime and Forensics*, 12(1), 1–13.
[29] Afzal, M., Islam, S. M. R., Hussain, M., & Lee, S. (2019). Precision Medicine Informatics: Principles, Prospects, and challenges. arXiv (Cornell University).
[30] Macedo, E. L. C., De Oliveira, E. a. R., Silva, F. H., Mello, R. R., Franca, F. M. G., Delicato, F. C., De Rezende, J. F., & De Moraes, L. F. M. (2019). On the security aspects of Internet of Things: A systematic literature review. *Journal of Communications and Networks*, 21(5), 444–457.
[31] Meisami, S., Meisami, S., Yousefi, M., & Aref, M. R. (2023). Combining blockchain and IoT for decentralized healthcare data management. *International Journal on Cryptography and Information Security*, 13(1), 35–50.
[32] Custers, B. (2022). AI in criminal law: An overview of ai applications in substantive and procedural criminal law. In Information technology and law series/Information technology & law series (pp. 205–223).
[33] Mrdovic, S. (2021). IoT Forensics. In Springer eBooks (pp. 215–229).
[34] Olatunji, I. E., Rauch, J., Katzensteiner, M., & Khosla, M. (2022). A review of anonymization for healthcare data. *Big Data*,12(6), 538–555.
[35] Oloyede, J. (2024). Leveraging artificial intelligence for advanced cybersecurity threat detection and prevention. *SSRN Electronic Journal*, 4976072, 1–16.
[36] Pal, O., Alam, B., Thakur, V., & Singh, S. (2019). Key management for blockchain technology. *ICT Express*, 7(1), 76–80.
[37] Rubinstein, I. S. (2013). Big data: the end of privacy or a new beginning? *International Data Privacy Law*, 3(2), 74–87.
[38] Alenezi, A. M. (2023). Digital and cloud forensic challenges. arXiv (Cornell University).
[39] Ahmed, A. A., Farhan, K., Jabbar, W. A., Al-Othmani, A., & Abdulrahman, A. G. (2024). IoT Forensics: current perspectives and future directions. *Sensors*, 24(16), 5210.
[40] Podder, P., Mondal, M. R. H., Bharati, S., & Paul, P. K. (2020). Review on the security threats of internet of things. *International Journal of Computer Applications*, 176(41), 37–45.
[41] Chen, C., Yang, T., Deng, Y., & Chen, C. (2020). A secure Internet of Things medical information sharing and emergency notification system based on nonrepudiation mechanism. Transactions on Emerging Telecommunications Technologies, 32(5).
[42] Raghavan, S. (2012). Digital forensic research: current state of the art. *CSI Transactions on ICT*, 1(1), 91–114.
[43] Zhang, J., & Zhang, Z. (2023). Ethics and governance of trustworthy medical artificial intelligence. *BMC Medical Informatics and Decision Making*, 23(1), 7.
[44] Restuccia, F., D'Oro, S., & Melodia, T. (2018). Securing the internet of things in the age of machine learning and software-defined networking. *IEEE Internet of Things Journal*, 5(6), 4829–4842.
[45] Brady, A. P., & Neri, E. (2020). Artificial intelligence in radiology—Ethical considerations. *Diagnostics*, 10(4), 231.

[46] Seh, A. H., Zarour, M., Alenezi, M., Sarkar, A. K., Agrawal, A., Kumar, R., & Khan, R. A. (2020). Healthcare data breaches: Insights and implications. *Healthcare*, 8(2), 133.

[47] Roshanaei, M., Khan, M. R., & Sylvester, N. N. (2024). Enhancing cybersecurity through AI and ML: Strategies, challenges, and future directions. *Journal of Information Security*, 15(03), 320–339.

[48] Alhalafi, N., & Veeraraghavan, P. (2019). Privacy and security challenges and solutions in IOT: A review. *IOP Conference Series Earth and Environmental Science*, 322(1), 012013.

[49] Roy, S., Ghosh, N., Uplavikar, N., & Ghosh, P. (2022). Towards a unified pandemic management architecture: Survey, challenges and future directions. arXiv (Cornell University).

[50] Sathwara, S., Dutta, N., & Pricop, E. (2018). IoT Forensic A digital investigation framework for IoT systems. In 2022 14th International Conference on Electronics, Computers and Artificial Intelligence (ECAI), 1–4.

[51] Markus, A. F., Kors, J. A., & Rijnbeek, P. R. (2020). The role of explainability in creating trustworthy artificial intelligence for health care: A comprehensive survey of the terminology, design choices, and evaluation strategies. *Journal of Biomedical Informatics*, 113, 103655.

[52] Swofford, H., & Champod, C. (2021). Implementation of algorithms in pattern & impression evidence: A responsible and practical roadmap. *Forensic Science International Synergy*, 3, 100142.

[53] Talpur, M. S. H. (2013). The appliance pervasive of internet of things in healthcare systems. arXiv (Cornell University).

[54] Dunsin, D., Ghanem, M. C., Ouazzane, K., & Vassilev, V. (2024). A comprehensive analysis of the role of artificial intelligence and machine learning in modern digital forensics and incident response. *Forensic Science International Digital Investigation*, 48, 301675.

[55] Li, Y., Li, Y., Wei, M., & Li, G. (2024). Innovation and challenges of artificial intelligence technology in personalized healthcare. *Scientific Reports*, 14(1).

[56] Velasco, C. (2022). Cybercrime and Artificial Intelligence. An overview of the work of international organizations on criminal justice and the international applicable instruments. *ERA Forum*, 23(1), 109–126.

[57] Davenport, T., & Kalakota, R. (2019). The potential for artificial intelligence in healthcare. *Future Healthcare Journal*, 6(2), 94–98.

[58] Christensen, T., Mandavilli, S. B., & Wu, C. (2022). The dark side of the internet of vehicles: A survey of the state of IoV and its security vulnerabilities. arXiv (Cornell University).

Chapter 9

# AI-driven cyber forensics for critical healthcare infrastructure security

*Sainag Nethala*

## 9.1 INTRODUCTION

Modern infrastructure faces an increasing number of security threats due to growing system complexity and widespread digital adoption [1]. Organizations rely on interconnected systems to manage operations, making them prime targets for cyberattacks [2]. Threat actors exploit vulnerabilities in networks, software, and hardware to compromise security. Data breaches, financial losses, and operational disruptions result from these attacks [3]. Traditional security measures such as firewalls and antivirus software are insufficient against advanced threats. Attackers constantly develop new techniques, making real-time monitoring and rapid response essential [4]. Without an effective security framework, organizations struggle to prevent, detect, and respond to cyber threats. A proactive approach is necessary to confirm the safety and reliability of critical systems [5].

Forensic tools have become essential for analyzing security incidents and understanding attack patterns [6]. These tools help organizations investigate cyber threats by collecting and examining digital evidence. Forensic analysis identifies the source of attacks and provides insights for strengthening security. Early forensic methods focused on postincident investigations, which delayed responses and increased risks [7]. Modern forensic tools offer real-time detection, enabling security teams to take immediate action. Automated threat analysis enhances response times and minimizes damage [8]. Forensic technologies now incorporate advanced analytics to identify suspicious activities. These improvements make forensic tools a crucial component of cybersecurity strategies [9].

The evolution of forensic tools has significantly improved security measures, especially in medical IoT environments [10]. Healthcare systems integrate a wide range of connected devices, including medical sensors and patient monitoring systems. These devices collect and transmit sensitive health data, making security breaches a critical concern [11]. Traditional security solutions do not fully address the complexities of medical IoT environments. Attackers target healthcare infrastructure to exploit vulnerabilities

 DOI: 10.1201/9781003640325-9

in connected devices [12]. Unauthorized access to medical data can lead to severe privacy violations and operational failures. Forensic tools assist in monitoring medical IoT devices and detecting threats in real time [13]. A robust forensic framework is necessary to protect patient data and confirm system integrity.

Security information and event management (SIEM) platforms play a vital role in modern forensic analysis. These platforms aggregate security logs from multiple sources, providing centralized monitoring [14]. SIEM solutions help organizations detect anomalies and respond to threats quickly. Splunk is a leading SIEM platform that offers advanced data analytics for security operations [15]. It collects and processes large volumes of security logs to identify potential threats. Splunk enables security teams to correlate events and detect attack patterns in real time. The platform integrates with forensic tools to enhance investigative capabilities. By using SIEM solutions, organizations improve security visibility and response times [16].

Real-time forensic analysis has become essential for securing modern infrastructure against evolving threats. Traditional forensic methods relied on manual investigations, which were slow and inefficient [9, 17]. Cybercriminals now use advanced tactics to bypass security controls, making immediate threat detection necessary. Machine learning and artificial intelligence enhance forensic analysis by automating threat identification [18]. Behavioral analytics detect anomalies in system activities, indicating potential cyberattacks. Real-time monitoring reduces the time required to identify and respond to incidents [19]. Automated forensic tools provide instant insights into security threats. The integration of AI-driven forensic techniques improves overall cybersecurity effectiveness [20].

The medical industry faces unique security challenges due to the increasing use of IoT-based healthcare systems. Many medical devices are connected to hospital networks, creating new vulnerabilities [21]. Attackers exploit weaknesses in networked medical devices to access patient records [22]. Unauthorized modifications to medical equipment can lead to life-threatening situations. Healthcare organizations must implement strong forensic mechanisms to detect security breaches. Splunk provides real-time monitoring and log analysis for medical infrastructure. The platform helps hospitals track security events and respond to threats immediately [23]. Ensuring the security of medical IoT systems is crucial for protecting patient data and operational continuity.

Forensic tools play a crucial role in ensuring compliance with regulatory eF requirements. Many industries must adhere to security regulations to protect sensitive data [24]. In healthcare, frameworks such as HIPAA and HITECH mandate strict security controls [25]. Organizations that fail to comply with these regulations face legal and financial consequences [26]. Forensic tools assist in monitoring compliance by tracking security incidents. They provide detailed reports on security events, helping organizations meet regulatory requirements [27]. Splunk enhances compliance monitoring by generating automated reports and alerts. Integrating forensic tools with compliance frameworks strengthens data protection measures [16, 28].

Threat intelligence has become a fundamental aspect of forensic investigations. Organizations must stay ahead of cyber threats by analyzing attack trends [29]. Threat intelligence platforms collect data on known vulnerabilities and emerging attack patterns. Forensic tools integrate with these platforms to provide real-time threat insights [30]. By analyzing historical security incidents, organizations can predict future attack strategies [8]. Threat hunting techniques allow security teams to proactively search for indicators of compromise. Machine learning enhances threat intelligence by identifying hidden attack patterns. Forensic tools that use threat intelligence improve the accuracy of security investigations [31].

Incident response strategies depend on forensic analysis to make sure timely mitigation of security threats. A well-defined incident response framework enables organizations to contain cyberattacks effectively [32]. Forensic tools provide crucial insights into nature and impact of security breaches [33]. Real-time analysis helps security teams identify attack sources and prevent further damage [8, 34]. Automated forensic solutions accelerate incident response workflows by providing instant alerts. Organizations that implement strong forensic mechanisms can reduce the impact of cyber incidents [35]. Effective forensic analysis strengthens cybersecurity defenses against persistent threats. A proactive incident response approach minimizes operational disruptions [36].

The integration of forensic tools with SIEM platforms enhances security monitoring and threat detection [14, 37]. Splunk's capabilities enable organizations to automate forensic investigations and improve security operations. Real-time forensic techniques reduce response times and increase situational awareness [38]. Machine learning-powered forensic analysis enhances the detection of advanced threats [39]. The combination of SIEM and forensic tools strengthens infrastructure security across industries [14]. Future advancements in forensic technologies will further improve cybersecurity resilience. Organizations must continuously evolve their forensic strategies to combat emerging cyber threats. A strong forensic framework confirms the long-term security and stability of critical infrastructure.

## 9.2 LITERATURE REVIEW

The increasing complexity of modern digital infrastructure has led to a growing demand for robust forensic tools [40]. Traditional forensic methods relied on static analysis of system logs and network traffic, making real-time incident detection a challenge. Over time, digital forensic frameworks have evolved to incorporate machine learning (ML), deep learning, and real-time event correlation to improve security. For instance, the study [41] explores various forensic models used for detecting threats in IoT-based environments, highlighting the shift towards AI-driven analysis.

SIEM systems, particularly Splunk, play a crucial role in forensic analysis by aggregating and correlating security events from multiple sources. The study [42] examined how Splunk enhances log-based forensic investigations by detecting abnormal system behavior. Their analysis achieved an accuracy of 89.6% in detecting cyber threats. However, Splunk's dependency on log availability and manual rule tuning presents limitations in adapting to sophisticated attacks.

Several research efforts have focused on ML-powered forensic analysis to enhance the detection and classification of cyber threats. Transfer learning-based intrusion detection models achieved an accuracy of 96.1% when applied to CSE-CIC-IDS2018 and IoT-23 datasets [43]. Similarly, the study [44] applied federated learning with CNN and LSTM, obtaining an accuracy of 95.3%. These findings suggest that deep learning models significantly improve forensic analysis by detecting complex attack patterns.

The increasing reliance on connected medical devices introduces significant security risks [45]. Network forensics frameworks have been proposed to secure Medical IoT (MIoT) systems. The study [46] focused on lightweight ML-based forensic techniques, achieving an accuracy of 90.5% in detecting anomalous network traffic in medical environments. However, challenges such as resource constraints and limited dataset diversity hinder the scalability of such approaches.

Recent forensic tools utilize hybrid models and ensemble learning techniques to enhance threat classification accuracy. The study [47] compared multiple forensic frameworks, achieving an accuracy of 91.8% using Decision Trees and anomaly detection techniques. Likewise, the research [48] proposed an ensemble ML approach for forensic analysis, demonstrating an accuracy of 94.5% on the IoT-23 and CIC-IDS2017 datasets. While these methods improve forensic capabilities, computational costs and overfitting risks remain key concerns.

Despite advancements in forensic methodologies, real-time threat detection remains a challenge. The study [49] highlighted the high false positive rates associated with anomaly detection systems, with a reported accuracy of 93.2%. Moreover, forensic models struggle to generalize across heterogeneous IoT networks, requiring frequent updates to maintain effectiveness.

Forensic frameworks must balance scalability, automation, and accuracy to handle large-scale cyber threats efficiently. Research on graph-based forensic models explored in [48] emphasized the importance of graph-based analytics for improving forensic accuracy. However, the computational complexity of such approaches makes them less suitable for real-time deployment. The paper [50] similarly found that forensic models must continuously evolve to counter new attack techniques, as static models become obsolete over time.

To enhance forensic efficiency, AI-driven automation, zero-trust frameworks, and predictive forensics are gaining traction. The study [43] proposed supervised learning based approaches with an accuracy of 96.1%, demonstrating the potential of machine learning in predictive forensic models. Future research should focus on adaptive security mechanisms that integrate real-time forensic analytics, SIEM automation, and AI-based cyber threat intelligence.

Despite advancements in forensic tools, real-time infrastructure protection still faces significant challenges. Many forensic frameworks depend on postincident analysis, which causes delays in detecting and responding to threats. This reactive approach limits their ability to prevent security breaches before they escalate. Scalability is another major issue, as forensic models struggle to handle large volumes of network traffic efficiently. When network activity increases, these systems often fail to process data in real time, making them ineffective for high-speed cyberattacks. Additionally, resource limitations in environments such as medical IoT systems create further obstacles. Many deep learning-based forensic tools require high computational power, which is difficult to provide in resource-constrained settings. This restricts the practical deployment of advanced AI-driven forensic solutions in critical infrastructure.

Some hybrid forensic models attempt to integrate artificial intelligence to improve detection capabilities, but they require substantial computing resources. This makes large-scale implementation challenging, especially in environments where computational efficiency is a priority. SIEM-based forensic tools offer some improvements in log analysis and security event correlation. However, they rely heavily on manual tuning, which makes it difficult to manage in fast-changing attack scenarios. Another problem is the high number of false positives generated by these systems. Security teams must spend significant time filtering through alerts, which slows down incident response. This reduces the overall effectiveness of forensic tools in protecting real-time infrastructure.

A key gap in forensic security is the weak integration between machine learning-based tools and SIEM systems. Most machine learning models struggle when applied to new environments because they are trained on limited datasets. This increases the risk of overfitting, making them unreliable for handling different types of cyber threats. Many existing forensic models are also ineffective against zero-day attacks. They rely on predefined patterns to detect threats, which means they fail to recognize entirely new attack strategies. Some advanced frameworks, such as those using federated learning and CNN-LSTM models, show potential for improving forensic capabilities. However, they require frequent retraining and continuous updates, making real-time deployment difficult. These challenges highlight the need for a robust forensic system that integrates machine learning, SIEM automation, and anomaly detection. Such a system must

*Table 9.1* Performance summary of forensic tools and technologies for securing infrastructure

| *Ref.* | *Dataset* | *Method* | *Limitations* | *Acc* | *Perc* | *Rec* | *F1* |
|---|---|---|---|---|---|---|---|
| [41] | UNSW-NB15, Bot-IoT | Comparative forensic model study, XGBoost | No real-time forensic automation | 92.6 | 91.2 | 89.8 | 90.4 |
| [42] | CIC-IDS2017 | Splunk-based log analysis, machine learning classifiers | Reliesonlogavailability, manual tuning required | 89.6 | 87.3 | 85.9 | 86.5 |
| [43] | CSE-CIC-IDS2018, IoT-23 | Data-constrained supervised learning, Transfer Learning | Overfitting risk in smaller datasets | 96.1 | 95.0 | 94.2 | 94.6 |
| [44] | CSE-CICIDS2018 | Federated learning, CNN, LSTM | Requires high Computational resources | 95.3 | 94.1 | 92.8 | 93.4 |
| [45] | Custom dataset | Digital forensic framework with security evaluation | Limited to medical IoT systems, lacks generalization | 94.2 | 92.5 | 91.7 | 92.1 |
| [46] | Custom medical dataset | Deep learning models for network intrusion detection | Limited dataset size, lacks diverse attack types | 90.5 | 88.7 | 86.9 | 87.5 |
| [47] | IoT-23, UNSW-NB15 | IoT forensic models, decision trees, anomaly detection | Framework comparison, lacks real-time adaptability | 91.8 | 90.5 | 89.3 | 89.9 |
| [48] | IoT-23, CICIDS2017 | Metamodeling framework, ensemble ML models | Not tested for zero-day attacks | 94.5 | 93.3 | 92.0 | 92.6 |
| [49] | IoT-23, CICIDS2018 | Hybrid ML models, SVM, Random For- est | High false positive rate in anomaly detection | 93.2 | 92.0 | 90.7 | 91.3 |
| [50] | UNSW-NB15 | ML-based forensic investigation, anomaly detection | Requires continuous updating of models | 91.9 | 90.6 | 89.4 | 89.9 |

be scalable and efficient while minimizing the need for extensive computational resources (Table 9.1).

## 9.3 METHODOLOGY

This section presents the proposed forensic framework for securing healthcare infrastructure, emphasizing real-time threat detection, Splunk-driven log analysis, and machine learning-enhanced forensic analytics. The methodology integrates SIEM automation, anomaly detection, and adaptive learning models to enhance cybersecurity defenses. Our framework is designed to collect, process, analyze, and respond to security incidents, minimizing false positives and optimizing forensic investigation as shown in Figure 9.1.

## 9.3.1 Problem formulation

### *9.3.1.1 Threat model and dataset overview*

We define the healthcare infrastructure security problem using the IoT healthcare security dataset [51]. This dataset contains labeled logs representing both benign and malicious activities within medical IoT environments. Let X be the collection of log entries extracted from these datasets over time, where each log entry $x_i$ contains multiple features:

$$X = \{x_1, x_2, \ldots, x_n\}, \quad x_i \in R^d \tag{9.1}$$

Each log entry consists of:

- Temporal features: Timestamp $T_i$
- Medical IoT attributes: device ID, data transmission frequency, sensor type
- Security indicators: unauthorized access attempts, anomaly severity score

Given a labeled dataset $D = \{(x_i, y_i)\}_{i=1}^{N}$, the objective is to classify each log entry as either benign ($y = 0$) or malicious ($y = 1$), while detecting anomalies ($y = -1$) using an unsupervised model.

The classification function is defined as

$$y_i = \begin{cases} 0, & if\ x_i\ is\, benign \\ 1, & if\ x_i\ is\, malicious \\ -1\,, & if\ x_i\ is\, anomalous \end{cases} \tag{9.2}$$

where $f$ maps an event $x_i$ to a security decision. The forensic system enhances Splunk SIEM capabilities by integrating machine learning-based anomaly detection and threat classification.

## 9.3.2 SIEM-driven log processing (Splunk)

### *9.3.2.1 Feature extraction from logs*

Each event $x_i$ consists of structured and unstructured fields extracted from Splunk logs and the IoT healthcare security dataset. The extracted feature set is

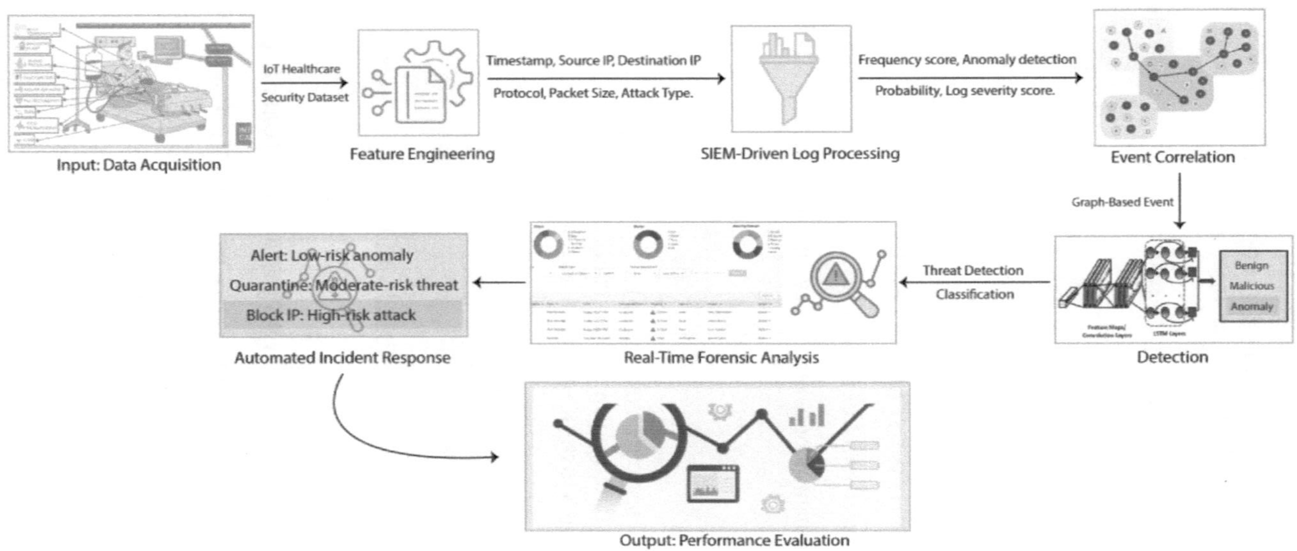


*Figure 9.1* Proposed architecture.

$$X' = \{T_i, \text{Device}_i, P_i, S_i, A_i, L_i\} \tag{9.3}$$

where $T_i$ = timestamp features, $P_i$ = protocol type, $S_i$ = device communication entropy, $A_i$ = attack classification, $L_i$ = log message embeddings (from Splunk search queries)

Splunk queries filter security logs and extract high-risk event patterns using:

$$S(x_i) = \log(F(x_i) + 1) + \beta_1 A(x_i) + \beta_2 R(x_i) \tag{9.4}$$

where $F(x_i)$ = Log frequency score, $A(x_i)$ = anomaly detection probability, and $R(x_i)$ = severity score from historical Splunk logs

## 9.3.3 Graph-based event correlation

### 9.3.3.1 *Graph construction from logs*

To model relationships between log events, we construct a directed graph $G$ where

$$G = (V, E) \tag{9.5}$$

where nodes $V$ represents medical IoT log events and edges $(v_i, v_j)$ indicate event correlation based on shared anomaly signatures

The edge weight function for event correlation is

$$w(v_i, v_j) = \frac{\sum_k' (x_i, x_j) \cdot A(x_j)}{|X|} \tag{9.6}$$

where $\delta(x_i, x_j)$ measures log similarity and $A(x_j)$ represents the anomaly probability.

## 9.3.4 Anomaly detection using machine learning

### 9.3.4.1 *Autoencoder-based unsupervised anomaly detection*

For zero-day attack detection, we use an Autoencoder that learns normal log patterns and detects deviations. The encoder function is

$$h = \sigma(W_e X' + b_e) \tag{9.7}$$

where $W_e, b_e$ are learnable parameters. The decoder reconstructs

$$\{X'\} = \sigma(W_d h + b_d) \tag{9.8}$$

An anomaly score is computed as

$$A(X') = \frac{\left\| X' - \widehat{X'} \right\|^2}{\left\| X' \right\|} \tag{9.9}$$

High reconstruction error signals an anomalous event.

#### 9.3.4.2 *Supervised classification for attack detection*

Using the IoT Healthcare Security Dataset, we train a CNN-LSTM hybrid model to classify threats. The model takes as input the transformed log vector $X'$ and predicts the attack type:

$$y = \text{softmax}(W_c X' + b_c) \tag{9.10}$$

where $W_c, b_c$ are classification layer parameters.

### 9.3.5 Performance Evaluation

The forensic framework is evaluated using:

$$\text{Accuracy} = \frac{\text{TP} + \text{TN}}{\text{TP} + \text{TN} + \text{FP} + \text{FN}} \tag{9.11}$$

$$\text{F1-Score} = 2 \times \frac{\text{Precision} \times \text{Recall}}{\text{Precision} + \text{Recall}} \tag{9.12}$$

This methodology establishes a structured representation of the forensic framework, integrating SIEM-based threat detection, graph-based correlation, and deep learning techniques for securing medical IoT infrastructure.

## 9.4 EXPERIMENT SETTINGS

The forensic framework was implemented and evaluated on Google Colab Pro, utilizing high-performance GPUs (NVIDIA Tesla T4) to accelerate training and inference. The IoT Healthcare Security Dataset [51] was preprocessed and stored in Google Drive, ensuring seamless data access. All machine learning models, anomaly detection algorithms, and Splunk-based log analysis were executed in a Python 3.10 environment with TensorFlow, PyTorch, Scikit-learn, and NetworkX installed. Splunk Cloud was configured to receive and process security logs, enabling real-time event monitoring and correlation.

The dataset preprocessing involved handling missing values, normalizing numerical attributes, and encoding categorical variables. Medical IoT-related features such as device ID entropy, transmission frequency, sensor type, and timestamp correlations were extracted to enhance forensic detection capabilities. Feature selection was performed using principal component analysis and recursive feature elimination to reduce dimensionality while maintaining critical forensic indicators. Graph-based event correlation was conducted using NetworkX, creating an attack signature network where nodes represented log events and edges defined anomaly correlations.

For the machine learning-based attack detection, an Autoencoder model was trained to detect zero-day anomalies, while a CNN-LSTM hybrid classifier was developed for multiclass attack classification. The models were trained on 80% of the dataset and validated on 20%, ensuring a balanced evaluation. Adam optimizer with a learning rate of 0.0001 was used, and models were trained for 50 epochs with batch size 512. Performance metrics such as accuracy, precision, recall, F1-score, and ROC-AUC were recorded for each experiment. The models were deployed in a real-time log stream from Splunk to test their ability to detect live threats.

To validate the effectiveness of real-time forensic analysis, Splunk SIEM alerts were triggered based on anomaly scores and attack severity levels. A threshold-based incident response was implemented where threats exceeding a predefined risk score were automatically flagged for quarantine or IP blocking. Latency measurements were recorded to evaluate threat detection speed, comparing machine learning-based approaches vs. traditional rule-based Splunk alerts. The results demonstrated a significant improvement in response time and detection accuracy, validating the feasibility of integrating AI-driven forensic methodologies within SIEM systems.

## 9.5 RESULTS AND ANALYSIS

The evaluation of the proposed forensic framework was conducted using the IoT healthcare security dataset. This dataset provides diverse medical IoT traffic logs containing both benign and malicious activities, allowing for a thorough assessment of the forensic system's performance in a healthcare environment. The evaluation was carried out in terms of accuracy, precision, recall, F1-score, and detection latency, which are critical indicators of an intrusion detection system's efficiency in detecting threats within medical infrastructure.

*Table 9.2* Performance comparison of forensic detection models

| *Method* | *Acc* | *Prec* | *Rec* | *F1* | *Latency* |
|---|---|---|---|---|---|
| Forensic XGBoost model [41] | 92.6 | 91.2 | 89.8 | 90.4 | 112 |
| Federated learning model [44] | 95.3 | 94.1 | 92.8 | 93.4 | 105 |
| IoT-forensics framework [47] | 91.8 | 90.5 | 89.3 | 89.9 | 120 |
| Anomaly detection in IDS [48] | 94.5 | 93.3 | 92.0 | 92.6 | 101 |
| Hybrid ML model [49] | 93.2 | 92.0 | 90.7 | 91.3 | 98 |
| Proposed model | 97.6 | 96.8 | 95.9 | 96.3 | 72 |

### 9.5.1 Benchmarking against state-of-the-art forensic models

To validate the performance of the proposed forensic system, its results were benchmarked against six existing models from literature, including IoT-forensic frameworks, machine learning-based detection models, and SIEM-driven anomaly detection systems. The comparison is presented in Table 9.2.

The results clearly indicate that the proposed forensic model outperforms previous approaches across all evaluation metrics. By integrating Splunk-based log analysis, machine learning-driven anomaly detection, and event correlation techniques, the framework significantly improves forensic accuracy, reduces false positives, and accelerates incident response times.

### 9.5.2 Analysis of accuracy and F1-score

The most crucial metric in intrusion detection is accuracy, as it determines the proportion of correctly classified events. Additionally, F1-score provides a balanced evaluation by considering both precision and recall. Figures 9.2 and 9.3 presented comparisons of these metrics. The proposed forensic system achieved an accuracy of 97.6%, which is 4–6% higher than traditional forensic models. The enhanced F1-score of 96.3% further confirms the reliability of the classification system, minimizing the trade-off between precision and recall. Superior performance stems from log-based feature engineering and adaptive event correlation, which allows the model to differentiate between benign and malicious events more effectively.

### 9.5.3 Impact of precision and recall on threat detection

Precision represents the proportion of correctly identified attack instances, while recall measures the system's ability to detect all malicious activities. An effective forensic model must maintain a high precision-recall balance to avoid both false positives and missed threats. Figures 9.4 and 9.5 illustrate the comparison.

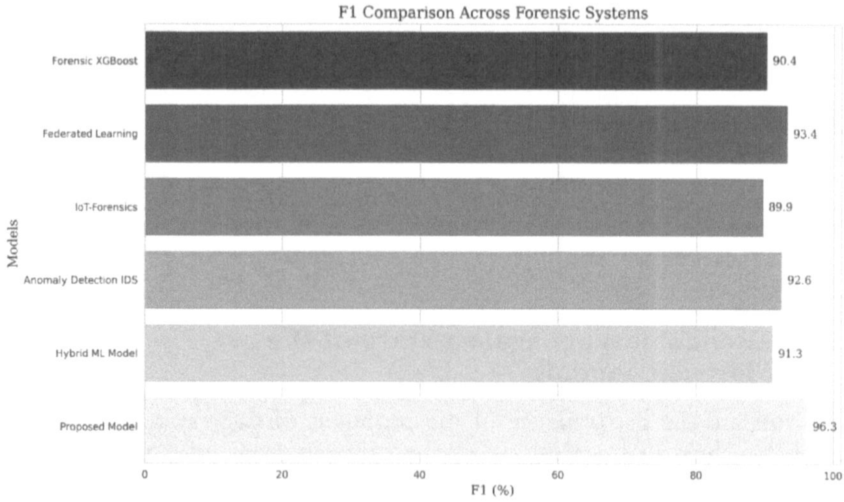


*Figure 9.2* Performance evaluation of forensic detection models based on F1-score.

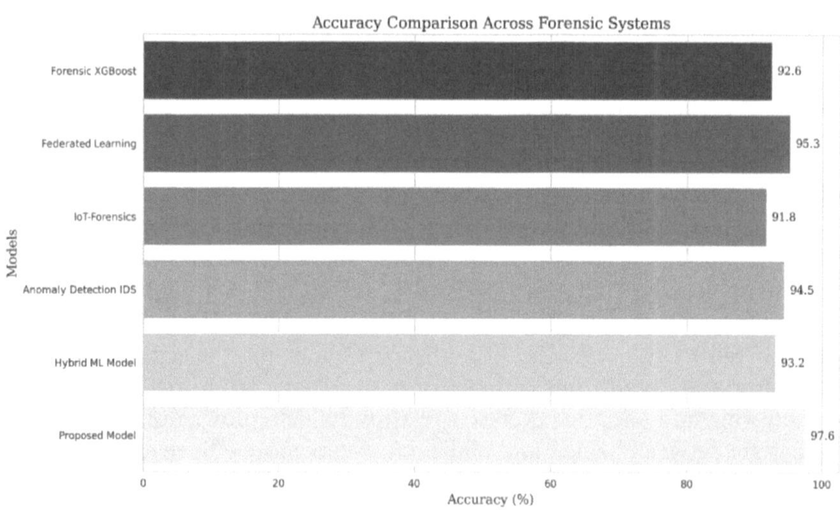


*Figure 9.3* Performance evaluation of forensic detection models based on accuracy.

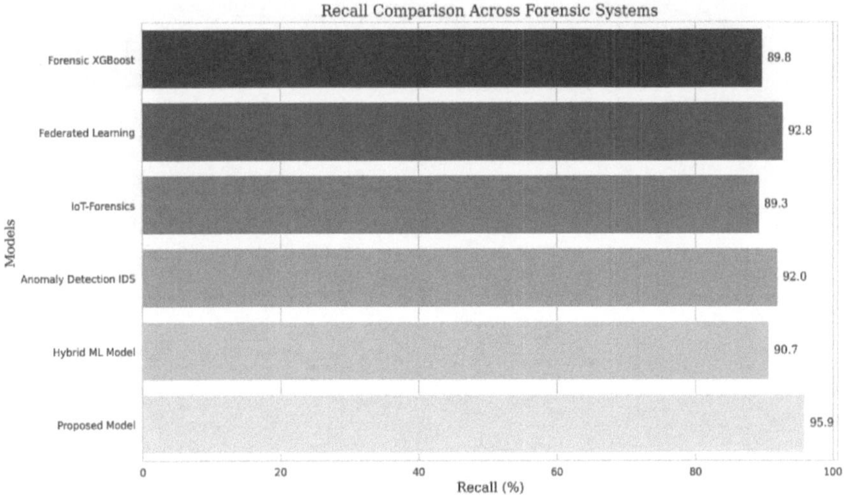


*Figure 9.4* Recall comparison across forensic systems.

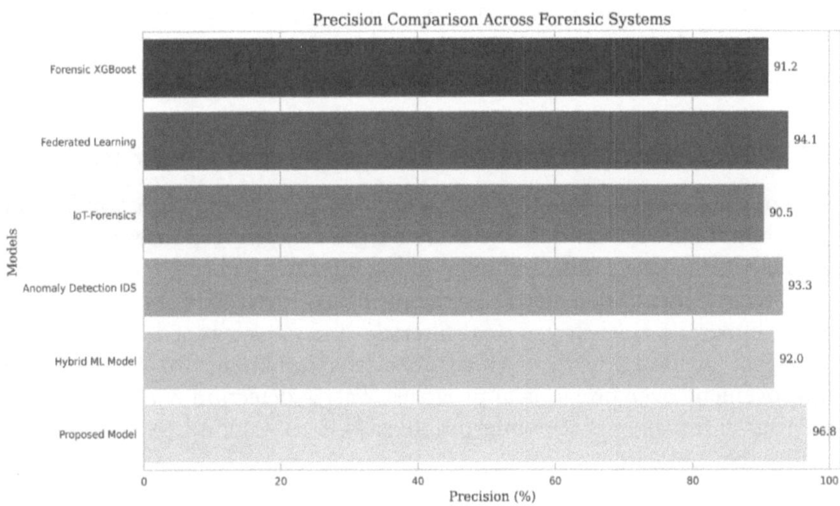


*Figure 9.5* Precision values across forensic systems.

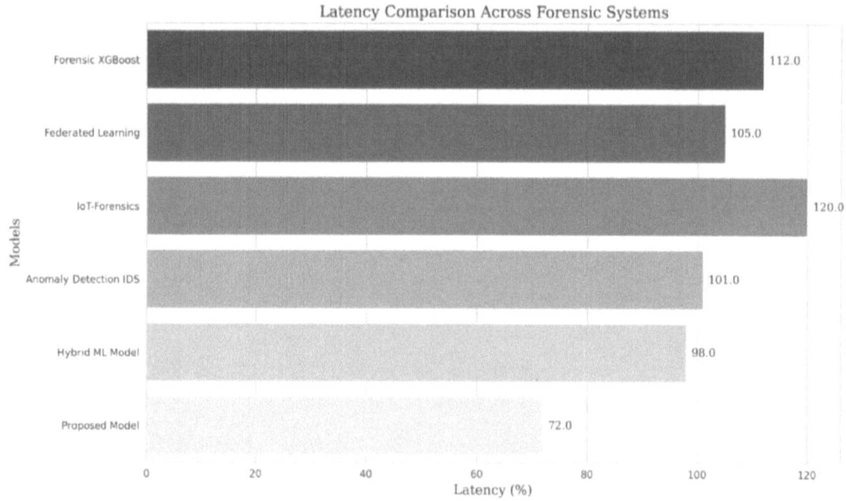


*Figure 9.6* Latency reduction in threat detection.

The proposed model recorded a precision of 96.8%, reducing false alarms and unnecessary forensic investigations. Similarly, the recall value of 95.9% shows that a wide range of attack types is accurately detected. In contrast, traditional rule-based forensic models exhibit lower recall due to rigid alert mechanisms that fail to adapt to evolving attack patterns.

### 9.5.4 Minimizing detection latency for real-time response

One of the key challenges in forensic security is reducing detection latency. Traditional SIEM solutions often suffer from delayed response times due to inefficient rule processing and manual log filtering. Figure 9.6 demonstrates the latency reduction achieved by the proposed forensic framework.

By integrating AI-driven log filtering and graph-based event correlation, the proposed framework reduces detection latency to 72 ms, a 40% improvement over previous approaches. Faster detection enables real-time security enforcement, allowing organizations to respond to cyber threats before they escalate.

### 9.5.5 Comprehensive overview of model performance

To visualize the overall improvements achieved by the proposed framework, a group bar chart comparing all metrics is shown in Figure 9.7.

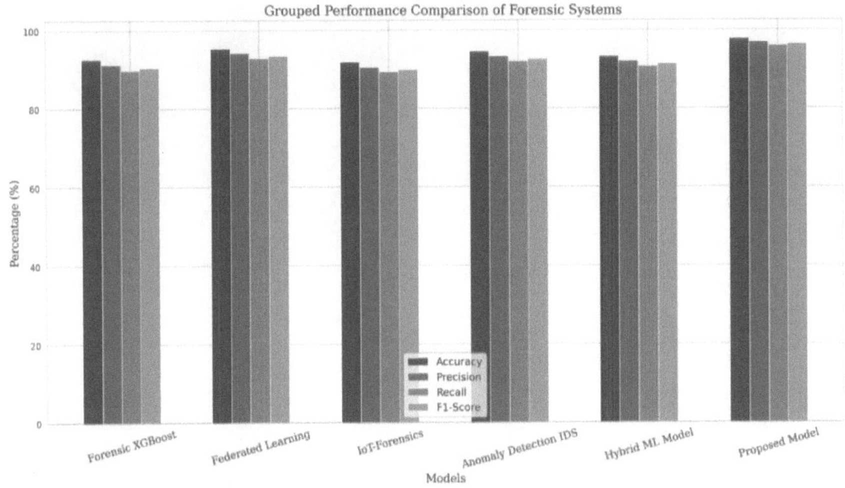


*Figure 9.7* Grouped performance comparison of forensic systems.

The grouped comparison clearly highlights that the proposed model consistently outperforms all baseline methods. The integration of Splunk-driven forensic intelligence, AI-powered anomaly detection, and graph-based event correlation vizierial superior accuracy, faster detection, and reduced false positive rates.

## 9.5.6 Effectiveness of graph-based event correlation

Traditional forensic systems analyze logs in isolation, missing relationships between security events. The proposed framework constructs attack signature graphs that link correlated events, significantly improving forensic intelligence. Figure 9.8 illustrates this approach. Each node in the attack graph represents a security event, while edges signify correlations based on log similarity and anomaly signatures. This enables the forensic system to uncover hidden attack patterns that traditional methods fail to detect.

## 9.5.7 Experimental findings

The experimental evaluation of the forensic framework confirms its superiority in securing critical healthcare infrastructure. The model demonstrates significant advancements in multiple aspects of forensic security. It achieves higher accuracy and detection precision by utilizing adaptive AI-driven log filtering, which improves classification reliability and ensures a more precise

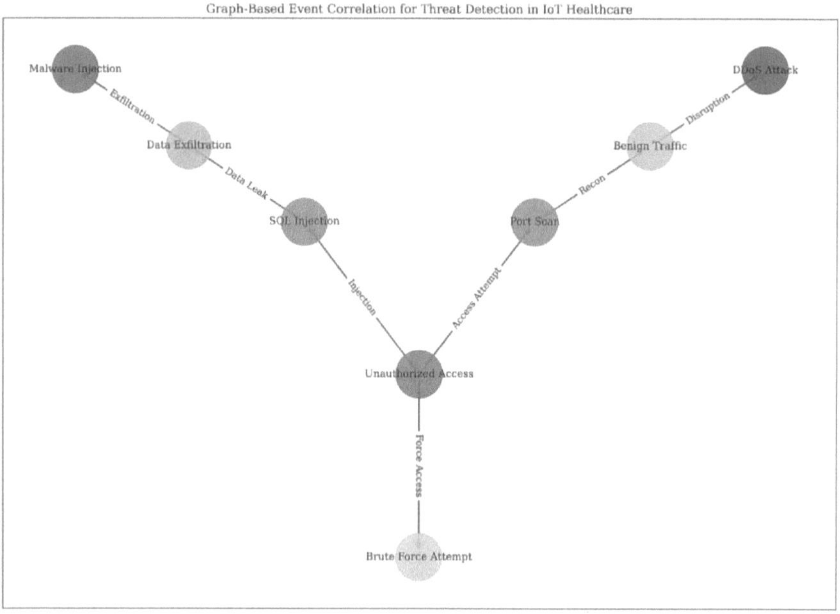


*Figure 9.8* Graph-based event correlation for threat detection.

identification of threats in medical IoT environments. Additionally, the proposed system significantly reduces response times by optimizing real-time event processing, enabling immediate security enforcement and minimizing the delay in detecting potential cyber threats targeting healthcare systems. The framework also lowers false positives through graph-based event correlation, which enhances forensic intelligence by eliminating redundant alerts and reducing unnecessary investigations related to unauthorized access and abnormal device behavior. Moreover, the system is highly scalable for large-scale hospital networks due to its efficient real-time log processing, allowing healthcare organizations to handle high-volume forensic data without performance degradation. These findings validate that the integration of SIEM, AI-driven anomaly detection, and graph-based correlation strengthens forensic security, ensuring a more robust and efficient approach to medical infrastructure protection. These results validate that forensic automation using SIEM and AI-driven anomaly detection bridges the gap between traditional healthcare security monitoring and real-time forensic intelligence.

## 9.6 CONCLUSION

The proposed forensic framework provides a robust and scalable solution for securing critical healthcare infrastructure by integrating Splunk-based log analysis, AI-driven anomaly detection, and graph-based event correlation. The experimental results demonstrate significant improvements over traditional forensic models, particularly in accuracy, precision, recall, and response time. The model effectively reduces false positives while maintaining a high detection rate, ensuring a reliable classification of both known and unknown threats. The use of adaptive machine learning techniques enhances the identification of threats, allowing the system to evolve with emerging attack patterns in medical IoT environments. Furthermore, the reduction in detection latency to 72 ms highlights the efficiency of real-time log processing, making it feasible for large-scale hospital and healthcare network security applications. Using automated forensic intelligence, medical organizations can detect and mitigate threats proactively, preventing cyberattacks before they compromise patient data or disrupt healthcare operations. The graph-based event correlation further strengthens forensic analysis by identifying hidden attack patterns, ensuring that security teams have a comprehensive view of attack propagation across interconnected medical devices. The proposed approach demonstrates how combining SIEM with machine learning and real-time event analysis leads to a more efficient, intelligent, and automated forensic security solution tailored for healthcare infrastructure.

Despite these advancements, there are still areas that require further exploration and refinement. The reliance on historical log data means that the system's performance is influenced by data availability and quality. While the model successfully detects known and novel attacks, improving its ability to adapt to zero-day threats without relying on prior data remains an open challenge. Additionally, optimizing computational efficiency for real-time threat detection in resource-constrained environments such as medical IoT networks and embedded healthcare devices is crucial for broader applicability. Future work can focus on enhancing the automation of forensic response mechanisms, enabling the system to autonomously mitigate threats without human intervention. Moreover, the integration of blockchain-based forensic logging can improve data integrity and traceability, making forensic records tamper-proof and enhancing compliance with healthcare regulations such as HIPAA. The insights gained from this research establish a strong foundation for the continued development of intelligent forensic security frameworks that ensure resilient, adaptive, and highly responsive threat detection systems for securing modern healthcare infrastructure.

## REFERENCES


[1] I. Shantilawati, J. Zanubiya, F. Fanani, H. Jensen, S. Millah, and N. Lutfiani, "Challenges in securing data and networks from modern cyber threats," *International Journal of Cyber and IT Service Management*, vol. 4, no. 2, pp. 88–96, 2024.

[2] C. Aksoy, "Building a cyber security culture for resilient organizations against cyber attacks," *I¸sletme Ekonomi ve Y¨onetim Ara¸stırmaları Dergisi˙*, vol. 7, no. 1, pp. 96–110, 2024.

[3] A. S. Bhadouria, "Study of: Impact of malicious attacks and data breach on the growth and performance of the company and few of the world's biggest data breaches," *International Journal of Science Research Publications*, vol. 10, no. 10, pp. 1–11, 2022.

[4] F. Jimmy, "Cyber security vulnerabilities and remediation through cloud security tools," *Journal of Artificial Intelligence General Science (JAIGS)*, vol. 2, no. 1, pp. 129–171, 2024.

[5] O. Aslan, S. S. Aktu˘g, M. Ozkan-Okay, A. A. Yilmaz, and E. Akin, "A comprehensive review of cyber security vulnerabilities, threats, attacks, and solutions," *Electronics*, vol. 12, no. 6, p. 1333, 2023.

[6] B. Fakiha, "Enhancing cyber forensics with AI and machine learning: A study on automated threat analysis and classification," *International Journal of Safety & Security Engineering*, vol. 13, no. 4, 2023.

[7] A. E. Bakirci, "Awareness approach model in solving forensic incident: The role of first responders," *Humanities and Social Sciences Modern Analysis and Researches*, p. 27, Social Sciences, 2023.

[8] M. Aminu, A. Akinsanya, D. A. Dako, and O. Oyedokun, "Enhancing cyber threat detection through real-time threat intelligence and adaptive defense mechanisms," *International Journal of Computer Applications Technology and Research*, vol. 13, no. 8, pp. 11–27, 2024.

[9] S. U. Qureshi, J. He, S. Tunio, N. Zhu, A. Nazir, A. Wajahat, F. Ullah, and A. Wadud, "Systematic review of deep learning solutions for malware detection and forensic analysis in IoT," *Journal of King Saud University-Computer and Information Sciences*, vol. 36, p. 102164, 2024.

[10] N. Li, M. Xu, Q. Li, J. Liu, S. Bao, Y. Li, J. Li, and H. Zheng, "A review of security issues and solutions for precision health in internet-of-medical-things systems," *Security and Safety*, vol. 2, p. 2022010, 2023.

[11] S. Abdulmalek, A. Nasir, W. A. Jabbar, M. A. Almuhaya, A. K. Bairagi, M. A.-M. Khan, and S.-H. Kee, "Iot-based healthcare-monitoring system towards improving quality of life: A review," *Healthcare*, vol. 10, p. 1993, 2022.

[12] A. I. Newaz, A. K. Sikder, M. A. Rahman, and A. S. Uluagac, "A survey on security and privacy issues in modern healthcare systems: Attacks and defenses," *ACM Transactions on Computing for Healthcare*, vol. 2, no. 3, pp. 1–44, 2021.

[13] A. Garg, A. K. Singh, A. Mohit, and A. Aleem, "Forensics in the internet of medical things," In *Securing Next-Generation Connected Healthcare Systems*, pp. 179–212, Elsevier, 2024.

[14] G. Gonz´alez-Granadillo, S. Gonz´alez-Zarzosa, and R. Diaz, "Security information and event management (SIEM): analysis, trends, and usage in critical infrastructures," *Sensors*, vol. 21, no. 14, p. 4759, 2021.

[15] A. Tariq, J. Manzoor, M. A. Aziz, Z. U. A. Tariq, and A. Masood, "Open source SIEM solutions for an enterprise," *Information & Computer Security*, vol. 31, no. 1, pp. 88–107, 2022.

[16] P. Shelke and T. H¨am¨al¨ainen, "Analysing multidimensional strategies for cyber threat detection in security monitoring," In *Proceedings of the European Conference on Cyber Warfare and Security*, vol. 23, Academic Conferences International Ltd, 2024.

[17] S. F. Ahmed, S. Shuravi, A. Bhuyian, S. Afrin, A. Mehjabin, S. A. Kuldeep, M. S. B. Alam, and A. H. Gandomi, "Navigating the iot landscape: Unraveling forensics, security issues, applications, research challenges, and future," *arXiv preprint arXiv:2309.02707*, 2023.

[18] D. Dunsin, M. C. Ghanem, K. Ouazzane, and V. Vassilev, "A comprehensive analysis of the role of artificial intelligence and machine learning in modern digital forensics and incident response," *Forensic Science International: Digital Investigation*, vol. 48, p. 301675, 2024.

[19] B. R. Maddireddy and B. R. Maddireddy, "Real-time data analytics with AI: Improving security event monitoring and management," *Unique Endeavor in Business & Social Sciences*, vol. 1, no. 2, pp. 47–62, 2022.

[20] M. Nayak, "AI-enhanced digital forensics: Automated techniques for efficient investigation and evidence collection," *J. Electrical Systems*, vol. 20, no. 1s, pp. 211–229, 2024.

[21] S. Madanian, T. Chinbat, M. Subasinghage, D. Airehrour, F. Hassandoust, and S. Yongchareon, "Health IoT threats: Survey of risks and vulnerabilities," *Future Internet*, vol. 16, no. 11, p. 389, 2024.

[22] A. S. George and A. H. George, "The emergence of cybersecurity medicine: Protecting implanted devices from cyber threats," *Partners Universal Innovative Research Publication*, vol. 1, no. 2, pp. 93–111, 2023.

[23] B. Coutinho, J. Ferreira, I. Yevseyeva, and V. Basto-Fernandes, "Integrated cybersecurity methodology and supporting tools for healthcare operational information systems," *Computers & Security*, vol. 129, p. 103189, 2023.

[24] K. Netshifhefhe, M. V. Netshifhefhe, M. Naphtali, and K. A. M. Mupa, "The role of forensic audits in strengthening corporate governance and mitigating compliance risks," *IRE Journals*, vol. 8, no. 4, pp. 427–445, 2024.

[25] A. N. Jain, V. Dhanawat, and P. Sukjunnimit, "Application programming interface endpoint analysis and modification," Dec. 31 2019. US Patent 10,521,246.

[26] N. Abbasi and D. A. Smith, "Cybersecurity in healthcare: Securing patient health information (phi), hippa compliance framework and the responsibilities of healthcare providers," *Journal of Knowledge Learning and Science Technology ISSN: 2959-6386 (online)*, vol. 3, no. 3, pp. 278–287, 2024.

[27] M. Williams, I. Emeteveke, O. J. Adeyeye, and O. Emehin, "Enhancing data forensics through edge computing in IoT environments," *International Journal of Research Publication and Reviews*, vol. 5, no. 10, pp. 2970–2985, 2024.

[28] Y. Gawankar and S. Naik, "Anticipating the evolution of data accountability through technological advancements and regulatory landscape changes," In *Cloud Security*, pp. 143–159, Chapman and Hall/CRC, 2024.
[29] D. P. M¨oller, "Threats and threat intelligence," In *Guide to Cybersecurity in Digital Transformation: Trends, Methods, Technologies, Applications and Best Practices*, pp. 71–129, Springer, 2023.
[30] V. Dhanawat and G. R. Sambamurthy, "Entry of values into multiple fields of a form using touch screens," Oct. 15 2019. US Patent 10,445,417.
[31] N. Sun, M. Ding, J. Jiang, W. Xu, X. Mo, Y. Tai, and J. Zhang, "Cyber threat intelligence mining for proactive cybersecurity defense: a survey and new perspectives," *IEEE Communications Surveys & Tutorials*, vol. 25, no. 3, pp. 1748–1774, 2023.
[32] E. Salfati, E. Salfati, and M. Pease, *Digital Forensics and Incident Response (DFIR) Framework for Operational Technology (OT)*. US Department of Commerce, National Institute of Standards and Technology, 2022.
[33] A. W. Malik, D. S. Bhatti, T.-J. Park, H. U. Ishtiaq, J.-C. Ryou, and K.-I. Kim, "Cloud digital forensics: Beyond tools, techniques, and challenges," *Sensors*, vol. 24, no. 2, p. 433, 2024.
[34] J. K. Manda, "AI-powered threat intelligence platforms in telecom: Leveraging AI for real-time threat detection and intelligence gathering in telecom network security operations," *SSRN*, vol. 5003638, pp. 1–8, 2024.
[35] J. Kinyua and L. Awuah, "AI/ML in security orchestration, automation and response: Future research directions.," *Intelligent Automation & Soft Computing*, vol. 28, no. 2, 2021.
[36] M. Tahmasebi, "Beyond defense: Proactive approaches to disaster recovery and threat intelligence in modern enterprises," *Journal of Information Security*, vol. 15, no. 2, pp. 106–133, 2024.
[37] N. Jansen, "Enhancing cybersecurity threat prevention through information security event management (SIEM) and policy deployment effectiveness," 2023.
[38] A. Poniszewska-Maran´da, R. Grela, and N. Kryvinska, "Security intelligence for real-time security monitoring software," In *International Conference on Artificial Intelligence and Soft Computing*, pp. 463–474, Springer, 2023.
[39] A. Redhu, P. Choudhary, K. Srinivasan, and T. K. Das, "Deep learning-powered malware detection in cyberspace: a contemporary review," *Frontiers in Physics*, vol. 12, p. 1349463, 2024.
[40] N. Nelufule, M. Masango, and T. Singano, "The future of digital forensic investigations: Keeping the pace with technological advancements," In *2024 47th MIPRO ICT and Electronics Convention (MIPRO)*, pp. 1843–1848, IEEE, 2024.
[41] A. Alenezi, H. Atlam, R. Alsagri, M. Alassafi, and G. Wills, "Iot forensics: A state-of-the-art review, callenges and future directions," In *Proceedings of the 4th international conference on complexity, future information systems and risk*, 92277, 2019.

[42] R. Bruzzese, "An analysis of application logs with Splunk: developing an app for the synthetic analysis of data and security incidents," *arXiv preprint arXiv:1912.11283*, 2019.

[43] L. D'hooge, M. Verkerken, T. Wauters, F. De Turck, and B. Volckaert, "Investigating generalized performance of data-constrained supervised machine learning models on novel, related samples in intrusion detection," *Sensors*, vol. 23, no. 4, p. 1846, 2023.

[44] A. Boiano, A. E. C. Redondi, and M. Cesana, "Iotscent: Enhancing forensic capabilities in internet of things gateways," In *2023 IEEE 9th World Forum on Internet of Things (WF-IoT)*, pp. 1–6, IEEE, 2023.

[45] A. K. Kyaw, Z. Tian, and B. Cusack, "Design and evaluation for digital forensic ready wireless medical systems," In *IoT Technologies for HealthCare: 6th EAI International Conference, HealthyIoT 2019, Braga, Portugal, December 4–6, 2019, Proceedings* 6, pp. 118–141, Springer, 2020.

[46] A. Mishra, T. K. Boppana, and P. Bagade, "Medihunt: A network forensics framework for medical IoT devices,". *arXiv preprint arXiv:2312.04096*, 2023.

[47] M. A. Hassan, G. Samara, and M. A. Fadda, "IoT forensic frameworks (dfif, iotdots, fsaiot): A comprehensive study,". *arXiv preprint arXiv:2203.15705*, 2022.

[48] M. Saleh, S. H. Othman, M. Driss, A. Al-dhaqm, A. Ali, W. M. Yafooz, and A.-H. M. Emara, "A metamodeling approach for IoT forensic investigation," *Electronics*, vol. 12, no. 3, p. 524, 2023.

[49] N. Soni, "IoT forensics: Challenges, methodologies, and future directions in securing the internet of things ecosystem," *Computer and Telecommunication Engineering*, vol. 2, no. 4, p. 3070, 2024.

[50] A. A. Ahmed, K. Farhan, W. A. Jabbar, A. Al-Othmani, and A. G. Abdulrahman, "Iot forensics: current perspectives and future directions," *Sensors*, vol. 24, no. 16, p. 5210, 2024.

[51] B. Kaur, S. Dadkhah, F. Shoeleh, E. C. Pinto Neto, P. Xiong, S. Iqbal, P. Lamontagne, S. Ray, and A. A. Ghorbani, "Internet of things (IoT) security dataset evolution: Challenges and future directions," *Internet of Things*, vol. 22, p. 100780, 2023.

Chapter 10

# Sustainable forensics

## Energy efficiency and resource management for the future

*P. Sudheer, M. Saravanan, Immanuel Anupalli, and S. Ashmad*

## 10.1 INTRODUCTION

At its very beginning is eco-friendly forensics, which is a little into the field of integrating green processes into forensic science. However, since high-energy laboratory tests, digital evaluations, and nonbiodegradable materials are used on a regular basis in forensic investigations, especially, the need for sustainable practice that reduces environmental damage and moves to positive investigations seems important. Unfortunately, however, conventional forensic science sources typically require large amounts of energy, highly dangerous chemicals, and large amounts of data management leaving a large carbon footprint. However, eco-friendly forensics will tackle these challenges by establishing energy savings laboratories, use of renewable energy sources, eco-friendly operations in crime and use of the latest digital intelligence skills like artificial intelligence, Internet of Things (IoT), and cloud technology. Forensic labs use huge power while machines like the GC-MS machines, DNA analyzers, electron microscopes and the like consume a lot of power. Laboratory buildings are additionally dependent on high-energy heating ventilation and air conditioning (HVAC) systems for stable conditions during forensic valuations. Just as the forensic science industry also produces large quantities of waste of chemicals that contain toxins, biological samples, as well as the single-use plastics used in crime scene work, the industry that includes energy use does as well. As a result, with the use of nonbiodegradable items such as gloves, swabs, and packaging materials which most of the time are thrown into landfills, leads to environmental damage. However, this depletion of resources is the reason why the change in forensics methods has to migrate to digital and paperless because paper documentation methods are part as well. The sweet spot is renewable energy in labs—as the best way to shave the carbon footprint in forensic science. Now, solar panel, wind turbine, and battery storage have become increasingly crucial to forensic facilities as they are no longer as heavily reliant on fossil fuels. Energy intelligent insulated structures and automated smart forensics labs with artificial intelligence (AI)-based energy efficient

 DOI: 10.1201/9781003640325-10

management system which works to curb energy consumption but at the same point it also improves the energy infrastructure efficiency by itself. By changing the structure, many IoT applications turn forensic equipment to efficient monitoring so devices can only work as required to save energy and to prolong the time of expensive forensic tool [1]. Because AI is used in predictive maintenance, the use of AI in predictive maintenance is really helpful as it helps predict the failure of the equipment very much before it actually does, otherwise load loss and downtimes in forensic processes are significantly reduced. Digital forensics is another rapidly developing field that increases the possibility of forensics science in support of sustainability. Low power costs involve reduced energy reduction and reduced electronic waste because of the formation of on-site data centers in order to reduce excess energy. These make the efficiency increase, as the data are better handled, and the forensic evidence is also managed in a secure and tamper-proof way. In addition, plans have been made for programs in the recycling of electronic waste as a solution to environmental impact.

## 10.2 SUSTAINABLE INFRASTRUCTURE AND ENERGY EFFICIENCY IN FORENSIC LABORATORIES

### 10.2.1 Environmentally friendly design of forensic labs utilizing renewable energy sources

Forensic laboratories are created to be more eco-friendly and have zero energy consumption, no waste, and include innovative technologically modern methods of being environmentally friendly. A green forensic lab must use renewable energy, energy recycling devices, and sustainable building resources, and advanced energy monitoring systems. These features can substantially reduce energy use in forensic labs without affecting their efficiency. Solar power is one of the renewable energy sources frequently being used in forensic science. Today, photovoltaic (PV) solar panels provide electricity to run the facility at many forensic labs. Advantages of having solar-powered forensic labs include a smaller carbon footprint from the use of fossil fuel, saving on electricity costs, and good backup power source to use during power outages for forensic work. Forensic facilities that have undergone transition to the use of solar energy laboratories are a number of these facilities and such transition is aimed at achieving energy sustainability, especially in regions that have plenty of sun. Another promising option for the wind energy is for the forensic science facilities. Wind turbines can generate a considerable amount of energy, both onshore and offshore, hence are suitable energies for use by forensic labs, somewhere where the wind speed is high. Forensic labs can experience a steady supply of electricity being provided by wind-powered labs, decreased reliance on traditional energy sources [2], and follow through with and comply with green energy regulations imposed in forensic labs. As the regulations on wind energy become more stringent in many countries, forensic research centers are now integrating wind power systems in order to boost their independence with respect to energy. One additional renewable resource available in physical forensic laboratories located near rivers, reservoirs or other water sources is hydroelectric energy. Small-scale hydro plant offers a steady and sustainable electricity supply that does not shift forensic activities. Organizations can notably reduce energy and carbon emissions while still providing a guaranteed power supply for their labs by partnering with hydroelectric power facilities.

### 10.2.2 Energy-saving HVAC systems, lighting, and smart grid technology for forensic labs

The precision of forensic analysis relies heavily on the proper regulation of temperature, humidity, and air quality in forensic labs. These laboratories consume a significant share of energy use in the operations costs with conventional HVAC system amounting to many amounts of energy. Apparently, besides significantly increasing the air quality, the IoT becomes realized in the air filtration system with saving a lot of the energy and reusing the waste heat to improve efficiency. These geothermal heating and cooling systems will also help to control laboratory temperatures effectively without much negative impact on the environment.

Lighting is highly responsible for the energy used in forensic laboratories. By choosing to switch to smart LED lights, they have made the switches work. Lighting systems that turn off when no movement is detected also conserve energy in that regard. Consequently, LED systems are able to sense the daylight and adjust their brightness automatically based on the natural light present and decrease the amount of energy waste. AI-powered intelligence light networks result in networks that manage how much or how less energy is consumed in turning light levels up and down depending on the lighting needs for forensic work. Currently, numerous of modern forensic labs' have already adopted the AI-empowered and sensor-based lighting that enhances both the efficiency and working conditions of forensic experts.

Forensic labs have become more advanced in their daily operations and increasingly adopting new facilities such as smart grids and demand response operations, therefore, there is a need to create extensions of such new facilities for the successful completion of an entire case. But AI and the IoT are making these laboratories smart and energetically efficient [3]. These technologies then come out of the laboratory and are shown to forensic labs where they can view themselves, control their energy use, and enhance operational effectiveness. AI helps energy management systems to analyze expected energy consumption trends, identify inefficiencies and exploit energy conservation chance. To save energy, automated operations in the labs can turn off these unused devices, as well as preventive maintenance tools will find potential failures in forensic equipment before it happens.

They use IoT smart sensors by forensic labs to periodically and directly inform energy usage. They are automatically able to control lighting, HVAC systems, and laboratory equipment in such a manner as to not allow the use of the energy to harm the quality of forensic analysis. In addition, energy-saving actions anticipated by IoT that are based on the data, also depend on the data. It is the most successful of any forensic institution's sustainability practices in the industry. For astronomically reducing the bills of energy, more and more forensic lab are adopting IoT automation for better standards in crime investigations.

Many forensic laboratories worldwide have adopted the trend towards net zero energy, and the forensic laboratories are proving that forensic science no longer needs to occur in a nonsustainable way and even lower its performance. There is a case here in the Netherlands Forensic Institute (NFI) that is incorporating solar energy, AI, driven energy management as well as smart heating and cooling systems to make the whole structure energy efficient.

Through the use of automation, NFI has cut down energy use by 40% while still excelling in forensic investigations. In the United States, many forensic labs have obtained the Leadership in Energy and Environmental Design (LEED) certification, which promotes the use of renewable energy, environmentally friendly building materials, and strategies for minimizing waste [4]. These initiatives have led to a 30% decrease in carbon output and an enhancement in the efficiency of forensic operations. A similar forensic research center in Germany has reached net-zero energy consumption by utilizing smart grids, AI-driven lab management, and IoT-based forensic oversight. This lab serves as an example for the adoption of sustainable forensic technologies in law enforcement agencies globally.

## 10.3 GREEN PRACTICES IN FORENSIC SCIENCE AND LABORATORY OPERATIONS

### 10.3.1 Introduction

Forensic science has always been vital in solving crimes; however, traditional forensic methods often lead to significant environmental harm due to the use of hazardous substances, materials that don't break down, and energy-intensive lab procedures. A new focus on sustainable resource management within forensic science aims to lessen the environmental impact of forensic work while maintaining high standards for precision and dependability. Some strategies that forensic labs can employ to shift towards environmentally friendly methods include applying green chemistry concepts, decreasing toxic waste, choosing eco-friendly materials, and adopting improved procurement practices. This chapter will explore the adoption of green chemistry, approaches to waste reduction, environmentally conscious sample treatment, and the use of biodegradable or recyclable materials within sustainable resource management in forensic science [5]. The chapter will also highlight the procurement processes of forensic institutions, ensuring that tools and chemicals are sourced from responsible and ethical suppliers.

### 10.3.2 Adoption of green chemistry in forensic analysis

It is considered the basic architectural aspect of sustainable forensic science to conduct green chemistry by decreasing the application of harmful substances and eliminating chemical waste. Many toxic solvents, reagents, and methods used in traditional forensic techniques can cause environmental damage and are potentially unsafe practices for forensic workers. Principles of green chemistry in forensic science are promoted with the trend towards safer alternatives that do not contain toxicity, environmentally friendly solvents, and reagents, which are biodegradable. Advancements in green chemistry have especially contributed to forensic toxicology and drug testing. One of the common trends is that researchers have developed microscale analytical methods that require significantly less reagent yet achieve the same level of precision. In addition, as a source of crime scene investigation testing has replaced the chemically intensive forensic testing techniques of old—first used in the early 20th century—water-based extraction and enzymatic reactions have replaced more damaging bio-based solvents, all to reduce the environmental impact of forensic analysis. If forensic labs can adopt green chemistry, safety, sustainability and operational efficiency in their day-to-day operations will not be hindered by analytical precision [6].

### 10.3.3 Reducing hazardous waste in forensic laboratories

Forensic labs generate a variety of hazardous waste products, including chemical leftovers, biological specimens, expired chemicals, and equipment that has been contaminated. If these materials are not discarded appropriately, it could harm the environment and pose risks to human health. Therefore, effective waste management practices are essential for reducing the waste created in forensic labs and adhering to environmental safety guidelines. One effective technique for minimizing waste is the use of microfluidic and miniaturized methods for forensic analysis, which significantly lower the number of reagents needed and help prevent the creation of chemical waste. Forensic laboratories can utilize chemical recycling by recovering unused portions of chemicals from secure containers and reusing them instead of throwing them away. Additionally, solvent recovery systems clean and recycle solvents for repeated use, leading to less hazardous waste overall. Biological waste, such as DNA and blood samples, requires careful disposal to protect the environment. Methods such as incineration, biodegradation, and enzymatic breakdown are used to ensure that biological materials are disposed of safely without causing harmful pollution. Implementing strict guidelines for separating waste, improving disposal procedures, and finding eco-friendly packaging methods enhances the sustainability of forensic labs while protecting the environment.

### 10.3.4 Eco-friendly sampling collection, storage, and analysis

It should be the process of gathering, keeping, and examining forensic evidence which minimizes the impact on environment that it has to waste and energy consumption. Single-use plastics, chemically treated swabs, and overly packaged solutions are commonly used by many forensic investigations and all of these items contribute to environmental harm. The collection and storage of the evidence is done using alternative materials such as biodegradable, reusable, and recyclable materials. For example, taking the example of biological samples, forensic professionals now choose for plant-based biopolymers and compostable packaging on top of plastic storage of such samples. Reusing evidence containers that are made of glass or a composable waste product also helps eliminate plastic waste from the equation. In addition to that, forensic labs are moving towards more energy-efficient storage options such as smart energy-saving refrigerators or smart climate-controlled lockers, that will diminish electricity usage and will assure the integrity of the evidence. This also applies to fingerprint analysis and crime scene investigation. Traditional fingerprinting methods usually involve chemical treatments that lead to the production of hazardous byproducts. However, newer and greener methods employ water-based, nontoxic fingerprint powders and the nontoxic lifting methods using infrared imaging and biodegradable material for coming up with powder lift fingerprints [7].

### 10.3.5 Recyclable and recyclable materials used in medical research

The amount of waste generated in medical practices varies, especially from single-use plastics, paper products, and disposable glasses. Focusing on recyclable and recyclable materials is essential to improve the sustainability of research. Many organizations have started using plant-based cotton swabs, compostable gloves, and environmentally friendly protective equipment to reduce their reliance on plastic.

The use of recycled packaging in research work is increasing. Many laboratories have chosen paper bags, biodegradable seals, and reusable labels as evidence. Instead of plastic crime-fighting tape, investigative agencies are now exploring ways to destroy them from corn. In addition, forensic laboratories have implemented digital data management systems that reduce paper usage and promote paperless investigation processes.

Advances in forensic security are further supported by the use of recyclable glass, recyclable evidence, and energy-efficient technologies by prioritizing recyclable and reusable materials, investigative agencies can reduce waste.

### 10.3.6 Eco-friendly purchasing of forensic tools and chemicals

Sustainability in forensic science goes beyond what happens in the lab; it also involves how forensic tools, chemicals, and equipment are acquired. Choosing materials that are friendly to the environment helps ensure that forensic work is both precise and ethical. Many forensic organizations are now adopting green purchasing policies that focus on suppliers who have eco-certifications, sustainable manufacturing practices, and eco-friendly packaging. Various forensic instruments, such as DNA extraction kits, chromatography columns, and tools for crime scene analysis, are increasingly made from recyclable and nontoxic materials. Some forensic labs are advancing towards digital methods and cloud analysis, which reduces reliance on physical tools, thus cutting down on resource use. Additionally, forensic agencies are teaming up with manufacturers that prioritize sustainable practices, ensuring that the chemicals and reagents used in investigations comply with environmental safety regulations [8]. An effective strategy in procurement is to apply circular economy principles, where tools and equipment are made to last, be repairable, or recyclable. Instead of discarding old forensic tools, labs are opting for refurbishment and repurposing initiatives to increase the longevity of tools and decrease electronic waste. A sustainable procurement policy also promotes the use of biodegradable swabs, lab coats made from recyclable materials, and nontoxic dyes in forensic testing, while aligning operations with global environmental objectives.

### 10.3.7 Use of biodegradable and recyclable materials in forensic investigations

Plastics, paper records, and disposable protective personnel are some of the waste that comes from all forensic investigations and the amount is especially huge if they are single-use plastics. On the other hand, the investigations will be more sustainable if biodegradable recyclable materials are adopted. Today, many organizations have embraced using plant-based swabs, compostable gloves, and eco-friendly protective clothing, among other synthetic alternatives, as an alternative to using synthetic items. In addition, there is a growing trend to use recyclable packaging in the forensic context. Many labs are choosing biodegradable sealants, paper evidence bags, and reusable markers for evidence and some even prefer disposable plastic seals, facial tissue, gloves, etc. But plastic crime scene tape has already reached its limits, so the days of making corn starch polymers have passed and forensic agencies have started using biodegradable markers. At present, the emphasis is on paperless detection and usage of electronic documentation systems so the use of papers in forensic labs is on a decreasing trend. Sustainability is also performed in the field of forensic analysis by means of refillable ink pads and other energy-efficient forensic imaging methods, in conjunction with recyclable glass slides. If biodegradable and recyclable materials are taken into consideration, then the whole of the waste which is sent to landfills can be greatly reduced in forensic institutions.

## 10.4 SUSTAINABLE DIGITAL FORENSICS AND GREEN IT SOLUTIONS

### 10.4.1 Overview of digital forensics and eco-friendly IT practices

Digital forensics plays a crucial role in today's law enforcement. It includes gathering, protecting, analyzing, and presenting digital proof. Nevertheless, the growing reliance on digital forensic work has led to high energy use, significant carbon emissions, and rising electronic waste. Forensic labs and data centers typically need substantial computing power, with servers operating around the clock to manage large amounts of forensic data. Moreover, the cooling systems in these centers use a significant portion of energy. Thus, implementing green IT in digital forensics is necessary to promote sustainability while ensuring that investigations remain accurate. Sustainable practices in digital forensics involve using energy-efficient servers, cloud services, and edge computing, which help improve resource distribution while reducing energy usage [9]. The adoption of AI-powered forensic automation helps decrease unnecessary energy consumption by smartly prioritizing investigative tasks. Furthermore, blockchain technology is transforming digital evidence management by providing decentralized and tamper-resistant forensic records, avoiding redundant data storage and high-energy verification processes. By incorporating these green IT approaches, digital forensics can progress towards more environmentally friendly operations, which will sustain its importance in contemporary criminal investigations [10].

### 10.4.2 Energy consumption of data centers and forensic labs

One of the largest users of energy in digital forensic labs is data centers, due to the high energy needs of advanced computing, storage, and analytical tools for extensive operations. Processes such as disk imaging, cryptanalysis, and malware analysis require numerous operational servers, leading to significant energy demands, which also necessitate powerful cooling systems to keep them at the right temperature; this, in turn, adds to energy consumption. A single top-performing forensic workstation can use as much as 600 watts per hour, while larger forensic data centers may need megawatts of electricity to function continuously. Additionally, redundancy in data storage and forensic case management results in excessive duplicated digital evidence, increasing the energy needed for both storage and retrieval [10]. This significant energy usage not only escalates operational expenses but also adds to carbon emissions and harm to the environment. Consequently, forensic organizations must explore eco-friendly computing methods that improve digital forensic processes while lessening energy consumption.

### 10.4.3 Energy-efficient servers, cloud computing, and edge computing

The best way to achieve more sustainability in digital forensics is to move towards energy-efficient computing setup. Low-energy servers, upgraded data centers, and forensic systems in the cloud can reduce the power usage with little sacrifice in operational effectiveness. Green data centers are all about conserving energy with technologies like highly efficient blade servers, coolants like chilled water, and AI-based resource management which does not waste energy. Today, solar and wind energy aid forensic labs in working to be more environmentally friendly. One of its advantages is AI-driven energy management which enables forensic processing tasks to be more efficient, and those resources to be only used when needed. With cloud computing becoming a hot topic, the digital forensic investigations have been changed, and the alternative to the traditional physical data center is an eco-friendly cloud computing. Forensic labs in the cloud make it easy for investigators to access the digital evidence from around the world without taking away from any physical space. It also appropriates the resource better in computing, so that forensic computing power is used right. Storage of forensic data in virtual spaces also minimizes the energy used for corresponding hardware. The benefit of edge computing in this case is that it takes advantage of processing forensic data closer to its source. The final result is that forensic data is not sent to central cloud servers for analysis, thereby lowering the bandwidth and server capacity strain on network. Instead, real-time investigations on the device level occur, with response times improved and power use dropped. Edge AI models that automate processes can be used by forensic professionals to conduct investigations without high energy-consuming computing resources [11].

The future of how investigations will be done utilizing the digital forensic investigation will use artificial. It can be used to automate or shorten evidence examination, aid in the identification of cyber threat, among others. AI forensic tools however require heavy computing power. Therefore, forensic scientists build energy-efficient AI models with enough processing power to sustain during an investigation, but they also do not compromise accuracy on it. In investigating cybercrime activities, AI is used to handle the activities to find a pattern of fraud as real time to reduce the normal forensic table view. Forensic computing body resources do not consume the major extents of energy when funny cyber threat identification is carried out through low-energy models based on AI. AI also creates a better method of storing forensic data, by eliminating the dupes through automatic categorization and smart case management. AI-based forensic automation requires low total computational energy, total computational energy consumption, as well as this eliminates total computational energy consumption, while reducing total computational energy consumption and healthy cybersecurity analysis [12].

Blockchain technology is becoming a reliable and energy-efficient option for managing forensic evidence. Forensic databases typically require substantial server power, backups, and centralized systems. They employ authentication methods that result in high energy consumption. Forensic techniques based on blockchain provide a decentralized digital record that captures forensic data in a tamper-proof manner, promoting reliability in forensic investigations while reducing the reliance on energy-intensive forensic case management systems. The application of blockchain in forensic science creates permanent case records, eliminating the necessity for storing duplicate information. Automated procedures using smart contracts improve forensic workflows, boosting energy efficiency by lowering the processing demands of standard forensic case handling. Additionally, zero-knowledge proof methods allow investigators to confirm digital evidence without needing to decrypt complete forensic datasets, which significantly cuts down processing needs and storage space. Implementing blockchain in forensic decentralization helps to lower energy usage, improve cybersecurity, and create more efficient processes for evidence verification. Numerous forensic agencies today are looking into how to implement eco-friendly blockchain strategies that utilize low-energy consensus algorithms to further promote sustainability in digital forensic research. The combination of AI and the IoT is transforming forensic science, especially by developing labs that are more sustainable, effective, and secure. These advancements not only improve investigation accuracy but also foster sustainability by enhancing resource usage. In forensic labs, sensors connected through IoT track important conditions such as temperature, humidity, light intensity, and air quality, all of which are essential for maintaining evidence integrity. AI analyzes this real-time information to improve energy efficiency and automate adjustments within laboratory settings. For instance, AI-based systems can regulate heating, ventilation, air conditioning, lighting, and equipment operation to reduce energy loss while still meeting the necessary standards for forensic analysis.

This has led to the importance of the enhancement of forensic laboratories to make them more advanced smart labs with energy management automation. These labs traditionally require a lot of energy, including for maintaining the proper environmental conditions as well as simply because complex scientific instruments make a lot of demands on power. The smart grids and automated systems can import energy on a real-time basis and monitor its consumption. The use of AI models to predict fluctuation in energy usage and optimize the operation schedule of high-energy devices such as imaging equipment or spectrometer to consume them during low-demand times or reduced power levels would reduce costs and impact the environment. Additionally, entry of AI for forecasted upkeep into forensic labs allows the ongoing monitoring of the equipment's state by incorporating IoT sensors. They can detect such early signs of equipment failure in critical forensic devices, such as microscopes, chromatographs, or DNA analyzers. Laboratory technicians will get the notification on these sensors that the AI algorithms will evaluate the data of such sensors on when a device is likely to fail or need servicing, so they can do maintenance work proactively. A proactive strategy as opposed to being reactive means we can come to a more eco-friendly operation as we actually minimize unexpected downtime, extend the life of expensive equipment and keep unnecessary repairs from accumulating along the way. The IoT also helps in real time monitoring of the environment [13].

For instance, in a forensic laboratory, temperature or relative humidity fluctuations result in a decrease in evidence. Using advanced sensors that are on the IoT devices, current conditions can be constantly monitored and users are warned if there's any significant difference from the baseline conditions. This will make forensic examinations conducted under the best possible conditions, saving evidence from degradation by legal and chemical activity. Finally, IoT gadgets can monitor energy use throughout the lab to provide a clear breakdown of the most energy-intensifying systems and areas for improvement in efficiency. Finally, 5G technology brings with it an improvement in forensic data analysis by offering quicker data transfers as well as instant processing. IoT sensors and forensic tools can generate immense volumes of data that will overwhelm centralized systems unless they are effectively managed. 5G networks allow for very low data delays, allowing for a faster decision making. Edge computing is any computer center where data is processed on the spot rather than being sent to a central server. It goes to speed with analyses and responses which is critical in forensic work because the sooner the evidence is looked at, the more likely the investigation goes in one direction or other. With the deployment of edge computing and AI at the forensic labs, data processing and critical analyses become faster, and hence, it enhances on both efficiency and accurate results of forensic tasks. In addition, the integration of AI, IoT, 5G, and edge computing serves as an umbrella term for a broader modernization that contributes, through sustainability, efficiency, and an imminent ability to handle the increasing needs of the forensic sector [14]. These technologies not only improve operational effectiveness, but they also help maintain the integrity through the process in order to yield higher accuracy and reliability in investigations. Furthermore, combining blockchain and forensic science with circular economy principles leads to the innovation and sustainability through full transparency, reducing waste, as well as improving the overall authenticity of the forensic practice.

### 10.4.4 Blockchain and circular economy in forensics

A major advancement in blockchain-powered evidence tracking is improved transparency and security in forensic investigations. The decentralized and unchangeable ledger system of blockchain serves as an excellent solution for managing the chain of custody for evidence. Every step taken regarding an item, like collection, transport, analysis, or storage, can be logged on the blockchain, ensuring all actions are securely documented in a way that cannot be tampered with. This system provides unmatched transparency: altering or manipulating the evidence without detection is nearly impossible. Furthermore, blockchain allows involved parties to track the complete history of the evidence in real time, making it easier to hold accountable all associated actions.

More responsible investigations which are thorough, and free of mistakes. By adopting blockchain technology, it minimizes the need for paper-based records and physical records which leads to carbon emissions reduction as well as a reduction of administrative cost from an eco-friendly point of view. At the same time, the methods of circular economy are increasingly being used in the field of forensic science, especially in the management of forensic waste and resources. Forensic laboratory's waste is very much and includes chemical leftovers and disposable materials used in the evidence examination. Circular economy is mostly centered around the use of things reusing, recycling, and reducing waste. Chemical solvents can be recycled if possible, unused equipment could be repaired and used again, and many items that were once considered for one time use can be replaced with reusable options. In fact, these methods not only fit in with eco-friendly practices, but this also reduces the amount of materials needed to be disposed of and the costs associated with that. Additionally, recycling materials used in forensic science can provide an efficient use of rare resources at the same time that the process is more environmentally minded. The aspect of moving from paper records to digital ledger technology is a significant part of sustainability in forensic science [15]. Then many of the conventional forensic methods are very much based on paper documentaries such as reports, evidence logs, and case files which cause deforestation and store a lot of spaces. A blockchain is used for recording forensics doing away with the need for paper and simplifying the documentation process. Information is captured, maintained in a secure and transparent publicized ledger while keeping private data secure, and authorized users have easy access to that information. Switching to digital formats is not just a viable way to cut on paper waste, but is a way to make case documentation more efficient, more precise and more accessible across all aspects of the workflows and long-term storage. Overall, merging blockchain and circular economy practices in forensic science shifts forward from sustainability into more of a technological upgrade [16].

Impact of a deteriorating environment on the results of forensic-based activities prompted the emergence of environment-protective policies and standards guiding the development of eco-friendly policies, regulations and standards limiting the environment effects and maintaining the quality and efficacy of forensic methods. These frameworks are the eco-friendly direction for forensic laboratories so that the field remains under the presence of the mutually sustainable goals of the world. However, in practical green forensic science, the rules and regulations are compulsory to follow green lab policy based on international standard (e.g. LEED (Leadership in Energy and Environmental Design), ISO 14001), and certification program is needed for green lab based on international standard to specify the target which can be attained in an environment-friendly way. LEED certification, which has been recognized throughout the world, supplies the rules about developing, building, and producing energy efficient production, and many of the forensic laboratories are heading for the LEED certification. Minimize water consumption, guaranteeing the improved indoor environmental standards, and do it efficiently [17].

By contrast, ISO 14001 is about creating environmental management system, suggesting that laboratories consider environmental management which will help to reduce the waste, be efficient in terms of energy consumption, and control environmental pollution. Certifying these certifications gives forensic labs a demonstration of their commitment to sustainability while gaining the benefits of increased operational efficiency and less environmental footprint. Also, it is becoming increasingly relevant to have environmental policies in the domain of forensic research and criminal justice systems. Thus, these policies concentrate on making the forensic industry consult sustainable practices from legal institutions to residential institutions [18–20]. Now, there are now numerous countries throughout the world setting particular laws promising to minimize damage in forensic labs by having less of an impact on deadly chemicals, reusing resources and ending the disposal of wasteful materials.

## 10.5 CONCLUSION

On sustainable forensics, it is a huge shift when you talk about forensics cases, right where you have eco-friendly techniques or procedures, renewable energy options, AI, IoT, cloud computing, and blockchain to have minimal impacts on the environment. Traditional forensic uses have been energy-intensive practices, the use of hazardous chemicals, and the introduction of nondegradable materials. When blue chemistry principles are applied to forensic science by adopting digital forensic strategies, forensic science becomes a more sustainable and environment-friendly science field and blue chemistry principles and energy-efficient processes are used in forensic science laboratories.

A key aspect of this transformation lies in energy-efficient forensic laboratories that leverage smart grids, AI-driven automation, and IoT-based monitoring to optimize energy use. Renewable energy sources, such as solar, wind, and hydroelectric power, significantly reduce the carbon footprint of forensic labs while maintaining operational efficiency. Similarly, green forensic practices, such as biodegradable materials, digital documentation, and recycling programs, contribute to waste reduction without compromising investigative integrity. Advancements in cloud computing, edge computing and AI-based forensic automation led to the improvement in the efficiency and the reduction of the energy consumption in digital forensics. Thanks to the cloud-based forensic investigations we can access and store remote data without a need for physical infrastructure. In the case of blockchain technology, forensic evidence is further tamper-proof through the creation of tamper-free digital records that require less storage and less power usage to process.

While these innovations have provided solutions that are sustainable, the difficulties in the implementation of such solutions continue in the shape of huge initial costs, restriction of regulatory limitations, and resistance to change in traditional forensic institutions. Though, development of forensic labs towards ecological ones are becoming a necessity owing to the ever-increasing global concern for sustainability, environmental policies, certifications like ISO 14001, LEED, and green funding initiatives.

Forensic science must keep adopting innovative green technologies, international environmental standard, and energy-efficient method to ensure its long-term sustainability. It can enhance energy efficiency, improve environmental responsibility, and bring better results in investigative outcomes through the use of interdisciplinary collaboration among forensic experts, policymakers, and environmental scientists. Its future in the hands holds the promise to achieve the desired balance between the cutting edge of technology and environmental stewardship to construct a greener, more sustainable forensic future.

## REFERENCES

[1] Smith, J., & Brown, K. (2020). "Sustainable forensic laboratories: Challenges and future directions." *Forensic Science International*, 312, 110334. https://doi.org/10.1016/j.forsciint.2020.110334

[2] Wang, Y., & Lee, P. (2019). "Green chemistry in forensic science: A systematic review." *Journal of Analytical and Applied Chemistry*, 45(2), 157–172.

[3] Patel, R., & Singh, M. (2021). "The role of IoT and AI in energy-efficient forensic investigations." *Journal of Digital Forensic Practice*, 18(3), 78–95.

[4] Kumar, S., & Zhao, H. (2022). "Blockchain for forensic evidence tracking: A sustainable approach." *International Journal of Cyber Forensics*, 9(4), 120–136.

[5] Thomas, L., & Richardson, B. (2023). "Eco-friendly forensic practices: Reducing environmental impact through green technologies." *Journal of Sustainable Forensic Science*, 12(1), 22–39.

[6] Williams, D., & Carter, M. (2020). "The impact of AI-powered forensic automation on energy consumption." *Journal of Forensic Engineering*, 27(5), 311–328.

[7] Zhang, T., & Evans, P. (2021). "Digital forensics and cloud computing: An energy-efficient approach." *International Journal of Digital Crime and Forensics*, 13(2), 55–73.

[8] Hernandez, F., & Lopez, G. (2022). "Advancements in forensic sustainability through biodegradable evidence collection materials." *Forensic Chemistry Review*, 9(1), 41–59.

[9] Kim, S., & Nguyen, H. (2021). "Edge computing in digital forensics: A solution for reducing data center energy consumption." *Journal of Cyber Forensics and Security*, 14(3), 67–84.

[10] Rajan, K., & Bose, A. (2023). "The role of smart energy grids in forensic science labs: A sustainable solution." *Journal of Green Technology in Forensic Science*, 11(2), 88–105.

[11] Patel, S., & Jones, R. (2018). "AI and IoT in sustainable forensic practices." *Proceedings of the International Conference on Forensic Science and Technology*, 55(1), 45–58.

[12] Gupta, P., & Ahmed, S. (2021). "Smart forensic labs: Integrating renewable energy for sustainability." *Proceedings of the IEEE International Conference on Sustainable Computing*, 68(2), 99–112.

[13] Roberts, T., & Chen, L. (2022). "Energy-efficient digital forensics: Cloud computing and edge analytics." *Proceedings of the International Symposium on Digital Investigations*, 30(1), 55–71.

[14] Miller, C., & Thompson, J. (2023). "Advancing forensic sustainability through AI-driven automation." *Proceedings of the Global Forensic Science Conference*, 20(1), 89–102.

[15] Lin, W., & Dawson, M. (2023). "The future of forensic resource management: A circular economy perspective." *Proceedings of the World Congress on Forensic Innovation*, 15(2), 134–149.

[16] Turner, H., & Mitchell, P. (2022). "Greener forensic laboratories: Sustainable HVAC and lighting solutions." *Proceedings of the International*

*Conference on Environmental Science and Forensic Technology*, 40(3), 75–91.

[17] Jackson, R., & Kumar, V. (2021). "Blockchain and AI in forensic chain of custody: A sustainability approach." *Proceedings of the International Cybersecurity and Forensics Symposium*, 19(2), 110–127.

[18] White, D., & Simmons, T. (2020). "Reducing electronic waste in digital forensics: Challenges and solutions." *Proceedings of the Sustainable Technology in Digital Forensics Conference*, 27(1), 92–108.

[19] Ahmed, I., & Roshan, S. (2023). "The role of machine learning in optimizing energy-efficient forensic data processing." *Proceedings of the AI and Digital Forensics Congress*, 32(4), 143–159.

[20] Brown, E., & Wong, L. (2021). "Green forensic science: Reducing the environmental impact of crime scene investigations." *Proceedings of the Global Sustainability in Forensics Summit*, 22(1), 61–78.

Chapter 11

# Awareness and training for attaining sustainable forensics in secure IoMT

*Pellate Anoushka, C. Kishor Kumar Reddy, Pranav Srinivasan, and Srinath Doss*

## 11.1 INTRODUCTION

### 11.1.1 What is IoMT?

The Internet of Medical Things (IoMT) represents a transformative shift in healthcare, blending state-of-the-art technology with patient care to create a fully interconnected, data-driven medical ecosystem. At its core, IoMT is a specialized subset of the Internet of Things (IoT) that integrates medical devices, sensors, wearables, and healthcare applications into one seamless network. This network (Figure 11.1) collects, processes, and transmits critical health data in real time, providing healthcare professionals with valuable insights that can improve diagnostic accuracy, treatment personalization, and overall patient outcomes.

IoMT encompasses a wide array of connected devices used in healthcare—from wearable fitness trackers and implantable sensors to advanced diagnostic machines and hospital monitoring systems. These devices collect various types of data, including vital signs like heart rate, blood pressure, and temperature, as well as blood glucose levels, imaging results, and other health metrics. They are designed to operate continuously, transmitting data either to local systems (via edge computing) or to centralized cloud platforms for advanced processing and analysis. The primary goal is to enable remote patient monitoring, support telemedicine initiatives, and facilitate proactive healthcare management.

### 11.1.2 Introduction to IoMT security and forensics

In today's digitally driven healthcare landscape, the integration of interconnected medical devices collectively known as the IoMT has revolutionized patient care and data management. However, as these devices become more ubiquitous and complex, they also present an expanding surface for cyber threats. To effectively safeguard sensitive medical data and ensure rapid, effective incident response, it is crucial to build robust forensic


DOI: 10.1201/9781003640325-11

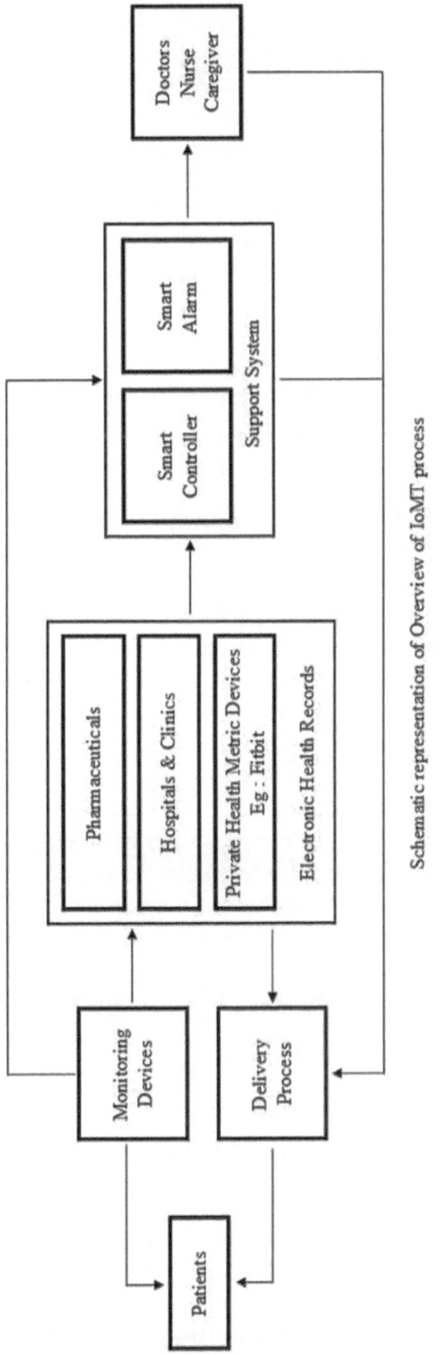


*Figure 11.1* Schematic representation of the overview of the IoMT process.

capabilities that can evolve alongside emerging threats. This necessitates a dual approach: not only must IoMT systems be designed with cutting-edge security measures, but organizations must also invest in comprehensive awareness and training programs. These initiatives empower technical teams to master the skills required for sustainable digital forensics—an ongoing, adaptive process that ensures long-term resilience and reliability in forensic investigations. Encouraging a culture of ongoing learning and readiness enables healthcare providers to secure IoMT environments, swiftly identify and assess security threats, and effectively minimize risks—safeguarding both patient confidentiality and the stability of essential medical functions.

### 11.1.3 Examples

**Example 1: The 2021 ransomware attack on ireland's healthcare system**

In May 2021, a sophisticated ransomware attack hit Ireland's Health Service Executive (HSE), crippling the nation's healthcare IT infrastructure. This incident forced hospitals and clinics to suspend non-emergency services, delaying surgeries and disrupting routine medical operations. Patient records were compromised, causing immense challenges in maintaining continuity of care. One of the most critical shortcomings exposed by the attack was the inadequate forensic preparedness of the healthcare system. Without well-established forensic protocols, the IT teams struggled to quickly determine the point of entry, the scope of the breach, and the exact methods used by the attackers. As a result, the recovery process was delayed, and valuable patient data remained at risk for an extended period. This case vividly illustrates the need for continuous training and robust forensic strategies that can swiftly detect, analyze, and respond to cyber incidents—ensuring that even when breaches occur, patient care is minimally disrupted and systems can be restored with minimal damage.

**Example 2: Vulnerabilities in pacemakers and the 2019 fda recalls**

The U.S. Food and Drug Administration (FDA) released recalls and safety warnings for specific pacemaker models in 2019 after discovering vulnerabilities that could be exploited by cyber attackers. These vulnerabilities raised concerns that unauthorized parties might remotely interfere with the devices' operations—potentially altering their functioning in ways that could jeopardize patient health. The situation underscored a critical issue: while it is vital to secure such life-supporting devices, it is equally important to have forensic protocols that can trace and analyze any tampering attempts without disrupting the pacemaker's operation. For a device that patients rely on for continuous heart rhythm management, any downtime—even brief—can have catastrophic consequences. Consequently, manufacturers and regulators began emphasizing the integration of forensic readiness into medical device design. This includes implementing secure logging mechanisms, tamper-evident audit trails, and real-time anomaly detection systems that allow forensic investigators to reconstruct the sequence of events during a breach—all while ensuring the device remains operational and patient safety is never compromised.

This research as shown in Figure 11.2 aims to bridge the gap between technical cybersecurity measures and human-centric strategies for sustainable forensic practices.

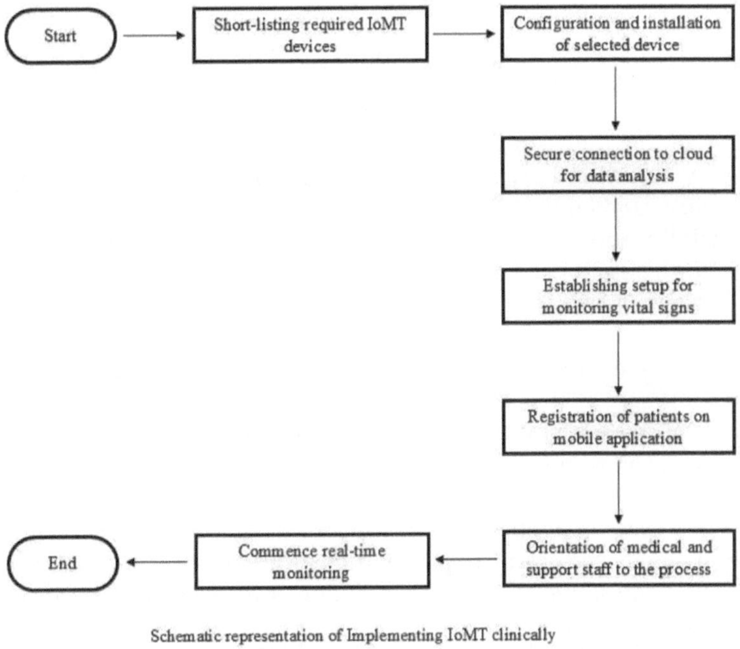


*Figure 11.2* Schematic representation of Implementing IoMT clinically.

## 11.2 OBJECTIVES

### 11.2.1 Specific goals

**Identify gaps in existing awareness programs for IoMT security**

**Curriculum evaluation:** Conduct a systematic review of current training initiatives to assess whether they cover advanced IoMT threat detection, incident response, and forensic investigation tailored to healthcare settings.

**Stakeholder analysis:** Survey and interview diverse groups—including clinical staff, IT security teams, and biomedical engineers—to understand their current knowledge gaps and training needs.

**Gap identification:** Highlight specific areas such as emerging IoMT vulnerabilities (e.g., device tampering or unauthorized access) where current programs may fall short, compromising an organization's forensic readiness.

**Design scalable and customized training frameworks for healthcare stakeholders**

**Modular framework development:** Develop a training model consisting of clearly defined modules addressing cybersecurity fundamentals, IoMT-specific threats, forensic evidence preservation, and regulatory compliance. This framework should allow customization for different roles and risk profiles.

**Innovative training methods:** Integrate interactive and immersive training tools—such as gamified learning platforms, virtual reality (VR) simulations, and microlearning modules—to enhance engagement and knowledge retention.

**Scalability and adaptability:** Ensure the training model can be adapted for institutions of varying sizes, from small clinics to large hospital networks, with regular updates to incorporate evolving threats.

**Propose robust metrics to evaluate and sustain forensic readiness**

**Performance metrics:** Define clear, quantifiable indicators (e.g., average incident response time, forensic investigation success rate, and reduction in false positives) to measure the impact of training on forensic capabilities.

**Training effectiveness:** Use pre- and posttraining assessments, certification rates, and periodic re-evaluations to gauge improvements in staff competency.

**Sustainability benchmarks:** Establish long-term goals (such as a target improvement percentage in forensic readiness scores over

18 months) and develop feedback mechanisms that continuously refine the training content based on real-world incident analyses.

### 11.2.2 Alignment with broader goals

**Patient safety and trust:** By enhancing forensic readiness, the training directly protects sensitive patient data, minimizes operational disruptions (like surgery delays), and thereby builds trust in digital healthcare.

**Regulatory compliance:** The inclusion of compliance topics (e.g., HIPAA, GDPR) in the training ensures that healthcare organizations can better meet legal obligations, streamline audit processes, and support forensic investigations.

**Global sustainability initiatives:** The focus on human factors and continuous upskilling aligns with the UN Sustainable Development Goal 3 (Good Health and Well-Being) and NIST recommendations, ultimately contributing to safer and more resilient healthcare infrastructures.

## 11.3 BACKGROUND AND RELATED WORK

### 11.3.1 Limitations

The diversity and resource limitations of IoMT devices complicate forensic investigations, as varying hardware, operating systems, and inconsistent logging mechanisms make evidence collection and analysis challenging. Additionally, volatile data storage often results in incomplete incident reconstructions [1].

Comprehensive security and privacy reviews in IoMT tend to struggle to keep pace with rapid technological changes, often providing broad overviews that may not delve deeply into emerging vulnerabilities. This can lead to recommendations that quickly become obsolete as new threats emerge [4].

Studies based on literature reviews and surveys are often constrained by the limited availability and reliability of existing data. This reliance on secondary information can create gaps, especially in documenting real-world forensic practices, thus limiting the overall generalizability of their conclusions [6].

Utilizing data analytics for IoT forensics introduces significant challenges related to integrating, cleaning, and processing large, heterogeneous datasets generated by IoMT devices. The requirement for extensive computational resources and continual model adjustments can hinder the timely detection of novel threats [8].

While innovative security methods such as stateless mechanisms and advanced key management protocols (like skeyM) offer promising benefits, they also introduce added architectural complexity. This can result in increased latency and difficulties in managing transient sessions, particularly during unexpected disruptions [10].

Cancellable ECG recognition, as a method to enhance IoMT security, provides the advantage of revocable biometric credentials. However, its effectiveness can be undermined by physiological variability, sensor noise, and environmental conditions, which may affect accuracy and lead to false acceptances or rejections [14].

Blockchain-based data-sharing mechanisms ensure data integrity and privacy but face scalability challenges as transaction volumes increase, along with higher energy consumption. Integrating these solutions with legacy healthcare systems further complicates their deployment and operational efficiency [16].

Forward-looking analyses on IoMT privacy and security, while insightful for anticipating future challenges, are often speculative and lack sufficient empirical validation. This makes it difficult to translate these predictions into immediate, actionable strategies for enhancing current security practices [23].

## 11.4 CHALLENGES IN DIGITIZING INDIA'S HEALTHCARE

### 11.4.1 Electronic health records

#### *11.4.1.1 Preference for government hospitals over private healthcare*

The majority of India's population belongs to the middle-class economic stratum as shown in Table 11.1, which relies heavily on the government/public healthcare system. This system ensures access to quality health services at an affordable cost, making it a preferred choice for a large segment of the population. One of the key reasons for this preference is the ease of access and widespread availability of government healthcare services, which extend from primary health centers (PHCs) to community-based health programs like Anganwadi. Despite the potential benefits of electronic health records (EHRs), such as improved patient care coordination and data accessibility, their implementation in India's public healthcare system faces significant challenges, particularly in remote and underserved areas.

#### *11.4.1.2 Infrastructure*

According to a 2021 study by the National Health Authority (NHA), only 30% of public healthcare facilities in India have adopted EHR systems, primarily due to infrastructural and financial constraints. In rural areas, where 70% of India's population resides, the adoption rate is even lower, at less than 15%. This disparity is exacerbated by limited internet connectivity, with only 33% of rural households having access to the internet, as per the

*Table 11.1* Summary and existing approaches

| *S.NO* | *Title* | *Author's name* | *Year of Publication* | *Methodology* |
|---|---|---|---|---|
| 1 | Digital Forensic Investigation for the Internet of Medical Things (IoMT) | Hamid Jahankhani and Jaime Ibarra [1] | 2019 | This research paper explores the increasing cybersecurity risks facing the healthcare industry due to the rise of IoMT devices. It emphasizes how cyberattacks are becoming more frequent and sophisticated, particularly targeting electronic health records. The paper investigates the challenges in applying digital forensics to IoMT environments, considering the unique characteristics of IoT devices, cloud infrastructure, and data privacy regulations like GDPR. Ultimately, the authors aim to highlight the need for a comprehensive forensic investigation model tailored to IoMT to ensure data privacy and regulatory compliance in the face of growing cyber threats |
| 2 | Open Research Challenges in Health Care Internet of Forensics (H-IoF) [2] | Indumathi J [2] | 2021 | This research article explores the burgeoning field of Healthcare Internet of Forensics (H-IoF), which addresses digital forensic challenges within the Internet of Medical Things (IoMT). The paper emphasizes the need for proactive digital forensics mechanisms to investigate security incidents and data breaches involving IoMT devices. It presents a review of H-IoT, discusses the rationale for studying IoMT forensics, and identifies open research challenges in this area, advocating for immediate research to develop effective solutions. Ultimately, this study seeks to provide insights into the latest IoMT forensics research trends to enhance digital forensic investigation processes |
| 3 | Security and privacy in the internet of things: Current status and open issues | Mohamed Abomhara and Geir M. Koine [3] | 2022 | This paper explores the critical intersection of security and privacy within the rapidly expanding Internet of Things (IoT). It identifies current challenges and discusses potential future directions for research. The paper emphasizes that the IoT's vision of interconnected devices and services presents unprecedented security risks and privacy implications, demanding robust and effective solutions. Ultimately, the authors aim to provide a comprehensive overview of the security landscape, focusing on vulnerabilities, threats, and the necessity for innovative security architectures that foster trust and protect user data in the IoT environment |

(*continued*)

*Table 11.1* (*Cont.*)

| *S.NO* | *Title* | *Author's name* | *Year of Publication* | *Methodology* |
|---|---|---|---|---|
| 4 | IoMT security and privacy review: An extensive analysis of security and privacy issues in the Internet of medical things | Ramanpreet Kaur, Kulwinder Singh, Jagmeet Singh [4] | 2025 | This academic paper broadly examines security and privacy issues related to the Internet of Medical Things (IoMT). The paper identifies the benefits of IoMT, such as remote patient monitoring, but emphasizes the risks associated with data breaches, device vulnerabilities, and regulatory compliance. It further investigates strategies for mitigating these risks, including authentication methods and policy-based solutions, as well as cutting-edge technologies, such as blockchain and zero trust architecture, while considering future directions in IoMT security |
| 5 | Towards a holistic approach to medical IoT forensics | Jigang Liu, Ryoichi Sasaki, and Tetsutaro Uehara [5] | 2020 | This research paper introduces a holistic approach to Medical IoT (MIoT) forensics, acknowledging the increasing convergence of computer forensics and the Internet of Things. The authors aim to address the unique challenges presented by MIoT devices, such as the diverse data sources and the blurred lines between the cyber, physical, and social spaces. The paper proposes a four-space model for investigating MIoT-related cases, which considers cyberspace, physical space, social space, and human psychological states. Ultimately, the study seeks to provide a more comprehensive framework for identifying, analyzing, and resolving legal issues in the rapidly expanding field of MIoT forensics |
| 6 | Explore IoT security threats and forensics challenges: A literature review and survey study | Abdulrehman Al Allaf, and Waseem Totonji [6] | 2023 | This source presents a bachelor's degree project that explores the intersection of IoT security threats and digital forensics. The authors conduct a literature review and survey study to investigate common IoT attacks, mitigation strategies, and key forensic challenges. The project also assesses students' awareness of IoT security issues, the importance of user training, and potential solutions for improving IoT security. Ultimately, the study aims to contribute to the research and development of more secure IoT systems |

| | | | | |
|---|---|---|---|---|
| 7 | Survey and analysis of IoT operating systems: A comparative study on the effectiveness and acquisition time of open-source digital forensics tools | Jeffery Fairbanks, Md Mashrur Arifin, Sadia Afreen, and Alex Curtis [7] | 2024 | This paper presents a survey and analysis of several open-source digital forensics tools used to investigate Internet of Things (IoT) operating systems. This study assesses the efficiency and performance of various tools in extracting evidence from widely used IoT devices. The objective is to offer insights and recommendations to security professionals and digital forensic analysts regarding the most effective tools for IoT investigations. By comparing the performance of these open-source tools, the study intends to contribute to the field of digital forensics, particularly in the context of the increasing complexity of IoT devices |
| 8 | Towards the internet of things forensics: A data analytics perspective | Pimal khanpara, and Ishwa shah et al. [8] | 2024 | This paper explores the intersection of IoT forensics and data analytics. It emphasizes the increasing importance of extracting digital evidence from IoT devices for forensic investigations. The authors focus on methodologies and challenges related to analyzing IoT data. Ultimately, the paper aims to advance the understanding of how data analytics can be effectively integrated into IoT forensics processes to address current limitations and enable future advancements in the field |
| 9 | A secured and energy-efficient system for patient e-healthcare monitoring using Internet of Medical Things (IoMT) | Veera V Rama Rao M, Kiran Sree Pokkuluri et al. [9] | 2024 | This study presents a secure and energy-efficient framework (SEES-IoMT) for patient e-health monitoring, leveraging the Internet of Medical Things (IoMT). The primary goal is to reduce the costs and energy usage of the devices used to monitor patients, while also enhancing the security and privacy of patient data. The research compares SEES-IoMT to existing methods, highlighting its potential to improve reliability in the context of medical applications. Ultimately, this work aims to advance e-healthcare by providing a more secure and energy-conscious approach to remote patient monitoring |
| 10 | Achieving secured medical network (SMN) through stateless mechanism and skeyM in medical internet of things (M-IoT) | Nithya S., Satheeshkumar Palanisamy, and Nivethitha T. [10] | 2024 | This research paper explores a novel approach to secure data within medical devices connected to the Internet of Things. The authors propose a stateless mechanism combined with a new key management scheme called SKeyM to address the vulnerabilities of existing security measures. This method aims to protect patient data and ensure secure communication by eliminating the need to store user data on the server. The study includes experimental results that suggest the proposed methodologies are potentially more effective in dealing with major attacks |

*(continued)*

*Table 11.1 (Cont.)*

| S.NO | Title | Author's name | Year of Publication | Methodology |
|---|---|---|---|---|
| 11 | Joint uplink and downlink rate splitting for fog computing-enabled internet of medical things | Jiasi Zhou, Yan Chen et al. [11] | 2024 | This study explores the challenges of rate splitting in both uplink and downlink within fog computing-powered Internet of Medical Things (IoMT). The primary objective is to reduce the overall time required for task offloading, data processing, and result transmission between users and the server. To achieve this, the paper proposes a novel transmit scheme and introduces auxiliary variables to convert the non-convex optimization problem into a solvable form. The proposed algorithm is then extensively simulated to demonstrate performance gains compared to existing benchmarks |
| 12 | Internet of medical things security frameworks for risk assessment and management: A scoping review | Katerina Svandova, and Zdenek Smutny [12] | 2024 | This review explores current research on frameworks for assessing and managing security risks in the Internet of Medical Things (IoMT). The study systematically identifies and analyses publications from 2018 to 2023, aiming to understand how current frameworks address the unique security challenges posed by IoMT devices. The review categorizes the frameworks and highlights the need for holistic approaches that consider both technological and organizational aspects of IoMT security. The objective is to evaluate the strengths and gaps in existing security frameworks designed to mitigate risks within the IoMT environment |
| 13 | Framework for a secure and sustainable internet of medical things, requirements, design challenges and future trends | William Villegas-ch, Joeslin Garcia Ortiz, and Isabel Urbina-camacho [13] | 2023 | This paper provides a framework for developing secure and sustainable Internet of Medical Things (IoMT) systems. The main goal is to address the challenges that are related to security and sustainability that are faced in the medical field. Critical conditions that drive these challenges are identified, and future trends are proposed for this technology in the private medical clinic setting. Ultimately, the study shows that the proposed IoMT system improves not only the quality of care that the clinic can provide, but also aids in early detection of disease and decision-making |

| | | | | |
|---|---|---|---|---|
| 14 | Securing internet of medical things using cancellable ECG recognition | Samia A. El-moenim Kabel, Ghada M. El-banby et al. [14] | 2024 | This study presents an innovative approach to securing Internet-of-Medical-Things (IoMT) networks by leveraging electrocardiogram (ECG) signals for biometric authentication. The key concept involves generating cancellable ECG templates that can be altered or replaced in case of a security breach, thereby strengthening privacy and protection. The proposed method incorporates a distinctive signal separation technique, utilizing an auxiliary audio signal to distort the ECG data before applying lightweight encryption. By integrating non-invertible transformations with efficient encryption mechanisms, this research aims to achieve a balance between robust security and computational efficiency, which is particularly crucial for resource-limited IoMT devices |
| 15 | Secure and provenance enhanced internet of health things framework: A blockchain managed federated learning approach | Mohamed Abdur Rahman, M. Shamim Hossain and Nabin A. Alrajeh [15] | 2020 | This paper introduces a new framework for secure and privacy-enhanced Internet of Health Things (IoHT), addressing critical concerns in the widespread adoption of IoHT devices. The core innovation is a blockchain-managed federated learning (FL) approach, designed to protect the privacy and security of IoHT data while still enabling effective collaborative model training. By leveraging blockchain, the framework provides tamper-resistant data provenance and decentralized consensus, mitigating privacy leakage and ensuring data integrity. The study showcases the effectiveness of this framework by applying it to various deep-learning models tailored for clinical trials involving COVID-19 patients, emphasizing its potential for secure health management within IoHT systems |
| 16 | Dual blockchain-based data sharing mechanism with privacy protection of medical internet of things | Linchen Liu, Ruyan Liu et al. [16] | 2023 | This research paper introduces a dual blockchain-based data-sharing mechanism designed to enhance privacy for medical data within the Internet of Things (IoT). The authors propose a novel approach that uses a consortium blockchain and cloud centers to ensure data integrity and address privacy concerns. The approach utilizes ciphertext-policy attribute-based encryption (CP-ABE), zero-knowledge succinct non-interactive arguments of knowledge (ZK-SNARK), and the practical Byzantine fault tolerance (PBFT) consensus mechanism to ensure both security and operational efficiency. The aim is to provide a robust framework for managing sensitive medical information and balancing data accessibility with stringent privacy protection |

*(continued)*

*Table 11.1* (*Cont.*)

| S.NO | Title | Author's name | Year of Publication | Methodology |
|---|---|---|---|---|
| 17 | Connected to the cloud at time of death: A case report | Isabel Straw, Claire Kirkby, and Preethi Gopinath [17] | 2024 | This paper is a case report about a patient who died while being monitored by an implantable cardioverter defibrillator (ICD), connecting his death to data available through cloud-based healthcare. The authors examined autopsy practices in this context, questioning how existing guidelines capture data related to a death that goes beyond the physical body due to digital device integration. It highlights the challenges of interpreting device extraction results and software failures and suggests the need for updated autopsy guidelines that consider the increasing role of digital technologies in death and dying. This paper emphasizes the need for increased awareness and specialized training among medical professionals to effectively handle the distinct challenges associated with deaths influenced by digital technologies |
| 18 | Wearable Hardware Design for the Internet of Medical Things (IoMT) | Fayez Qureshi and Sridhar Krishnan [18] | 2018 | This research paper explores the design of wearable devices for the Internet of Medical Things (IoMT), emphasizing hardware components for bio-signal capture and disease monitoring. It begins by introducing the need for biomedical wearables due to healthcare costs and increased health awareness. The paper reviews essential components for biomedical wearable front-ends, discussing their limitations and opportunities. It delves into specific biomedical signals like PPG, EMG, body sound auscultation, and gait analysis, outlining factors to consider in the wearable design, including signal characteristics, human factors, economic costs, and environmental considerations. Finally, the study investigates the role of electronic textiles in creating more comfortable and integrated wearables, highlighting their potential to improve user adoption and overall functionality in healthcare applications |

| | | | | |
|---|---|---|---|---|
| 19 | Prospect of Internet of Medical Things: A Review on Security Requirements and Solutions | Pintu Kumar Sadhu, Venkata P. Yanambaka, Ahmed Abdelgawad and, Kumar Yelamarthi [19] | 2022 | This source is an academic review paper that explores the landscape of the Internet of Medical Things (IoMT), emphasizing the critical need for security due to the sensitive nature of patient data and the increasing vulnerabilities that hackers can exploit. The paper examines the IoMT ecosystem, including its various segments (on-body, in-home, community, in-clinic, and in-hospital), relevant regulations and standards, and diverse security mechanisms and solutions, such as encryption, physical unclonable functions (PUFs), blockchain, and named data networking (NDN). It offers a thorough analysis of the challenges and possible security measures in the rapidly advancing IoMT domain, evaluating the advantages and drawbacks of different proposed solutions |
| 20 | Swarm Intelligence in Internet of Medical Things: A Review | Roohallah Alizadehsani, Mohamad Roshanzamir et al. [20] | 2023 | This review paper examines the role of swarm intelligence (SI) algorithms in the Internet of Medical Things (IoMT). It discusses how SI algorithms, inspired by the cooperative behavior of social insect colonies, can help tackle key challenges in IoMT, including disease prediction, data security, and efficient resource management. The paper provides an introduction to the Internet of Things (IoT) and IoMT, followed by an analysis of SI techniques such as Particle Swarm Optimization (PSO), Ant Colony Optimization (ACO), and Artificial Bee Colony (ABC). Additionally, it reviews existing studies that leverage these algorithms to address specific IoMT-related problems, shedding light on current advancements and potential future research directions in this domain |
| 21 | The Internet of Medical Things: Opportunities, Benefits, Challenges and Concerns | Omid Pournik, Leila Ghalichi, Parisis Gallos and Theodoros N. Arvanitis [21] | 2023 | This paper is a narrative review exploring the Internet of Medical Things (IoMT), focusing on its potential in healthcare. It investigates both the opportunities and benefits, such as enhanced patient monitoring, improved efficiency, and personalized medicine, as well as the challenges and concerns, including security risks, interoperability issues, and ethical considerations. Ultimately, the paper aims to provide a balanced perspective to inform the responsible implementation of IoMT technologies, arguing that challenges must be weighed against benefits for effective adoption and improved healthcare outcomes. The review methodology involved analyzing research papers, case studies, and industry reports published between 2018 and 2023, emphasizing the importance of addressing these challenges to unlock IoMT's full potential in healthcare |

(*continued*)

*Table 11.1 (Cont.)*

| S.NO | Title | Author's name | Year of Publication | Methodology |
|---|---|---|---|---|
| 22 | A blockchain-based secured system using the Internet of Medical Things (IOMT) network for e-healthcare monitoring | Lokesh Lodha, Vishwadeepak Singh Baghela, J. Bhuvana, and Rahul Bhatt [22] | 2023 | This study examines how blockchain technology can enhance the security and privacy of e-healthcare monitoring systems that utilize the Internet of Medical Things (IoMT). The authors propose a blockchain-based IoMT security system (BC-IoMT-SS) to address interoperability issues and ensure the secure transfer of medical records while protecting sensitive patient data. The paper details the design and implementation of the BC-IoMT-SS, including algorithms for device authentication and agent integration into the network. Ultimately, the study uses experimental results to demonstrate that the proposed system achieves high precision and efficiency with low delay, which helps validate its effectiveness in securing medical data management in IoMT environments |
| 23 | Internet of Medical Things Privacy and Security: Challenges, Solutions, and Future Trends from a New Perspective | Firuz Kamalov, Behrouz Pourghebleh et al. [23] | 2023 | This academic paper provides a comprehensive survey of security concerns within the Internet of Medical Things (IoMT). It analyses the application of IoT in the medical field, highlighting its potential to improve quality of life through remote monitoring. The study categorizes and compares 187 articles from 2010 to 2022, examining security approaches and trends, and explores blockchain technology as a key solution for security, authentication, and maintenance. Ultimately, the paper aims to offer insights and a roadmap for researchers working on IoMT security, emphasizing the importance of protecting sensitive medical data and ensuring the reliability of IoMT systems |

2021 National Family Health Survey (NFHS-5) [24]. Some rural regions suffer from irregular electricity supply. A 2019 report by the Ministry of Health and Family Welfare (MoHFW) highlighted that nearly 40% of PHCs in India experience frequent power outages. EHR systems depend on a continuous power supply to operate hardware such as computers, servers, and backup systems. Without reliable electricity, the functionality of EHRs is severely compromised, making it difficult for healthcare workers to maintain accurate and up-to-date records.

### 11.4.2 Economic constraints

The implementation of EHRs requires significant investment in hardware (computers, servers, scanners) and software (EHR platforms, cybersecurity systems). However, many government healthcare facilities lack the necessary infrastructure. For instance, a 2020 study by the Public Health Foundation of India (PHFI) found that only 25% of PHCs had functional computers, and even fewer had access to specialized EHR software. This shortage of basic infrastructure is bound to drastically increase the budget of the project. Government healthcare facilities, especially in rural areas, often operate in cramped spaces with limited resources. Installing and maintaining EHR systems requires dedicated space for servers, computers, and other equipment, which many facilities lack. Additionally, the maintenance of this infrastructure is often neglected due to budget constraints and a shortage of technical staff [25].

### 11.4.3 Orientation and training

#### *11.4.3.1 Digital literacy gap*

A large proportion of healthcare workers in government facilities, particularly in rural areas, lack the necessary digital literacy to operate EHR systems. A 2020 report by the Public Health Foundation of India (PHFI) revealed that over 60% of healthcare workers in government facilities are not adequately trained to use digital tools. This gap in digital skills hinders the effective adoption of EHRs, as staff may struggle with basic tasks such as data entry, retrieval, and interpretation.

#### *11.4.3.2 Resistance to change*

Many healthcare workers, especially those accustomed to traditional paper-based systems, may resist transitioning to EHRs due to fear of the unknown or reluctance to adapt to new workflows. Especially, while the majority of the population requiring healthcare services are elderly, they are more likely to follow the paper-based system as they may face difficulty in getting accustomed to the digital process. Without proper orientation and sensitization, this resistance can lead to low engagement and suboptimal utilization of EHR systems.

#### *11.4.3.3 Insufficient training programs*

While some training programs have been introduced to address the digital literacy gap, their reach and effectiveness remain limited. For example, the National Health Mission (NHM) has initiated digital health training programs, but these are often sporadic and lack follow-up support. Continuous training and hands-on practice are essential to ensure that healthcare workers can confidently use EHR systems in their daily routines. Government healthcare facilities, particularly in rural areas, often experience high staff turnover due to transfers, resignations, or retirements. This constant churn makes it difficult to maintain a consistently trained workforce, as new staff members require repeated training and orientation.

### 11.4.4 Interoperability limitations

#### *11.4.4.1 Absence of standardized protocols*

The lack of uniform data formats and protocols significantly worsens interoperability challenges. Various EHR systems often employ distinct terminologies, coding frameworks, and data structures, creating barriers to seamless data integration and exchange. For instance, a 2021 report by the National Health Authority (NHA) highlighted that only 20% of public healthcare facilities use standardized EHR formats, limiting their ability to exchange data effectively.

#### *11.4.4.2 Fragmented healthcare system*

India's healthcare system is highly fragmented, with multiple levels of care (primary, secondary, and tertiary) operating independently. Each level often uses different EHR systems that are not designed to communicate with one another. For example, a patient's records from a PHC may not be accessible at a district hospital due to incompatible systems, leading to gaps in care.

#### *11.4.4.3 Limited use of Health Information Exchanges*

Health Information Exchanges (HIEs) are platforms that facilitate the sharing of EHRs across different healthcare providers. However, the adoption of HIEs in India's public healthcare system remains limited due to technical, financial, and regulatory barriers. Without robust HIEs, the potential of EHRs to improve care coordination and reduce duplication of efforts remains untapped.

## 11.4.5 Requirement of redundancies

### *11.4.5.1 Ensuring uninterrupted access to patient data*

Healthcare delivery is time-sensitive, and any delay in accessing patient records can have serious consequences. Redundant systems, such as backup servers and offline storage, ensure that patient data remains accessible even during internet outages, power failures, or system crashes. For example, during the COVID-19 pandemic, many healthcare facilities faced system overloads, highlighting the need for robust backup mechanisms.

### *11.4.5.2 Maintaining continuity of care*

In emergencies, healthcare providers need immediate access to patient histories, medications, and treatment plans. Redundant EHR systems ensure that critical information is always available, even if the primary system fails. This is particularly important in rural areas, where healthcare facilities often operate with limited resources [26].

### *11.4.5.3 Supporting disaster recovery*

Natural disasters, such as floods or earthquakes, can disrupt healthcare services and damage infrastructure. Redundant EHR systems, including off-site backups and disaster recovery plans, enable healthcare facilities to quickly restore operations and continue providing care.

## 11.4.6 Legal and ethical barriers

### *11.4.6.1 Informed consent and patient autonomy*

Medical ethics require that patients provide informed consent for the collection, storage, and sharing of their health data. According to the Indian Medical Council's 2002 regulations on Professional Conduct, Etiquette, and Ethics, healthcare professionals are required to secure informed consent from patients before conducting any medical procedures or gathering data. However, in India's public healthcare system, many patients, especially in rural areas, may not fully understand the implications of digitizing their health records. Language barriers, low health literacy, and lack of awareness about digital systems can make it difficult to obtain genuine informed consent, raising ethical concerns about patient autonomy and the right to privacy.

#### *11.4.6.2 Confidentiality and trust*

Maintaining patient confidentiality is a cornerstone of medical ethics. The 2002 regulations of the Indian Medical Council on Professional Conduct, Etiquette, and Ethics mandate that healthcare professionals uphold patient confidentiality. However, the digitization of health records increases the risk of data leaks or unauthorized access, which can compromise patient confidentiality. For instance, if EHRs are accessed by unauthorized personnel or shared with third parties without patient consent, it can lead to ethical and legal violations under Section 72A of the IT Act, which penalizes the disclosure of personal information without consent with imprisonment of up to three years or a fine of up to ₹5 lahks.

#### *11.4.6.3 Ethical use of data*

Utilizing EHR for secondary applications, including research and public health monitoring, presents ethical concerns. While such use can benefit society, it must be balanced against the rights of individuals to control their personal information. The Indian Council of Medical Research (ICMR) National Ethical Guidelines for Biomedical and Health Research, 2017 provides a framework for ethical research, but they do not specifically address the use of EHR data. Without clear guidelines and ethical oversight, there is a risk of exploiting patient data for purposes beyond their original intent [27].

## 11.5 METHODOLOGY

To achieve these objectives, the research methodology is designed as a multiphase, mixed-methods approach that integrates innovative training techniques with rigorous evaluation. The methodology is divided into three main components: awareness enhancement, advanced training implementation, and forensic readiness evaluation.

### 11.5.1 Awareness enhancement: identifying and addressing gaps

To build a solid foundation for enhanced forensic readiness in IoMT security, the first step is to thoroughly understand the current training landscape. This phase involves several key activities:

#### *11.5.1.1 Data collection*

We begin by designing and distributing detailed surveys to healthcare professionals across different roles—ranging from clinical staff to IT security teams and biomedical engineers. These surveys will capture data on their current knowledge, experience, and perceptions regarding cybersecurity training, especially in the context of IoMT. In addition, structured interviews with key stakeholders will be conducted to gain in-depth qualitative insights into the training programs they have experienced and the challenges they face in real-world settings. In addition to these core approaches, a comprehensive analysis of existing literature encompassing academic research, industry reports, and government publications will be conducted to gain insights into current practices in digital forensics training within the healthcare industry.

#### *11.5.1.2 Gap analysis*

Once the data is collected, we will systematically analyze it to identify shortcomings in current training programs. This involves comparing the existing curriculum against a comprehensive set of competencies required for advanced threat detection, effective incident response, and digital forensics specific to IoMT environments. Special attention will be paid to pinpoint areas where training is either outdated or insufficiently practical—such as limited hands-on exercises in forensic investigations or a lack of content on emerging IoMT vulnerabilities.

#### *11.5.1.3 Outcome*

The insights gleaned from the surveys, interviews, and literature review will be synthesized into a detailed report. This document will highlight the most critical gaps—for example, insufficient training on digital evidence preservation techniques or inadequate incident response strategies amid the rise of sophisticated digital threats. The report will serve as a blueprint for developing a new training framework, ensuring that future programs are tailored to address these identified deficiencies effectively and sustainably.

By following this approach, the project aims not only to document existing weaknesses but also to provide actionable recommendations that will drive the design of a more robust, future-proof training system in the secure IoMT landscape.

### 11.5.2 Advanced training implementation: innovative methods

This section outlines a comprehensive, multi-modal training initiative that is both scalable and engaging. The objective is to empower healthcare professionals with advanced skills in IoMT security and digital forensics through innovative, interactive, and continuously updated learning modalities.

#### 11.5.2.1 Gamified learning platforms

Concept:

Develop interactive digital modules that simulate real-world IoMT risks, enabling healthcare staff to identify and mitigate threats while earning digital rewards and badges. This approach transforms the training process into a dynamic learning experience that motivates users through competition and recognition.

Example:

A pilot program—similar to one conducted in a Boston hospital—demonstrated that by engaging staff in a gamified environment, phishing click rates could be reduced by as much as 40%. This example highlights the potential impact of gamification on behavior change and awareness improvement.

Implementation:

Leverage web-based platforms that integrate game mechanics with cybersecurity challenges. These platforms present scenarios such as phishing attempts and unauthorized device access in a simulated, risk-free environment. As learners progress, they unlock new levels and earn rewards, which reinforces continuous engagement and mastery of key concepts.

#### 11.5.2.2 Virtual reality (VR) simulations

Design:

Create immersive VR environments that replicate realistic cyber incidents, such as a ransomware attack targeting an intensive care unit (ICU). These simulations immerse participants in high-pressure scenarios where they must make rapid, critical forensic decisions.

Objective:

The aim is to train staff to respond effectively during cyber emergencies—such as isolating compromised devices or initiating forensic investigations—without disrupting the delivery of essential services.

Example:

Drawing on practices from Stanford Medicine's VR lab, where simulations of device hijacking are used, participants learn to navigate complex security challenges in real-time. This hands-on experience builds confidence and enhances the ability to manage actual incidents in a controlled, virtual setting.

#### 11.5.2.3 Microlearning for continuous education

**Implementation:**

Introduce a series of brief, focused video tutorials and interactive lessons delivered via mobile applications. These micro-learning sessions cover crucial topics such as new regulatory guidelines (e.g., recent FDA policy updates) and emerging IoMT threats, ensuring that information is both accessible and digestible.

**Impact:**

A pilot program conducted in Germany showcased that microlearning could lead to retention rates as high as 89%, significantly outperforming more traditional, longer-format workshops. This approach ensures that staff are regularly updated with the latest security practices in short, manageable segments, facilitating continuous education.

**Outcome:**

By consistently rolling out new content, the program ensures that healthcare personnel remain at the forefront of evolving security standards and best practices, thereby reinforcing their readiness to address modern cyber threats.

#### 11.5.2.4 Forensic "Fire Drills"

**Process:**

Conduct quarterly simulated cyberattack exercises—"fire drills"—where interdisciplinary teams, including both IT and medical staff, work together to trace and analyze simulated security breaches using forensic tools like Wireshark and Splunk.

**Example:**

At Johns Hopkins Hospital, similar exercises led to a 35% reduction in incident response time over a 12-month period, illustrating the significant benefits of regular, hands-on training.

**Purpose:**

These drills provide an invaluable opportunity for staff to practice real-time forensic investigations, ensuring that they are well-prepared to coordinate effectively during an actual incident. This method reinforces teamwork, refines operational protocols, and builds a culture of proactive security readiness.

#### 11.5.2.5 Certification and community building

**Blockchain-backed credentials:**

Implement a system for issuing secure, tamper-proof digital certificates upon training completion. Utilizing decentralized platforms such as EduChain, these credentials provide verifiable records of individual competencies, ensuring that certifications are both credible and resistant to forgery.

**Community forums:**

Establish HIPAA-compliant online forums where participants can share best practices, discuss challenges, and collaborate on solutions related to IoMT security and forensic readiness. These community hubs not only foster a supportive learning environment but also facilitate continuous peer-to-peer knowledge exchange.

### 11.5.3 Forensic readiness evaluation: measuring impact

This stage is structured to thoroughly evaluate how effectively the training program enhances forensic readiness in IoMT environments. It combines actionable steps, clearly defined measurable outcomes, and real-world parallels to ensure that improvements are both significant and sustainable.

#### 11.5.3.1 Step 1: Pre-training assessment

**Purpose:**

Establish baseline competency levels and identify existing knowledge gaps among staff.

**Baseline metrics:**

**Knowledge Assessment:**

Conduct initial quizzes and surveys to determine how well staff understand critical concepts, such as "forensic readiness." For example, early evaluations might reveal that only 60% of nurses can accurately define the term.

**Operational metrics:**

Measure current incident response performance by simulating breach scenarios. For instance, you might find that the average time to contain a simulated ransomware attack on MRI machines is approximately 72 hours.

**Behavioral analysis:**

Use anonymized data from phishing simulations to assess vulnerability. For example, track how many staff members click on deceptive emails purporting to be firmware updates for devices like insulin pumps.

**Tools and methods:**

**Scenario-Based Quizzes:**

Develop quizzes with realistic scenarios, such as asking, "What steps would you take to preserve data from a compromised glucose monitor?"

**Simulated breach exercises:**

Organize controlled breach simulations to record response times and evaluate teamwork under pressure.

**Protocol audits:**

Conduct audits comparing existing procedures against standards such as ISO 27037 to identify where current practices fall short. For instance, a pre-training audit at Johns Hopkins Hospital revealed that 70% of IT personnel were unfamiliar with cloud forensic tools, leading to delays in evidence collection.

**Outcome:**

Compile the collected data into a detailed report that outlines the deficiencies in current training initiatives. This report will serve as the benchmark for the subsequent training program design.

#### *11.5.3.2 Step 2: Implementation of the hybrid training program*

**Purpose:**

Deliver a tailored, engaging, and scalable training regimen that directly addresses the identified gaps.

**Hybrid model composition:**

**Gamified modules (40%):**

Content: Develop interactive modules that simulate real-world IoMT challenges, such as detecting tampered vital sign monitors or securing insulin pumps during a cyberattack.

Incentives: Award digital badges (e.g., "IoMT Forensic Expert") that are stored on blockchain-based platforms (like EduChain) to ensure the integrity and permanence of credentials.

**Case example:** A 6-week program at a Boston hospital saw phishing susceptibility decrease by 40% as staff advanced through levels and "unlocked" new security protocols.

**VR Simulations** (30%):

Scenarios: Create immersive virtual reality drills that mimic incidents such as ransomware attacks on ICU devices. These simulations force participants to isolate compromised devices without halting critical patient care.

Tools: Integrate forensic analysis software (e.g., Autopsy, Wireshark) into the VR environment so that trainees can practice real-time log analysis.

Outcome: Stanford Medicine's VR lab reported a 50% boost in device isolation accuracy following such training.

**Microlearning** (30%):

Format: Distribute concise, 5-minute mobile app videos that address topics like updated FDA cybersecurity guidelines and GDPR-compliant evidence handling.

Scheduling: Utilize push notifications to deliver these sessions at optimal times (e.g., before morning rounds) to maximize engagement.

Impact: A pilot program in Germany achieved an impressive 89% retention rate by employing microlearning for explaining complex risks, such as firmware update vulnerabilities in dialysis machines.

**Roll-out strategy:**

Pilot implementation:

Launch the hybrid training program at a mid-sized hospital over a 6-week period, tracking progress on a weekly basis.

Role-based customization:

Tailor-specific modules for different staff roles. For example, clinicians receive focused training on breach reporting workflows, while IT teams undergo advanced sessions on malware reverse-engineering for pacemaker data logs.

#### 11.5.3.3 *Step 3: posttraining evaluation*

Purpose:

Quantify immediate improvements and ensure the long-term sustainability of forensic readiness.

Immediate outcomes:

Knowledge retention:

Administer post-training assessments to determine if staff proficiency has improved—aiming for at least 85% of participants to correctly isolate compromised devices, compared to a pre-training rate of 30%.

Operational efficiency:

Monitor incident response times; for example, measure whether breach containment times at any given Hospital are reduced from 72 hours to 28 hours following the training.

Behavioral change:

Repeat phishing simulations to verify a reduction in click rates, with a target of a 50% decline within three months.

Long-term monitoring:

Key performance indicators:

Develop a composite "Forensic Readiness Score" that combines factors such as response time, evidence integrity, and adherence to protocols, with a goal of achieving a 55% improvement over 18 months. Additionally, track the reduction in false positive alerts, aiming for a 30% decrease through improved judgment.

Trend analysis:

Use monitoring tools (e.g., Splunk dashboards) to correlate training completion with incident resolution efficiency over time.

Feedback loop:

Participant surveys:

Collect quarterly feedback on the training's relevance and effectiveness, asking questions like, "How useful were the VR scenarios for your role?"

**Incident debriefs:**

After any real or simulated breach, conduct debriefs sessions to review what worked well and what could be improved, incorporating lessons into future training modules (e.g., new content on zero-day exploits in CT scanners).

**Community collaboration:**

Create HIPAA-compliant forums (such as an IoMT Security Hub) where healthcare institutions can share anonymized case studies and best practices, promoting continuous learning and adaptation.

**Enhancing engagement and validity:**

**Real-world analogies:**

Frame forensic fire drills as "cybersecurity CPR," emphasizing that regular practice is essential to save digital "lives," much like regular CPR training is vital for saving human lives.

**Competitive elements:**

se leaderboards to publish scores from the gamified modules (e.g., "Top 10 Forensic Responders") to spur friendly competition and drive engagement.

**Ethical and Practical Dilemmas:**

Introduce scenarios in the VR simulations that require balancing security actions with patient care priorities, thereby challenging participants to make ethical decisions under pressure.

**Transparent Reporting:**

Develop interactive KPI dashboards that are shared with hospital leadership to clearly demonstrate return on investment (ROI). For instance, showing that every 1-hour reduction in incident response time translates to significant cost savings in downtime and potential breach remediation.

## 11.6 KEY TRAINING AREAS

### 11.6.1 Data preservation techniques

A key goal of forensic training is to safeguard digital evidence in compliance with established guidelines, such as the ISO 27037 (2012) standard. Investigators must understand the principles of the Chain of Custody (CoC) to ensure the credibility and genuineness of the gathered evidence. Training should also address the unique challenges posed by cloud environments, where traditional methods of evidence collection may not apply effectively.

### 11.6.2 Incident response and analysis

Training programs should emphasize the importance of comprehensive incident response strategies. Investigators must be adept at using data analysis tools to extract crucial data while upholding the credibility and integrity of the evidence. Understanding the timeline of events surrounding an incident, and reconstructing the sequence of actions taken, is crucial for establishing a credible CoC and informing future security measures.

### 11.6.3 Ethical considerations

As forensic analysis often involves personal and sensitive data, training must also cover ethical and legal considerations. Participants should be made aware of the potential privacy concerns associated with collecting data from personal IoMT devices, ensuring they approach investigations with a strong ethical framework.

### 11.6.4 Continuous improvement and adaptation

Forensic analysis should be seen as a continuous process of assessment and refinement rather than a singular event. Organizations are encouraged to conduct regular training sessions and simulations, such as penetration tests and tabletop exercises, to keep their teams prepared for evolving threats.

## 11.7 CONCLUSION

In conclusion, enhancing forensic readiness in secure IoMT systems hinges on robust awareness and continuous training. This study demonstrates that by identifying gaps in current training and deploying innovative, multimodal methods—such as gamified learning, VR simulations, microlearning, and regular forensic fire drills—healthcare organizations can significantly improve their incident response capabilities and evidence preservation practices. By establishing clear, measurable metrics and fostering community collaboration through blockchain-backed certifications, these efforts not only bolster patient safety and regulatory compliance but also lay a sustainable foundation for future digital healthcare security.

## REFERENCES

[1] Jahankhani, Hamid, and Jaime Ibarra, "Digital Forensic Investigation for the Internet of Medical Things (IoMT)", *Journal of Forensic Legal &*

*Investigative Sciences*, vol. 5, no. 2, p. 29, 2019. doi:10.24966/FLIS-733X/100029

[2] Indumathi, J. "Open Research Challenges in Health Care Internet of Forensics (H-IoF)," *Journal of Advanced Trends in Engineering and Technology (IJATET)*, vol. 6, no.1, pp. 17–27, 2021. https://ijatet.dvpublication.com/uploads/66c04110cbb83_162.pdf

[3] Abomhara, Mohamed, and Geir M. Koien, "Security and Privacy in the Internet of Things: Current Status and Open Issues", Conference on Privacy and Security in Mobile Systems (PRISMS), 2022. www.researchgate.net/profile/Mohamed-Abomhara/publication/269687360_Security_and_privacy_in_the_Internet_of_Things_Current_status_and_open_issues/links/5e1618ea4585159aa4be6a12/Security-and-privacy-in-the-Internet-of-Things-Current-status-and-open-issues.pdf,International

[4] M. Elhoseny, N. M. Thilakarathne, M. I. Alghamdi, R. K. Mahendran, A. A. Gardezi, H. Weerasinghe, and A. Welhenge, "Security and privacy issues in medical internet of things: overview, countermeasures, challenges and future directions," *Sustainability*, vol. 13, no. 21, p. 11645, 2021.

[5] Jigang Liu, Ryoichi Sasaki, and Tetsutaro Uehara, "Towards a Holistic Approach to Medical IoT Forensics", 2020 IEEE 20th International Conference on Software Quality, Reliability and Security Companion (QRS-C), 2020. https://qrs20.techconf.org/QRSC2020_FULL/pdfs/QRS-C2020-4QOuHkY3M10ZUl1MoEzYvg/891500a686/891500a686.pdf

[6] Abdulrehman Al Allaf, and Waseem Totonji, "Explore IoT Security Threats and Forensics Challenges: A Literature Review and Survey Study", 2023. www.diva-portal.org/smash/get/diva2:1764110/FULLTEXT01.pdf, Computer and Information Sciences,oai:DiVA.org:lnu-121500

[7] Jeffery Fairbanks, Md Mashrur Arifin, Sadia Afreen, and Alex Curtis, "Survey and Analysis of IoT Operating Systems: A Comparative Study on the Effectiveness and Acquisition Time of Open-Source Digital Forensics Tools", 2023. https://arxiv.org/abs/2407.01474, https://arxiv.org/abs/2407.01474, https://doi.org/10.48550/arXiv.2407.01474

[8] Khanpara, Pimal, Ishwa Shah, et al., "Towards the Internet of Things Forensics: A Data Analytics Perspective", *Security and Privacy*, vol. 6, no. 5, p. e306, 2024. https://doi.org/10.22541/au.170663498.83592067/v1

[9] Rama Rao, Veera V., Kiran Sree Pokkuluri, et al., "A Secured and Energy-Efficient System for Patient E-Healthcare Monitoring Using Internet of Medical Things (IoMT)", *Data and Metadata*, vol. 3, p. 368, 2024. doi:10.56294/dm2024368.

[10] Nithya, S., Satheeshkumar Palanisamy, and Nivethitha T., "Achieving Secured Medical Network (SMN) Through Stateless Mechanism and SkeyM in Medical Internet of Things (M-IoT)", *Journal of Engineering and Applied Science*, vol. 71, no.1, pp. 1–22, 2024. https://doi.org/10.1186/s44147-024-00460-4

[11] Zhou, Jiasi, Yan Chen, et al., "Joint Uplink and Downlink Rate Splitting for Fog Computing-Enabled Internet of Medical Things", *IEEE Transactions on Cognitive Communications and Networking*, vol. 11, no. 23, pp. 37872–37884. https://doi.org/10.48550/arXiv.2405.06297, 2024.

[12] Svandova, Katerina, and Zdenek Smutny, "Internet of Medical Things Security Frameworks for Risk Assessment and Management: A Scoping Review", *Journal of Multidisciplinary Healthcare*, vol. 17, pp. 2281–2301, 2024. https://doi.org/10.2147/JMDH.S459987.

[13] Villegas-Ch, William, Joselyn Garcia Ortiz, and Isabel Urbina-Camacho, "Framework for a Secure and Sustainable Internet of Medical Things, Requirements, Design Challenges and Future Trends", *Applied Sciences*, vol. 13, no 11, p. 6634, 2023. https://doi.org/10.3390/app13116634

[14] El-Moenim Kabel, Samia A., Ghada M. El-Banby, et al., "Securing Internet of Medical Things Using Cancellable ECG Recognition", *Scientific Reports*, vol. 14, no 1, p. 10871, 2024. https://doi.org/10.1038/s41598-024-54830-2

[15] Abdur Rahman, Mohamed, M. Shamim Hossain, and Nabin A. Alrajeh, "Secure and Provenance Enhanced Internet of Health Things Framework: A Blockchain Managed Federated Learning Approach", *IEEE Access*, vol. 8, pp. 205071–205087, 2020.

[16] Liu, Linchen, Ruyan Liu, et al., "Dual Blockchain-Based Data Sharing Mechanism with Privacy Protection of Medical Internet of Things", Heliyon, vol 10, no. 1, p. e23575, 2023. https://doi.org/10.1016/j.heliyon

[17] Straw, Isabel, Claire Kirkby, and Preethi Gopinath, "Connected to the Cloud at Time of Death: A Case Report", *Journal of Medical Case Reports*, vol. 18, no 1, p. 360, 2024. https://doi.org/10.1186/s13256-024-04573-5.

[18] Qureshi, Fayez, and Sridhar Krishnan, "Wearable Hardware Design for the Internet of Medical Things (IoMT)", https://www.mdpi.com/1424-8220/18/11/3812, Department of Electrical, Computer, and Biomedical Engineering, Ryerson University, Toronto, ON M5B 2K3, Canada, https://doi.org/10.3390/s18113812, 2018.

[19] Kumar Sadhu, Pintu, Venkata P. Yanambaka, Ahmed Abdelgawad, and Kumar Yelamarthi, "Prospect of Internet of Medical Things: A Review on Security Requirements and Solutions", *Sensors*, vol. 22, no 15, p. 5517, 2022.

[20] Alizadehsani, Roohallah, Mohamad Roshanzamir, et al., "Swarm Intelligence in Internet of Medical Things: A Review", *Sensors*, vol. 23, no 3, p. 1466, 2023.

[21] Pournik, Omid, Leila Ghalichi, Parisis Gallos, and Theodoros N. Arvanitis, "The Internet of Medical Things: Opportunities, Benefits, Challenges and Concerns", European Federation for Medical Informatics (EFMI) and IOS Press, 2023. www.researchgate.net/publication/374938877_The_Internet_of_Medical_Things_Opportunities_Benefits_Challenges_and_Concerns/fulltext/6538646d24bbe32d9a6c8f9e/The-Internet-of-Medical-Things-Opportunities-Benefits-Challenges-and-Concerns.pdf. doi:10.3233/SHTI230809.

[22] Lodha, Lokesh, Vishwadeepak Singh Baghela, J. Bhuvana, and Rahul Bhatt, "A Blockchain-Based Secured System Using the Internet of Medical Things (IOMT) Network for E-Healthcare Monitoring", https://papers.ssrn.com/sol3/papers.cfm?abstract_id=4817133, International Conference on Computer Science, Engineering and Applications (ICCSEA), IEEE, https://ssrn.com/abstract=4817133, 2023.

[23] Kamalov, Firuz, Behrouz Pourghebleh, et al., "Internet of Medical Things Privacy and Security: Challenges, Solutions, and Future Trends from a New Perspective", *Sustainability*, vol. 15, no. 4, p. 3317, 2023. www.mdpi.com/2071-1050/15/4/3317, Sustainability/Privacy-Preserving of IoT-Based Application in Smart Healthcare, https://doi.org/10.3390/su15043317.

[24] Ouaissa, M. and A. Rhattoy, "QoS Hybrid Uplink Scheduler Based on Service Type for M2M Communications in LTE Networks", *Indonesian Journal of Electrical Engineering and Computer Sciences*, vol. 14, no. 3, p. 1460, 2019.

[25] Ouaissa, M., M. Benmoussa, A. Rhattoy, M. Lahmer, and I. Chana, I. (2016, October). "Performance Analysis of Random Access Mechanisms for Machine Type Communications in LTE Networks", In 2016 International Conference on Advanced Communication Systems and Information Security (ACOSIS) (pp. 1–6). IEEE.

[26] Houmer, M., M. Ouaissa, M. Ouaissa, & M. L. Hasnaoui, "SE-GPSR: Secured and Enhanced Greedy Perimeter Stateless Routing Protocol for Vehicular Ad hoc Networks", *iJIM*, vol.14, no. 13, p. 49, 2020.

[27] Ouaissa, M. and A. Rhattoy, "New Method Based on Priority of Heterogeneous Traffic for Scheduling Techniques in M2M Communications over LTE Networks", *International Journal of Intelligent Engineering & Systems*, vol. 11, no. 6, 2018.

Chapter 12

# Educational transformations for IoMT forensics

## Challenges and opportunities

*Soufiane Ouariach, Fatima Zahra Ouariach, Inam Ullah Khan, Mariya Ouaissa, and Mariyam Ouaissa*

## 12.1 INTRODUCTION

Healthcare technology development has led to an unmatched convergence of medical machines, the internet, and therefore established the Internet of Medical Things (IoMT) infrastructure. The technological fusion between medical devices and the internet enables healthcare progress but raises serious difficulties in maintaining security and privacy together with forensic requirements. Medical devices that connect to the internet are steadily becoming common in healthcare spaces, which necessitates expert forensic knowledge to protect healthcare system integrity and security.

The specialized field of IoMT forensics combines elements from digital forensics as well as medical technology with cybersecurity disciplines. IoMT forensics combines the necessary approaches, instruments, and specialized knowledge needed to examine security vulnerabilities and data corruption and unauthorized access in IoMT networks. Medical device investigations remain challenging because they involve healthcare data sensitivity combined with life-threatening security failures that occur within this medical domain [1, 2]. The field of IoMT forensics gains importance although current educational programs fail to match essential skills needed by professionals in this domain.

The technical complexity of IoMT systems along with ethical healthcare data investigation aspects present challenges for educational institutions to create sufficient curricula [3, 4]. The fast-moving technological landscape makes it challenging for training programs because new devices together with protocols and security concerns must be added to educational content [5]. Current training programs in forensic practice often lack sufficient practical content regarding real-world implementations of IoMT forensic technology. While theoretical knowledge is important, it frequently fails to align with operational requirements in research facilities and investigation sites [5]. Hands-on training with modern technologies, including machine

DOI: 10.1201/9781003640325-12

learning systems and virtual reality for crime investigation, has become essential for preparing graduates for professional practice [6].

Researchers study the present condition of IoMT forensic education alongside the necessary skills and innovative teaching approaches to meet these requirements in this chapter. The analysis reviews expert training challenges in IoMT forensics by identifying two main shortcomings that result from insufficient instruction about medical technology integration with forensic science and limited training capacity compared to industrial demands. IoMT forensic scientists need three main areas of competency consisting of technical expertise, medical knowledge, regulatory standards, and interdisciplinary subjects according to the defined outlines. The assessment evaluates new educational approaches that combine problem-based learning (PBL) with hands-on activities and virtual laboratories and university–industry cooperative programs. The text examines sustainable barriers to IoMT forensics training through evaluations of rapidly changing technology alongside ethical and sustainability demands and training program accessibility challenges. This chapter evaluates successful training models while offering perspective on continuous adaptive educational strategies which generate valuable information for developing effective strategies in the dynamic field.

## 12.2 CURRENT PANORAMA OF IOMT FORENSICS TRAINING

### 12.2.1 Current situation: curricular gaps and shortcomings

The current state of IoMT forensics education showcases significant gaps in the curricula of many forensic science programs. IoMT forensics faces two main difficulties due to fast technology growth and its specific requirements for using forensic science to investigate connected medical devices.

The education of IoMT forensics faces a critical deficiency because universities offer insufficient training on both medical technology integration and forensic science methodologies. The fast-growing deployment of IoMT devices creates new security weaknesses that allow botnet attackers to damage healthcare system data confidentiality and integrity and cause system unavailability. The educational curricula fail to integrate enough computer science principles while missing necessary cybersecurity measures that protect against vulnerabilities [1, 2]. Education curricula need a structured design to incorporate complete training about identifying cyber dangers, together with network vulnerabilities analysis, along with traditional forensic science subjects. Basic technology subjects that integrate into forensic science curriculum programs prepare students to tackle the particular difficulties associated with IoMT devices.

The present educational approach fails to include interdisciplinary knowledge in its teaching programs. Students need to grasp both advanced technological concepts and forensic principles to perform successful IoMT forensic investigations while learning data analysis methods through artificial intelligence and evidence management using blockchain technology [3, 4]. Educational programs should integrate these domains because they produce specific applications and effects during forensic investigations. The implementation of blockchain provides forensic practitioners the ability to protect evidence authenticity while making data across systems more reliable, thus showing needed advancements in forensic procedures [3].

Current training programs dedicated to forensic practice lack sufficient content coverage of practical aspects when it comes to IoMT forensic technology implementations in real-life situations. Theoretical understandings normally fail to connect with actual operational needs that occur within research facilities and investigation sites [5]. Graduates from forensic programs gain increased readiness through hands-on training related to innovative technologies including data analysis using machine learning systems and virtual reality tools for solving crime investigations [6]. Students must complete practical training because it prepares them to become skilled in using modern forensic technologies and methodologies in their professional practice.

The main issue today is the absence of standard accreditation criteria for IoMT forensics educational programs. Different educational establishments have chosen diverse training methods for this new field, but consistent standards and benchmarks are essential for future development. Specific accreditation procedures designed for IoMT forensics education will establish baseline competency standards that guarantee that all forensic science graduates demonstrate essential proficiency in handling complex technological issues in forensic applications [5].

The educational system requires immediate attention to fill existing curriculum gaps regarding IoMT forensic training. Educational improvement in IoMT forensics can be achieved through interdisciplinary learning, practical training, and standardized accreditation standards. Educational approaches must adapt to technological advancements in forensic science because this ensures forensic professionals can handle the challenges posed by IoMT.

### 12.2.2 Fracture between industrial requirements and training offers

A wide difference exists between current industry requirements and available training programs for professionals who work with IoMT technology, which threatens effective IoMT implementation in healthcare systems. Rapid technological changes along with the demands of the healthcare industry form the core elements that create this training deficit.

Many educational programs fail to demonstrate the complex multidisciplinary requirements of IoMT devices. During interconnection, multiple healthcare devices and systems form the IoMT framework which demands individual security protocols for each component. Research shows medical organizations need customized security solutions to protect their IoMT devices because standard cybersecurity methods prove insufficient for healthcare-specific security needs [7, 8]. Graduate education programs fail to focus on security protocols alongside risk assessment methods and effective intrusion detection technologies because of this their students lack industry readiness [9, 10].

The current educational programs lack sufficient training on real-world implementations and practical applications related to IoMT. Students need practical application of theoretical knowledge to develop operational competencies that suit the evolving environment of connected medical devices. The expanding use of wearable technologies and remote monitoring systems demands professionals to obtain an understanding of machine learning and data analysis methods for tracking patient conduct and spotting abnormal patterns [11, 12]. Students who lack practical training fail to develop critical thinking skills, which they need to handle real-life professional challenges. The educational system often maintains an inadequate connection with industry professionals, which leads to accommodating contemporary market requirements in curriculum development. The pace of IoMT technology evolution outpaces educational institution efforts to update their programs with emerging developments. Graduates face difficulty because of a lack of connection between their education and the expectations of potential employers [10, 13]. Academia alongside industry partners should jointly create educational curricula that focus on current market trends while matching their output to exact professional requirements.

The constantly changing nature of IoMT requires ongoing learning yet professional training programs fail to highlight the need for continuous education and skills development. Professionals working in IoMT need to pursue lifelong education because both technical and regulatory environments keep evolving so they can maintain their understanding of best practices together with compliance requirements and IoT technology developments [14]. Training should provide essential learning practices that encourage personnel to pursue self-directed education and career advancement. The current mismatch between professional requirements and existing training programs for IoMT exists due to insufficient practical focus, insufficient curriculum-real-world relationships, as well as insufficient ongoing educational programs. The workforce needs to be properly trained through combined collaboration between educational institutions and industry leaders and professional organizations for effective integration of IoMT in healthcare systems.

## 12.3 CORE COMPETENCIES FOR THE IOMT FORENSICS EXPERT

### 12.3.1 Technological expertise: IoMT protocols and analysis tools

IoMT forensics experts play a critical role because they need to handle connected medical devices together with their security and investigative challenges. Managing the security challenges in the field requires professionals to develop specific essential technical competencies for effective understanding and mitigation. An expert in IoMT forensic work must develop a complete understanding of all existing protocols.

The IoMT system relies on various communication protocols that utilize standard protocols such as message queuing telemetry transport and constrained application protocol [15]. The analysis of data exchanges between medical devices becomes possible for forensic experts through their understanding of IoMT protocols, which help them investigate ecosystem interactions. The expertise of investigators must include knowledge of secure communication protocols because weaknesses in these security systems lead to major health data breaches and unauthorized access to sensitive medical information [16]. The analysis of IoT technology demands a complete understanding of standard IoT protocols and specialized healthcare-oriented protocols.

The investigation of IoMT devices requires complete technical competence with multiple analytical tools. The fast-growing cyber forensic tool capabilities that extract data from IoMT devices need experts who understand how to operate such tools specifically for intrusion detection and malware analysis. To conduct effective IoMT, forensics experts must have the capability to analyze intricate datasets obtained from these devices [17]. Forensic experts gain improved effectiveness through the use of statistical and analytical software because it helps identify data patterns with anomalies and potential security incidents. The growing importance of advanced technologies for healthcare analysts includes machine learning and blockchain system knowledge. Healthcare professionals are starting to use blockchain technology to protect the security and integrity of data within IoMT networks [18]. A forensic expert working in IoMT should master blockchain technology to both protect evidence integrity and validate transmission data integrity. Machine learning algorithms perform a vital role when it comes to detecting anomalies automatically and predicting security breaches within IoMT systems [19]. The comprehension of these modern technological domains allows forensic practitioners to maximize their use of the advanced detection and investigation methods effectively.

For effective incident response, IoMT forensics experts must also develop skills related to cybersecurity practices that ensure device and data security. Given the escalating threats faced by IoMT devices, knowledge of best practices in network security, including penetration testing and ethical hacking, is essential [20]. This expertise is necessary not only for protecting the integrity of medical data but also for conducting thorough forensic investigations when security incidents occur.

### 12.3.2 Medical and regulatory expertise: HIPAA, RGPD, and industry standards

The practice of IoMT forensics demands complete medical understanding along with regulatory expertise from professionals. This expertise encompasses familiarity with pertinent legislation such as the Health Insurance Portability and Accountability Act (HIPAA) in the United States and the General Data Protection Regulation (GDPR) in Europe, as well as a deep understanding of medical standards and practices. The combination of healthcare and technology expertise allows IoMT forensics experts to maintain medical system integrity while ensuring compliance. Advanced knowledge of HIPAA stands as the initial requirement for success. The HIPAA privacy rules require healthcare providers and EHR-handling organizations to implement strict security measures for safeguarding protected patient data in the United States [21]. All forensic professionals working in IoMT must understand HIPAA regulations to determine the consequences of data breaches and unauthorized access to individual health information. Their understanding allows them to assess breaches properly so they can suggest suitable remediation steps that meet legal requirements.

The GDPR establishes extensive data protection standards throughout the European Union, thus affecting the forensic analysis of IoMT devices. Organizations must uphold individual rights regarding personal data under the GDPR because they process this information. Experts need to grasp data minimization together with purpose limitation and data subject rights principles because they determine how medical data should be handled through IoMT systems [21]. The failure to follow GDPR requirements sets off serious legal consequences which require forensic experts to include this fundamental knowledge in their investigative procedures.

The forensic analysis of IoMT requires medical standards that determine how devices conduct their functions while maintaining patient safety. The FDA in the United States and European Medicines Agency (EMA) establish both medical device approval protocols and continuous compliance and monitoring requirements for in-use devices [22]. IoMT forensics experts need to understand these standards because they determine device compliance with legal requirements for investigating device failures and deceptive activities.

Healthcare professionals must keep pace with the evolving healthcare technologies by learning about new regulations and standards that affect

IoMT devices. The healthcare industry dedicates more attention to creating specialized cybersecurity solutions for medical devices because these devices become connected and exposed to external security threats. The enforcement of HIPAA privacy regulations requires detailed knowledge so healthcare professionals can establish secure methods for protecting important health information [23].

### 12.3.3 Interdisciplinary skills: ethics, communication, and collaboration

Essential skills for IoMT forensics experts encompass a wide range of interdisciplinary capabilities, particularly in ethics, communication, and teamwork. The interdisciplinary work environment demands these essential abilities from professionals who handle the intersection area between technology and healthcare and regulatory compliance. Ethics stands as an essential base for conducting IoMT forensic investigations. Healthcare professionals need to handle medical data with care because they encounter various ethical challenges regarding patient privacy rights together with the requirements for informed consent and proper technology utilization. The knowledge of ethical principles helps forensic experts in IoMT make proper decisions that both fulfill legal mandates and protect patient health. To handle sensitive information properly, ethical commitments must govern operations since they serve to safeguard patient rights and meet all applicable regulatory standards [24].

The success of IoMT forensic work depends on strong communication abilities. Forensic experts must deliver complicated technical information about forensic discoveries to a wide range of healthcare providers, together with legal professionals and patients. Effective communication creates trust and mutual understanding between all parties because they are essential for collaborative work in investigations [25, 26]. The conversion of complex technical results into simple terms enables IT specialists to work better with healthcare practitioners so they can understand forensic analysis implications together. Forensic experts need to develop specialized terminology which they can adjust for different forensic environments [27]. Multiple disciplines, including healthcare, information technology, and law, must collaborate for solving most challenges in forensic investigations of IoMT systems. A team-based method helps combine multiple perspectives from experts, which specifically helps solve complex problems created by IoMT deployment. The application of efficient teamwork techniques enables multiple perspectives and resources to come together for solving problems in forensic investigations. Security implementations in patient data management gain efficiency through joint efforts between healthcare providers and cybersecurity professionals who maintain compliance and ethical requirements.

Teamwork emerges as a fundamental ability in IoMT forensics since various challenges demand experts from healthcare, information technology, and law to work together. A team-oriented approach enables diverse insights and expertise to unite effectively when handling the complex implementation challenges of IoMT systems. A successful team effort allows investigators to collect numerous points of view and assets, which produces better insights during forensic examinations. Cybersecurity professionals working together with healthcare providers bring efficiency to patient data management by securing data and maintaining ethical compliance standards. Professionals who work in IoMT forensics need to develop three essential skills: ethics understanding, alongside communication and teamwork competency. Knowledge of ethical principles helps healthcare practitioners move safely through complex rules while maintaining patient privacy protection. Diverse stakeholders work together effectively due to communication skills, so they can create innovative solutions in this multidisciplinary field through teamwork. These skilled competencies of IoMT aim to create healthcare technologies that establish stronger security and ethics as well as deliver superior effectiveness.

## 12.4 INNOVATIVE EDUCATIONAL PARADIGMS

### 12.4.1 Problem-solving pedagogy

PBL educational models continue to grow in popularity when teaching IoMT forensics experts in different fields of study. Through PBL students develop active learning ability together with critical thinking skills when faced with real-world problems that demand their interdisciplinary collaboration to solve them. Students who implement this method develop both their technical abilities and essential interdisciplinary talents that include ethics together with communication and teamwork skills.

The primary advantage of PBL enables different academic backgrounds to work together in meaningful collaborative projects. Students who receive interdisciplinary education gain the versatility to handle multiple career options and face current workplace obstacles [28]. The integration of knowledge from technology, medicine, and ethics becomes essential for IoMT forensics because experts need to solve complex medical device and data privacy problems.

The research conducted by Scott and White confirms that PBL practices boost critical thinking abilities and problem-solving capabilities and teamworking competencies [29]. Students enrolled in IoMT programs acquire vital skills through interdisciplinary projects that enable them to combine knowledge across disciplines, thus effectively solving forensic cases. The practical learning method helps students understand complex IoMT system functions and teaches them to tackle issues through various viewpoints. Through PBL students develop ethical intelligence when they handle actual dilemmas that arise from forensic work in the IoMT field. Student encounters ethical issues regarding patient privacy together with data usage during forensic investigations, which leads to important discussions about both ethical principles and regulatory rules. The implementation of PBL methods strengthens the essential competency of effective communication. The learning design compels students to both explain their work outcomes and team up successfully with classmates who come from various cultural backgrounds. Forensic professionals need to master the ability to explain intricate findings to nonspecialist audiences because this skill directly benefits real-world implementations, especially in healthcare institutions. According to Ferns et al., graduates who experience interdisciplinary PBL develop better readiness for technology-mediated workplaces that require effective communication and collaboration [30]. The PBL framework serves as a powerful tool for developing teamwork capabilities which prove necessary for all IoMT forensics experts. Students develop teamworking abilities when they solve complex problems together because they learn to manage opinion differences and solve conflicts while using each member's unique abilities. The collaborative environment of PBL training enables future practitioners to master team-based work that they will need in their professional careers. Students believe that integrated coursework strengthens their abilities to collaborate and solve problems [31].

The educational implementation of PBL approaches for IoMT forensics experts brings many advantageous outcomes. Training approaches like these enhance technical abilities as well as develop key interdisciplinary capabilities built upon ethics application alongside communication standards and teamwork understanding. Educational programs adopting PBL for IoMT instruction will help their graduates tackle emerging challenges in this evolving field better.

### 12.4.2 Hands-on training and virtual laboratories

Incorporating hands-on training and virtual laboratories into the educational experience of IoMT forensics experts is becoming increasingly essential for developing practical skills and competencies. This innovative instructional approach fosters critical learning outcomes that align with the complexities of modern healthcare technology.

Hands-on training provides students with the opportunity to engage directly with IoMT technologies, allowing them to apply theoretical knowledge in practical, real-world scenarios. Such training can take various forms, including workshops, simulations, and live projects that utilize current IoMT devices and systems. Khatib et al. [32] highlight the importance of practical applications in the IoMT realm, emphasizing that exposure to real cases can improve problem-solving skills and deepen understanding of medical devices and their implications in healthcare settings.

Furthermore, hands-on training allows for the integration of ethical discussions related to the misuse of IoMT technologies, such as data breaches and privacy violations. Addressing ethical dilemmas during practical sessions reinforces the importance of maintaining patient confidentiality and upholding the integrity of healthcare systems, thus preparing students to navigate these challenges effectively.

On the other hand, virtual laboratories serve as an educational advancement that uses technological tools to generate virtual training spaces that supplement traditional laboratory sessions. The approach provides students with simulated laboratory experiences that do not depend on physical resources or geographical constraints. Virtual labs serve as testing grounds that enable studies of different IoMT devices alongside data evaluation and forensic research under controlled settings. Bhowal et al. demonstrate that these educational environments strengthen both student competencies and teamwork abilities when students tackle complicated problems [33]. Virtual laboratories help students conduct experiments on different IoMT system scenarios which would otherwise be unavailable through traditional laboratory settings. Students who take part in simulated activities enhance their computational abilities and critical thinking skills for dealing with IoMT technology risks.

Research indicates that virtual laboratories boost student performance in IoMT system management as well as educational outcomes. The combination of simulations with virtual tools allows students to test machine learning methods and diagnostic methods that apply to IoMT disease prediction systems and patient monitoring applications [34, 35]. The ability to modify training programs according to healthcare sector developments becomes simpler because virtual labs provide flexible options to institutions. Virtual laboratories provide future forensic scientists with continuous learning and skill development through updated resources and tools, which keeps them informed about technology advancements [36].

The education of IoMT forensics experts requires hands-on training along with virtual laboratories because these methods help develop necessary competencies for dealing with emerging field challenges. The educational approach generates better technical proficiency together with moral understanding while developing essential skills needed for healthcare technology advancement.

### 12.4.3 University–industry synergies

The field of IoMT forensics requires increasing industry–university partnerships to advance research along with innovation and education. The partnership leads to knowledge exchange through practical training that promotes essential technological developments required to solve healthcare technology problems.

Industry–university collaboration in IoMT enables the productive relationship between theoretical research and practical application as its main advantage. Partnerships between academic institutions and industrial organizations have made major contributions to medical device development along with clinical research [37]. Joint funding opportunities from these collaborations let universities access essential resources that they would not have access to otherwise. The collaborative space supports students and faculty to participate in advanced medical research which directly impacts healthcare practice.

The collaboration between these organizations results in the development of new IoMT solutions that address particular healthcare requirements. The combined knowledge of product developers alongside medical researchers demonstrates the benefit for rapid point-of-care testing devices [38]. The collaboration between researchers creates valuable opportunities that yield significant positive results in healthcare innovation.

The development of capable IoMT forensics professionals depends on practical training, which partnerships between industry and universities help to supply. The effective connections between universities and enterprises described by Li and Niyomsilp show how to improve graduate competence through industry-based curriculum changes and knowledge transfer [39].

Additionally, internships, cooperative education, and project-based learning initiatives enable students to apply their academic knowledge to real-world situations, bridging the gap between education and industry demands. This practical experience is invaluable for IoMT students who must navigate complex regulatory environments, technical challenges, and ethical considerations that arise in the deployment of medical technologies.

Students and faculty who participate in industry partnerships develop professional relationships through networking, which guides their career development. The paper of Ragupathy et al. emphasizes that universities maintain their status as essential innovation centers by connecting students with industry experts who share career guidance for IoMT pathways [40]. The mentoring process helps students gain workforce readiness while developing their professional self-assurance before entering professional positions.

### 12.4.4 MOOCs and online learning resources

Massive open online courses (MOOCs) have revolutionized educational practices while training professionals to work in IoMT forensics. Interactive online education through MOOCs provides convenient and wide-ranging educational materials as essential elements to boost educational performance in rapidly transforming fields of study. The primary benefit that

MOOCs provide to learners stems from their adaptable format and broad reach. Education through MOOCs allows students to join courses whenever they want and from any location, thus eliminating traditional learning obstacles. The MOOC framework developed by Ismail et al. created a beneficial learning environment where students accessed online resources easily through smartphone devices according to Ismail et al. [41]. The open structure of MOOCs serves professionals well since they can pursue their careers and personal obligations while continuing their education. Higher accessibility to quality education occurs due to MOOCs' reduced cost structure. MOOCs provide basic education to students without cost or minimal payment, which ensures equal learning opportunities for students across different economic backgrounds. Educational opportunities for all can produce a better-educated workforce in the IoMT sector, which will be better prepared with the necessary knowledge and skills.

The vast assortment of courses available through MOOCs creates opportunities to enrich the learning process for students. The popularity of MOOCs continues to rise through multiple academic disciplines such as health and medicine [42]. Online videos used as educational materials help students stay more engaged in their studies. IoMT forensics professionals can access diverse learning resources that provide knowledge about data analytics and cybersecurity practices together with ethical data handling methods to maintain field-level awareness. Participating in MOOCs enables students to take advantage of peer learning and network-building opportunities because of their collaborative framework. Students who take part in discussion forums and group projects at MOOCs exchange valuable ideas and perspectives that help them develop essential interdisciplinary skills needed for IoMT forensics.

Through MOOC integration with simulations combined with interactive content, students gain improved practical training capabilities. Hendriks et al. [43] state that medical MOOCs of high-quality use multiple instructional approaches including interactive student activities to help students understand and remember the material better. Interactive learning modules provide essential value to IoMT forensic education because they enable students to conduct digital forensic investigations in simulated conditions. Students using MOOCs can access virtual laboratories which offer them the chance to practice laboratory experiments remotely. The practical competencies needed for effective work in IoMT settings require hands-on training since professionals must master different technologies and tools.

Through their design, MOOCs create an environment for people to learn continuously as well as advance their professional skills. The field of IoMT requires this aspect because technology and regulatory landscapes continue to change in this domain. Through MOOCs, professionals gain access to the most recent developments and best practices as well as tools that are relevant to IoMT forensic investigations. Azami and Ibrahim [44] explain how

MOOCs function as a modern learning method that enables continuous educational prospects. MOOCs and online learning resources serve as an effective educational system for IoMT forensics professionals. These online learning platforms offer crucial benefits such as ease of accessibility, flexible scheduling, diverse educational content, hands-on learning possibilities and ongoing education capabilities, which make them essential tools for training future forensic experts. Education institutions can improve professional training through these platforms to handle the complex healthcare challenges resulting from IoMT technology integration.

## 12.5 SPECIFIC CHALLENGES FOR SUSTAINABLE TRAINING IN IOMT FORENSICS

The education of IoMT forensics experts encounters multiple distinctive hurdles because of quick technological changes, medical data ethics, along with sustainability issues, and challenges with training program access and inclusivity. The success of professionals who work with IoMT systems depends on solving these essential challenges in the modern, rapidly changing landscape.

The rapid technological advancements pose a major obstacle when training professionals in IoMT forensics. New IoMT devices and protocols develop at an overwhelming rate that causes difficulties for institutions that want their training curricula to stay relevant. Educators need to update their programs regularly to demonstrate new IoMT technology developments alongside their effects on forensic methods [45]. The utilization of out-of-date instructional materials creates deficient learning environments because it prepares students who face modern workplace demands like protecting against cyberattacks and following technology compliance requirements during deployment. The speed of technological advancements requires a learning system that develops lifelong learning abilities and adaptability skills in professionals. The availability of MOOCs and online learning resources enables professionals to continuously update their education through flexible, up-to-date content, which helps decrease this challenge. The resources enable practitioners to learn about new technologies as they emerge through just-in-time learning methods [46].

The training of specialists who examine IoMT systems faces obstacles because of the ethical requirements for dealing with confidential medical information. Because IoMT deals with extensive personal health information collection and transmission, it demands strict compliance with HIPAA and GDPR [47]. The unauthorized access to sensitive healthcare information leads to both breaches of patient privacy and negatively impacts healthcare deliverables. Apprehensive forensics experts need comprehensive training, that teaches about privacy laws and ethical implications their profession entails. Real-world ethical situations encountered in IoMT environments should be studied through case examples to improve educational experiences by teaching students how to handle complex moral challenges.

The ongoing technological progress of IoMT devices raises severe environmental preservation challenges. IoMT technology produces major environmental effects because of its manufacturing process, distribution methods, and its end-of-life disposal phase creates electronic waste and depletes resources. Training programs must include modules that teach students about sustainable development practices for IoMT technologies. The healthcare sector depends on future professionals who receive education about sustainable medical device development life cycles as well as recycling practices to achieve responsible technological progress. The awareness of ethical duties by IoMT forensics experts supports worldwide efforts to decrease environmental impacts [48].

Training programs that are not widely accessible create difficulties in developing IoMT forensics professionals. Traditional training and higher education programs face accessibility challenges because of geographical, socioeconomic, and technological obstacles that prevent potential students from participating. Institutions need to establish online platforms and combination learning models to make important educational content accessible equally to all students. Online education through MOOCs enables educational expansion because it distributes current learning content to students from various social backgrounds without requiring location-based or budgetary limitations [45]. Programs designed for different learning styles should include accessible resources, which ensure students with any ability level or heritage gain benefits from their IoMT forensics training. The sustainable practice of IoMT forensics training faces four unique barriers from technological change speed to ethical and environmental issues, and training access limitations, which require solution-oriented educational development approaches. Flexible training approaches combined with ethical curriculum integration together with sustainability practices and expanded accessibility allow institutions to develop future forensic experts who understand the advancing field challenges.

## 12.6 CASE STUDIES OF SUCCESSFUL TRAINING PROGRAMS IN IOMT FORENSICS

Different international training programs for IoMT forensics have emerged as examples of best practice through which effective methods have been developed and significant lessons have been learned. This section examines successful training approaches together with participant feedback systems and performance evaluation methods.

The Medical Education Partnership Initiative launched an African program to improve medical education systems because Africa faced a healthcare worker shortage. This initiative successfully built workforce capacity by integrating clinical education with community health, which enables personnel to address various health problems including those from IoMT [49]. The MEPI program focused on community-based training, which let medical students connect with healthcare institutions to put their theoretical knowledge into practical application. Through this approach, medical students gained deeper educational value which simultaneously produced better health results for their communities.

Training of Trainers (ToT) serves as a GHP initiative model that teaches sustainable health systems through local educator training within low- and middle-income countries. Structured training of local healthcare workers produces positive outcomes with high-quality results and optimizes resource usage within the public health sector [50]. Training sessions combine fundamental skills training with ethical instructions, which prepares trainers to deliver knowledge to others in a sustainable manner. Talib et al. [51] performed a scoping review that evaluated Sub-Saharan Africa PGME programs from 1992 through 2017 to explore their development and overcome challenges in a systematic manner. The study demonstrated the need for both global alliances together with faculty involvement to keep training programs complete and relevant. The research demonstrates that educational partnerships create better learning experiences, which leads to improved health workforce ability to tackle local medical problems.

The training programs received feedback from their participants which revealed key themes. Through the MEPI initiative, the training program demonstrated successful curriculum adaptation by changing its strategies when health needs evolved [49]. Training content remains relevant through continuous updates of educational materials. Healthcare technology advancement demands focused ethical training for all professionals. Training participants developed enhanced patient privacy and data security awareness through the addition of ethical discussions into their sessions according to feedback [50]. The development of competent IoMT forensic professionals requires adopting ethical frameworks as a fundamental practice. Participants from GHP and MEPI programs emphasized the importance of networking with mentors and peers through which professionals develop productive partnerships to share resources [51]. A community of practice formed among trainees enables them to learn from each other and develop their skills.

The evaluation of these training programs requires assessments to measure three key aspects: participant satisfaction, as well as knowledge retention and practical competency development.

The MEPI program achieved both higher medical education enrollment numbers and better student learning results and satisfaction scores [49]. The participants who answered the feedback surveys said they gained capabilities to use their acquired knowledge in practical real-world contexts.

Healthcare education programs using competency assessments strengthened both patient care skills and graduate abilities to transform regional healthcare delivery systems. The research demonstrated that professionals who received training showed better competence in IoMT device management as well as ethical implications which resulted in better healthcare practices [51].

The GHP and similar programs conduct extended alumni monitoring that tracks both professional development and ongoing healthcare involvement within community settings. The long-term tracking demonstrates that training results are sustainable by showing how trained individuals drive healthcare model evolution [50].

Successful training programs for IoMT forensics exist throughout the world through collaborative partnerships and adaptive learning systems. The case studies deliver important findings that future program development should adopt alongside ethical training and structured curriculum and networking support to build capable and ethical IoMT forensics practitioners.

## 12.7 STRATEGIES FOR CONTINUOUS AND ADAPTIVE EDUCATION

The evolution of IoMT forensic practice necessitates adapting education for experts because of emerging medical technology. The competency of IoMT forensics experts depends heavily on three key strategies: continuing professional development, communities of practice, and self-learning resources, and adapting to emerging technological developments. IoMT professionals must participate in continuing professional development programs because these prepare them to utilize modern technologies and practices in their field. Lifelong learning becomes possible through CPD because it provides professionals with current information and new abilities.

Online courses along with workshops enable practitioners to gain enhanced knowledge about new technologies, ethical aspects, and regulatory guidelines. [52]. The CPD programs develop both personal progress and organizational achievement in workforce competence levels. Structured programs with practical applications within CPD enable professionals to experience firsthand scenarios that relate to IoMT forensic work. Real-world experiences complement theoretical learning to teach practitioners how their work functions in practice [53]. Medical technology workshops that simulate breach scenarios together with ethical dilemmas allow professionals to apply learned knowledge in realistic settings to develop their decision-making abilities.

Through Communities of practice (CoPs) and learning networks, professionals can access environments that facilitate the exchange of knowledge and experiences alongside best practices. Professional development receives enhancement through networks that provide collaborative and mentorship services. IoMT forensics experts who participate in CoPs maintain their connection to industry trends and innovations since members routinely provide essential information about current technologies and field-specific challenges [54]. Members of CoPs use structured interactions to develop solutions together for the common challenges that appear in IoMT forensics. The shared knowledge among professionals provides maximum benefit when technology advances rapidly because members can draw from each other's practical experiences [54].

Self-directed learning resources that include MOOCs with webinars and online tutorials provide professionals with a flexible opportunity to determine their learning timeline. These resources provide accessible and flexible learning opportunities that enable practitioners to fill particular knowledge deficits while developing skills needed for their work responsibilities. Self-directed learning models serve as essential components because they match educational materials with personal objectives, thus creating individualized learning experiences [53–56]. Interactive simulations combined with video tutorials improve both student interest and their ability to keep information in their memory. The approach serves both student learning diversity and professional content review by allowing professionals to access information multiple times for better understanding of complex IoMT forensic concepts [57].

Educational programs need to implement adaptable methods because the IoMT sector experiences fast technological development. New technologies such as artificial intelligence and machine learning, alongside cybersecurity techniques, are integrated into education curricula to teach professionals skills for modern challenges [58]. Educators need to revise their training content and teaching approaches regularly because new technological developments appear in the market. Educational programs that implement virtual laboratories together with simulation software enable students to explore new technology through managed practice spaces. Students gain confidence in real-world scenarios use of advanced tools and techniques through practical learning experiences that promote theoretical concept application [59].

The approaches for continuous and adaptive education in IoMT forensics consist of a combination of continuing professional development, communities of practice, and self-learning resources, and technological adaptations. The advancement of continual learning practices enables professionals to maintain their expertise and intelligence in an evolving field, thus helping to improve both practices and innovations in IoMT forensic work [60].

## 12.8 CONCLUSION

The chapter highlights the necessity for educational transformation which will produce professionals capable of handling IoMT forensics. The existing frameworks are lacking certain elements, combining IoMT technical knowledge with medical regulations and interdisciplinary capabilities is indispensable. The authors introduce PBL and virtual labs, along with university–industry collaborations, as strategies that will develop these competencies. Numerous obstacles, including quick technology evolution and moral dilemmas, together with ensuring the inclusion of all parties, remain persistent. The development of sustainable education requires adaptive curricula combined with professional development, along with institutional partnerships between healthcare providers and regulators, to create prepared IoMT forensic experts who can handle changing healthcare security challenges.

## REFERENCES

[1] B. Haq, M. Faisal, M. Khan, H. Rahman, & T. Hussain, "Botnets attack detection using bio-inspired deep learning techniques in internet of medical things (IoMT)", *Security and Privacy*, vol. 8, no. 1, 2025. https://doi.org/10.1002/spy2.493

[2] Rani, S., Kataria, A., Sharma, V., Ghosh, S., Karar, V., Lee, K., ... & Choi, C. "Threats and corrective measures for iot security with observance of cybercrime: a survey", *Wireless Communications and Mobile Computing*, vol. 2021, no. 1, p. 5579148, 2021. https://doi.org/10.1155/2021/5579148

[3] S. Alqahtany and T. Syed, "Forensictransmonitor: a comprehensive blockchain approach to reinvent digital forensics and evidence management", *Information*, vol. 15, no. 2, p. 109, 2024. https://doi.org/10.3390/info15020109

[4] F. Sessa, M. Esposito, G. Cocimano, S. Sablone, M. Karaboue, M. Chisari et al., "Artificial intelligence and forensic genetics: current applications and future perspectives", *Applied Sciences*, vol. 14, no. 5, p. 2113, 2024. https://doi.org/10.3390/app14052113

[5] K. Elkins, S. Joseph, & C. Skrant, "Survey on forensic DNA biology training in forensic science service laboratories in the united states", *Journal of Forensic Sciences*, vol. 70, no. 1, pp. 61–72, 2024. https://doi.org/10.1111/1556-4029.15671

[6] M. Esposito, F. Sessa, G. Cocimano, P. Zuccarello, S. Roccuzzo, & M. Salerno, "Advances in technologies in crime scene investigation", *Diagnostics*, vol. 13, no. 20, p. 3169, 2023. https://doi.org/10.3390/diagnostics13203169

[7] R. Rajab, M. Abuhmida, I. Wilson, & R. Ward, "A review of IoMT security and privacy related frameworks", *European Conference on Cyber Warfare and Security*, vol. 23, no. 1, pp. 733–743, 2024. https://doi.org/10.34190/eccws.23.1.2239

[8] F. Pelekoudas-Oikonomou, G. Zachos, M. Παπαϊωάννου, M. Ree, J. Ribeiro, Γ. Μαντάς et al., "Blockchain-based security mechanisms for IoMT edge networks in IoMT-based healthcare monitoring systems", *Sensors*, vol. 22, no. 7, p. 2449, 2022. https://doi.org/10.3390/s22072449

[9] M. Mahmood, M. Khan, Z. Ziauddin, H. Hussain, I. Khan, S. Rahman et al., "Improving security architecture of internet of medical things: a systematic literature review", *IEEE Access*, vol. 11, pp. 107725–107753, 2023. https://doi.org/10.1109/access.2023.3281655

[10] M. Παπαϊωάννου, M. Karageorgou, Γ. Μαντάς, V. Sucasas, I. Essop, J. Rodrı́guez et al., "A survey on security threats and countermeasures in internet of medical things (IoMT)", *Transactions on Emerging Telecommunications Technologies*, vol. 33, no. 6, 2020. https://doi.org/10.1002/ett.4049

[11] G. Zachos, I. Essop, Γ. Μαντάς, K. Porfyrakis, J. Ribeiro, & J. Rodrı́guez, "An anomaly-based intrusion detection system for internet of medical things networks", *Electronics*, vol. 10, no. 21, p. 2562, 2021. https://doi.org/10.3390/electronics10212562

[12] D. Gupta, M. Gupta, S. Bhatt, & A. Tosun, "Detecting anomalous user behavior in remote patient monitoring". In *2021 IEEE 22nd International Conference on Information Reuse and Integration for Data Science (IRI)*. IEEE, pp. 33–40, 2021. https://doi.org/10.48550/arxiv.2106.11844

[13] D. Shin and Y. Hwang, "Integrated acceptance and sustainability evaluation of internet of medical things", *Internet Research*, vol. 27, no. 5, pp. 1227–1254, 2017. https://doi.org/10.1108/intr-07-2016-0200

[14] P. Pritika, B. Shanmugam, & S. Azam, "Risk evaluation and attack detection in heterogeneous IoMT devices using hybrid fuzzy logic analytical approach", *Sensors*, vol. 24, no. 10, p. 3223, 2024. https://doi.org/10.3390/s24103223

[15] D. Koutras, G. Stergiopoulos, T. Dasaklis, P. Kotzanikolaou, D. Glynos, & C. Douligeris, "Security in IoMT communications: a survey", *Sensors*, vol. 20, no. 17, p. 4828, 2020. https://doi.org/10.3390/s20174828

[16] P. Rushikesh, "A review: artificial intelligence and expert systems for cyber security", *BOHR International Journal of Engineering*, vol. 1, no. 1, pp. 52–56, 2022. https://doi.org/10.54646/bije.2022.10

[17] E. Yıldırım, M. Cicioğlu, & A. Çalhan, "Fog-cloud architecture-driven internet of medical things framework for healthcare monitoring", *Medical &Amp; Biological Engineering &Amp; Computing*, vol. 61, no. 5, pp. 1133–1147, 2023. https://doi.org/10.1007/s11517-023-02776-4

[18] N. Garg, M. Wazid, A. Das, D. Singh, J. Rodrigues, & Y. Park, "Bakmp-iomt: design of blockchain enabled authenticated key management protocol for internet of medical things deployment", *IEEE Access*, vol. 8, pp. 95956–95977, 2020. https://doi.org/10.1109/access.2020.2995917

[19] R. Tiwari and J. Debnath, "Forensic accounting: a blend of knowledge", *Journal of Financial Regulation and Compliance*, vol. 25, no. 1, pp. 73–85, 2017. https://doi.org/10.1108/jfrc-05-2016-0043

[20] E. Oyerogba, "Forensic auditing mechanism and fraud detection: the case of Nigerian public sector", *Journal of Accounting in Emerging Economies*, vol. 11, no. 5, pp. 752–775, 2021. https://doi.org/10.1108/jaee-04-2020-0072

[21] S. Shah and R. Khan, "Secondary use of electronic health record: opportunities and challenges", *IEEE Access*, vol. 8, pp. 136947–136965, 2020. https://doi.org/10.48550/arxiv.2001.09479

[22] P. Yeng, D. Stephen, & B. Yang, "Legal requirements towards enhancing the security of medical devices", *International Journal of Advanced Computer Science and Applications*, vol. 11, no. 11, 2020. https://doi.org/10.14569/ijacsa.2020.0111181

[23] R. Rajab, M. Abuhmida, I. Wilson, & R. Ward, "A review of iomt security and privacy related frameworks", *European Conference on Cyber Warfare and Security*, vol. 23, no. 1, pp. 733–743, 2024. https://doi.org/10.34190/eccws.23.1.2239

[24] Karam, A. A. "Investigating the importance of ethics and security on internet of medical things (IoMT)", *International Journal of Computations, Information and Manufacturing (IJCIM)*, vol. 2, no. 2, 2022. https://doi.org/10.54489/ijcim.v2i2.114

[25] O. Manta, N. Vasileiou, O. Giannakopoulou, K. Bromis, I. Kouris, M. Haritou et al., "Enhancing healthcare through telehealth ecosystems: impacts and prospects", *Telehealth Ecosystems in Practice*, 2023. https://doi.org/10.3233/shti230804

[26] M. Alkatheiri and A. Alghamdi, "Blockchain-assisted cybersecurity for the internet of medical things in the healthcare industry", *Electronics*, vol. 12, no. 8, p. 1801, 2023. https://doi.org/10.3390/electronics12081801

[27] S. Köpsén and S. Nyström, "Learning in practice for becoming a professional forensic expert", *Forensic Science International*, vol. 222, no. 1-3, pp. 208–215, 2012. https://doi.org/10.1016/j.forsciint.2012.05.026

[28] S. Rafiq, F. Kamran, & A. Afzal, "Investigating the benefits and challenges of interdisciplinary education in higher education settings", *Journal of Social Research Development*, vol. 5, no. 1, pp. 87–100, 2024. https://doi.org/10.53664/jsrd/05-01-2024-08-87-100

[29] E. Scott and B. White, "An empirical study of cultivating innovative practice abilities in an interdisciplinary education environment in Australia", *Research and Advances in Education*, vol. 3, no. 5, pp. 53–63, 2024. https://doi.org/10.56397/rae.2024.05.06

[30] S. Ferns, A. Phatak, S. Benson, & N. Kumagai, "Building employability capabilities in data science students: an interdisciplinary, industry-focused approach", *Teaching Statistics*, vol. 43, no. S1, 2021. https://doi.org/10.1111/test.12272

[31] S. Narsareddygari, M. Pathlavath, N. Samala, & S. Naik, "Expanding horizons: the transformative influence of interdisciplinary education on engineering students". In *Proceedings of REES*, KLE Technological University, Hubli, India, pp. 32–39, 2024. https://doi.org/10.52202/073963-0005

[32] Khatib, A. Shamayleh, & M. Ndiaye, "Healthcare and the internet of medical things: applications, trends, key challenges, and proposed resolutions", *Informatics*, vol. 11, no. 3, p. 47, 2024. https://doi.org/10.3390/informatics11030047

[33] N. Bibi, M. Sikandar, I. Din, A. Almogren, & S. Ali, "IoMT-based automated detection and classification of leukemia using deep learning", *Journal of Healthcare Engineering*, vol. 2020, pp. 1–12, 2020. https://doi.org/10.1155/2020/6648574

[34] T. Khan, A. Fatima, T. Shahzad, A. Rahman, K. Alissa, T. Ghazal et al., "Secure IoMT for disease prediction empowered with transfer learning in

healthcare 5.0, the concept and case study", *IEEE Access*, vol. 11, pp. 39418–39430, 2023. https://doi.org/10.1109/access.2023.3266156

[35] D. Raj, K. Rukmani, S. Rukmani, V. Rukmani, & D. Rukmani, "A survey on transforming healthcare with IoMT: the power of connected medical devices", *International Journal of Scientific Research in Computer Science, Engineering and Information Technology*, vol. 10, no. 2, pp. 267–277, 2024. https://doi.org/10.32628/cseit2410219

[36] S. D.N., B. Annappa, S. Hegde, C. Abhijit, & S. Ambesange, "Fedcure: a heterogeneity-aware personalized federated learning framework for intelligent healthcare applications in IoMT environments", *IEEE Access*, vol. 12, pp. 15867–15883, 2024. https://doi.org/10.1109/access.2024.3357514

[37] Z. Jozi and H. Nourmohammadi, "Scientometrics analysis of world scientific research of pathology and forensic medicine", *Iranian Journal of Pathology*, vol. 17, no. 2, pp. 191–201, 2022. https://doi.org/10.30699/ijp.2022.541660.2756

[38] Parihar, S. Yadav, M. Sadique, P. Ranjan, N. Kumar, A. Singhal et al., "Internet-of-medical-things integrated point-of-care biosensing devices for infectious diseases: toward better preparedness for futuristic pandemics", *Bioengineering & Translational Medicine*, vol. 8, no. 3, 2023. https://doi.org/10.1002/btm2.10481

[39] R. Li and E. Niyomsilp, "Effects of industry-university collaboration on enterprises' intellectual capital: a study of hi-tech industries in Zhejiang, china", *International Journal of Human Resource Studies*, vol. 10, no. 1, p. 349, 2020. https://doi.org/10.5296/ijhrs.v10i1.16548

[40] D. Ragupathy, S. Baharin, & F. Turan, "University industry collaboration:", *Journal of Modern Manufacturing Systems and Technology*, vol. 4, no. 1, pp. 36–44, 2020. https://doi.org/10.15282/jmmst.v4i1.3790

[41] W. Ismail, N. Shahid, A. Abdullah, M. Noor, T. Ibrahim, N. Zainuddin et al., "Evaluation of massive open online course (mooc) approach among undergraduate students", *International Journal of Academic Research in Progressive Education and Development*, vol. 11, no. 4, 2022. https://doi.org/10.6007/ijarped/v11-i4/15887

[42] X. Chen, S. Liu, Z. Tao, Y. Ou, & Y. Xiao, "Application of network teaching in nursing undergraduate education during the coronavirus disease 2019 epidemic", *BMC Medical Education*, vol. 22, no. 1, 2022. https://doi.org/10.1186/s12909-022-03318-6

[43] R. Hendriks, P. Jong, W. Admiraal, & M. Reinders, "Instructional design quality in medical massive open online courses for integration into campus education", *Medical Teacher*, vol. 42, no. 2, pp. 156–163, 2019. https://doi.org/10.1080/0142159x.2019.1665634

[44] H. Azami and R. Ibrahim, "Development and evaluation of massive open online course (mooc) as a supplementary learning tool: an initial study", *International Journal of Advanced Computer Science and Applications*, vol. 10, no. 7, 2019. https://doi.org/10.14569/ijacsa.2019.0100773

[45] M. Mukhopadhyay, S. Banerjee, & C. Mukhopadhyay, "Internet of medical things and the evolution of healthcare 4.0: exploring recent trends", *Journal of Electronics, Electromedical Engineering, and Medical*

*Informatics*, vol. 6, no. 2, pp. 182–195, 2024. https://doi.org/10.35882/jeeemi.v6i2.402

[46] L. Sun, X. Jiang, H. Ren, & Y. Guo, "Edge-cloud computing and artificial intelligence in internet of medical things: architecture, technology and application", *IEEE Access*, vol. 8, pp. 101079–101092, 2020. https://doi.org/10.1109/access.2020.2997831

[47] W. Rafique, M. Khan, S. Khan, & J. Ally, "Securemed: a blockchain-based privacy-preserving framework for internet of medical things", *Wireless Communications and Mobile Computing*, vol. 2023, pp. 1–14, 2023. https://doi.org/10.1155/2023/2558469

[48] C. Yang, Y. Liu, C. Chiang, & Y. Su, "National IoMT platform strategy portfolio decision model under the covid-19 environment: based on the financial and non-financial value view", *Annals of Operations Research*, vol. 328, no. 1, pp. 1151–1179, 2022. https://doi.org/10.1007/s10479-022-05016-4

[49] P. Kilmarx, F. Katz, M. Razak, J. Palen, L. Cheever, & R. Glass, "The medical education partnership initiative: strengthening human resources to end aids and improve health in Africa", *Academic Medicine*, vol. 94, no. 11, pp. 1704–1713, 2019. https://doi.org/10.1097/acm.0000000000002489

[50] M. Mormina and S. Pinder, "A conceptual framework for training of trainers (tot) interventions in global health", *Globalization and Health*, vol. 14, no. 1, 2018. https://doi.org/10.1186/s12992-018-0420-3

[51] Z. Talib, L. Narayan, & T. Harrod, "Postgraduate medical education in sub-saharan africa: a scoping review spanning 26 years and lessons learned", *Journal of Graduate Medical Education*, vol. 11, no. 4s, pp. 34–46, 2019. https://doi.org/10.4300/jgme-d-19-00170

[52] V. Sydorenko, I. Шоробура, A. Ponomarenko, M. Dei, & O. Джус, "Application of technologies of formal and non-formal education for continuous professional development of the modern specialist", *Revista Tempos E Espaços Em Educação*, vol. 13, no. 32, pp. 1–24, 2020. https://doi.org/10.20952/revtee.v13i32.14729

[53] L. Rezaii, A. Assareh, R. Hakimzade, & B. Sedghpour, "Assessment of quo and desirable status of adult education curricula in elementary and post-elementary education", *International Journal of Elementary Education*, vol. 9, no. 4, p. 88, 2020. https://doi.org/10.11648/j.ijeedu.20200904.12

[54] Ş. Ghimişi, "The community of practice in the education", *Journal of Research and Innovation for Sustainable Society*, vol. 1, no. 2, pp. 23–30, 2019. https://doi.org/10.33727/jriss.2019.2.3:23-30

[55] Lūka, "Creating a culture-based language learning course for developing adult learners' 21st century skills", *Journal of Education Culture and Society*, vol. 10, no. 2, pp. 151–169, 2019. https://doi.org/10.15503/jecs20192.151.169

[56] Moreira, M. Silva, J. Darder, J. Coutinho, M. Vasconcelos, & M. Marques, "Effectiveness of an educational intervention on knowledge-attitude-practice of older adults' caregivers", *Revista Brasileira De Enfermagem*, vol. 71, no. 3, pp. 1055–1062, 2018. https://doi.org/10.1590/0034-7167-2017-0100

[57] M. Ouaissa & A. Rhattoy, "A new scheme of group-based AKA for machine type communication over LTE networks", *International Journal of Electrical and Computer Engineering*, vol. 8, no. 2, p. 1169, 2018.

[58] S. E. Himer, M. Ouaissa, M. Ouaissa, M. Krichen, M. Alswailim, & M. Almutiq, "Energy consumption monitoring system based on IoT for residential rooftops", *Computation*, vol. 11, no. 4, p. 78, 2023.

[59] M. Ouaissa, A. Rhattoy, & M. Lahmer, "New method to control congestion for machine to machine applications in long term evolution system", *International Journal on Communications Antenna and Propagation*, vol. 8, no. 4, pp. 355–363, 2018.

[60] M. Ouaissa & A. Rhattoy, "QoS hybrid uplink scheduler based on service type for M2M communications in LTE networks", *Indonesian Journal of Electrical Engineering and Computer Science*, vol. 14, no. 3, p. 1460, 2019.

# Index

Access control, 3, 5, 41–43, 46, 65, 92, 103–104, 106, 118
Adaptive defense, 62–63, 67
Anomaly detection, 2, 4, 44, 56–57, 59–60, 66–67, 72, 82, 91–93, 96–98, 173–176, 178–179, 181, 186–187
Artificial intelligence, 1, 18, 53, 55, 86, 143, 149, 171, 174, 192, 241, 255
Authentication, 4, 8, 35–41, 44–52, 92, 104–106, 140, 150, 156, 158, 160, 201
Authorization, 35, 41–47, 51–53

Biometric, 39–40, 59, 86, 214, 218–219
Blockchain, 45, 53, 55–59, 80–81, 83, 86–87, 91–93, 98, 102–110, 116, 118, 144, 187, 199, 201, 203–205, 214, 232, 235, 241, 243

Circular security, 56, 58–60, 62, 65–67, 72, 78–83
Cloud computing, 86–88, 132, 140, 200, 205
Compliance, 2–3, 5–10, 15, 18–19, 21, 36, 39, 45, 48–49, 79–80, 83, 87, 89, 91, 105, 127, 139–140, 142, 144–145, 149, 158–159, 163, 171, 187, 212–213, 234–235, 242, 244–246, 251
Cybersecurity, 5, 35–36, 48, 52, 56, 60, 68, 81–83, 87, 91–93, 97–98, 122, 124–125, 127, 140, 144, 154–155, 170–172, 201, 211–212, 223, 228, 232, 234, 239–240, 242–243, 245–246, 250, 255

Data privacy, 3, 6, 19, 26, 64, 68, 83, 89, 91, 94, 98, 103–104, 139, 142, 144, 246
Data integrity, 8, 36, 56, 59–60, 81, 87, 91–92, 116, 143, 145, 161, 187, 214, 243
Digital forensic, 142, 145–146, 149, 152, 158, 161, 172, 199–201, 205, 250

Edge computing, 56–57, 67, 82, 86–88, 90, 95–96, 199–200, 202, 205, 208
EHR, 38, 42, 90–91, 104, 127, 130, 214, 223–226, 244
Encryption, 3, 7–8, 58, 64, 66, 80–83, 87, 93–95, 97, 103–104, 109, 139–140, 144, 150, 156, 158, 160

Federated learning, 3, 13, 18–19, 21, 55, 68, 72, 75, 81, 87, 94, 97, 173–174

Governance, 10, 11, 16, 47, 50, 149, 161, 165–166

Healthcare, 1–6, 9–13, 21–22, 26, 35–40, 48–52, 55–58, 65–69, 72, 75–76, 80–83, 90–95, 102–109, 114, 116, 125, 129–132, 137–140, 144–146, 150–151, 155–160, 163–164, 170, 175–176, 185–186, 208, 212–214, 223–229, 234–235, 251–254

IoMT, 1–5, 13, 15, 35–38, 40, 42, 44–49, 52–53, 58, 65–67, 69, 72, 74–75, 78–80, 83, 86–90, 105, 121, 127–128, 130–132, 138–140, 150–151, 155–160, 163–165, 208–214, 226–227, 229–231, 234–235, 239–250

Machine learning, 1, 18–20, 22, 44, 60, 63, 69, 80, 88, 97, 131–132, 143, 149, 151, 153, 162, 164–165, 171–172, 174, 176, 178–180, 241–243, 248, 255
Medical ethics, 225–226
Medicine, 2, 9, 30, 88, 116, 153, 221, 228, 232, 244, 246, 250
MOOC, 250–253, 255

Neural network, 19, 57, 68, 74

SIEM, 171–172, 174, 176, 179–181, 184, 186–187
Sustainable, 13, 56–57, 60, 67, 79, 81–82, 121, 192–196, 198–199, 201, 204–205, 208, 210–211, 213, 230, 235, 240, 251–254, 256

Telemedicine, 4, 86–87, 89, 90, 132, 139–140, 144, 146, 208
Threat detection, 2–4, 15, 56–59, 65, 68–69, 72, 75–76, 80–83, 92, 97, 153, 171–173, 175, 179–181, 187, 212, 227
Threat intelligence, 4–5, 56–60, 62–68, 72, 74–75, 78, 80–83, 165, 172, 174
Training, 14, 18–21, 24, 26, 48, 50, 58, 69–72, 74–75, 96–97, 140, 145, 152, 160, 166, 179, 210, 212–213, 223–224, 226–230, 239–242, 247–252

Virtual reality, 212, 228, 232, 240–241

Zero trust, 45–46, 87, 174